GUIDELINES FOR PULMONARY REHABILITATION PROGRAMS

SECOND EDITION

AMERICAN ASSOCIATION OF CARDIOVASCULAR & PULMONARY REHABILITATION

PROMOTING HEALTH & PREVENTING DISEASE

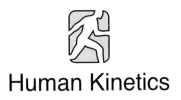

Human Kinetics

Library of Congress Cataloging-in-Publication Data

American Association of Cardiovascular & Pulmonary Rehabilitation.
      Guidelines for pulmonary rehabilitation programs / American
Association of Cardiovascular and Pulmonary Rehabilitation. -- 2nd
ed.
            p.   cm.
      Includes bibliographical references and index.
      ISBN 0-88011-863-6
      1. Lungs--Diseases, Obstructive--Patients--Rehabilitation-
-Standards.   2. Lungs--Diseases--Patients--Rehabilitation-
-Standards.   3. Respiratory therapy-Standards.   I. Title.
      [DNLM: 1. Lung Diseases, Obstructive--rehabilitation.
2. Rehabilitation--standards.   WF 600 A5117g 1998]
RC776.03A64   1998
616.2'403--dc21
DNLM/DLC
for Library of Congress   97-46467
                                                                      CIP
ISBN: 0-88011-863-6

Developmental Editor: Julie A. Marx
Assistant Editors: Laura Ward Majersky and Sarah Wiseman
Copyeditor: Amie Bell
Proofreader: Sarah Wiseman
Indexer: Theresa Schaefer
Graphic Designer: Stuart Cartwright
Graphic Artist: Judy Henderson
Cover Designer: Stuart Cartwright
Interior Photographer: Tom Roberts
Illustrator: Joe Bellis
Printer: United Graphics

Printed in the United States of America   10 9 8 7 6 5 4 3 2

Human Kinetics
Web site: http://www.humankinetics.com/

United States: Human Kinetics, P.O. Box 5076, Champaign, IL 61825-5076
1-800-747-4457
e-mail: humank@hkusa.com

Canada: Human Kinetics, 475 Devonshire Road, Unit 100, Windsor, ON N8Y 2L5
1-800-465-7301 (in Canada only)
e-mail: humank@hkcanada.com

Europe: Human Kinetics, P.O. Box IW14, Leeds LS16 6TR, United Kingdom
(44) 1132 781708
e-mail: humank@hkeurope.com

Australia: Human Kinetics, 57A Price Avenue, Lower Mitcham, South Australia 5062
(088) 277 1555
e-mail: humank@hkaustralia.com

New Zealand: Human Kinetics, P.O. Box 105-231, Auckland 1
(09) 523 3462
e-mail: humank@hknewz.com

The second edition of *Guidelines for Pulmonary Rehabilitation Programs* by the AACVPR is dedicated to the strong and courageous patients who live day to day and breath by breath with their chronic lung disease, and to the unique groups of health care professionals that work day to day with these challenging and inspiring patients.

Contents

Notice

The purpose of this publication is to represent a nationally derived consensus statement of guidelines applying to pulmonary rehabilitation programs. However, the book should not be deemed all-inclusive in its presentation of various guidelines, nor should it be considered exclusive of other methods or modalities for providing care. Ultimately the responsibility for delivering services in accordance with the standard of care lies with the facility and the professional staff. Moreover, circumstances may necessitate deviation from any particular guideline. Professionals must exercise independent judgment as to what is appropriate for individual patients or groups of patients under particular circumstances.

By developing and publishing this statement, the American Association of Cardiovascular and Pulmonary Rehabilitation; its officers, directors, agents and employees; and others involved in this publication do not assume any duty owed to any third party as a result of any use of this document. Any duty owing to third parties remains the responsibility of those who provide relevant services.

By reason of the development and publication of these guidelines the writing committee, the association and the publisher are not or shall not be deemed to be engaged in the practice of medicine or any allied health field. In performing and rendering services, professionals must engage the services of appropriately licensed individuals as required by state law.

Foreword

In 1993 the American Association of Cardiovascular and Pulmonary Rehabilitation (AACVPR) published the first edition of the *Guidelines for Pulmonary Rehabilitation Programs*. Since then appreciation for the value of rehabilitation for individuals with chronic lung disease continues to increase. A new definition for pulmonary rehabilitation was developed during an NIH Workshop:

> *Pulmonary rehabilitation is a multidimensional continuum of services directed to persons with pulmonary disease and their families, usually by an interdisciplinary team of specialists, with the goal of achieving and maintaining the individual's maximum level of independence and functioning in the community.* (p. 826)[1]

The American Thoracic Society published a new statement on the assessment and treatment of patients with chronic obstructive pulmonary disease that includes pulmonary rehabilitation in the algorithm of care.[2] The beneficial outcomes of pulmonary rehabilitation have been discussed in a comprehensive textbook on the topic.[3]

The Medical Advisory Panel of the national Blue Cross Blue Shield Association declared pulmonary rehabilitation to be a "reasonable technology" in February of 1996. A joint committee of the American College of Chest Physicians and the AACVPR produced an evidence-based practice guidelines statement supporting the value of pulmonary rehabilitation.[4]

This enhanced recognition of pulmonary rehabilitation is timely. Chronic illnesses cost an estimated $425 billion for direct health care in the United States in 1990.[5] With the addition of indirect costs, such as lost work days due to disability or death, the estimated cost grows to $659 billion. Chronic illnesses account for about 70% of direct health care costs in the United States. An estimated 100 million Americans suffer from one or more chronic conditions.

The World Health Organization estimates that by the year 2020 tobacco-related disease will cause one in every 10 deaths in the world (8.4 million in 2020 from tobacco use compared to 3 million from tobacco use in 1990). In 1990 COPD was the sixth leading cause of death in the world. It is currently the fourth leading cause of death in the U.S.[6]

Obstructive airway diseases account for the majority of patients participating in pulmonary rehabilitation programs. It is currently estimated that 14.2 million Americans have COPD (12.5 million with chronic bronchitis and 1.65 million with emphysema) and 10 million have asthma. Individuals with other chronic lung diseases, however, can also benefit from pulmonary rehabilitation.[7, 8]

We are doing a great job caring for people who are acutely ill, but we fail to adequately deal with the needs of patients (and their families) once they leave the hospital. Rehabilitation and better in-home support must be a top priority to help people learn to live with their chronic illnesses.[5]

I am pleased to have the opportunity to write the foreword for this new edition of AACVPR's *Guidelines for Pulmonary Rehabilitation Programs*. With the changes in health care coverage in the United States, pulmonary rehabilitation teams have modified the way treatment plans are developed and implemented. These changes have presented new challenges, but they have also introduced new opportunities. The committee that has worked diligently on this edition has comprehensively revised this document. We all owe a debt of gratitude to Gerilynn Connors, Lana Hilling, and each member of their committee for this monumental work.

John E. Hodgkin, MD
Medical Director of Respiratory Care and Pulmonary Rehabilitation
St. Helena Hospital, Deer Park, CA
Clinical Professor of Medicine
University of California, Davis

REFERENCES

1. Fishman, A.P. 1994. NIH workshop summary: Pulmonary rehabilitation research. *Am J Respir Crit Care Med* 149:825-33.

2. American Thoracic Society. 1995. Standards for the diagnosis and care of patients with chronic ob-

structive pulmonary disease (COPD). *Am J Respir Crit Care Med* 152 (Suppl. 5):S77-120.

3. Hodgkin, J.E. 1996. Benefits of pulmonary rehabilitation. In *Pulmonary rehabilitation*, edited by A.P. Fishman, 33-53. New York: Marcel Dekker.

4. Pulmonary rehabilitation: Joint ACCP/AACVPR evidence-based guidelines. 1997. Chest 112:1363-96.

5. Hoffman, C., D. Rice, and H. Sung. 1996. Persons with chronic conditions: Their prevalence and costs. *JAMA* 276:1473-79.

6. National Center for Health Statistics, U.S. Dept. of Health and Human Services, 1995.

7. Novitch, R.S., and H.M. Thomas III. 1996. Pulmonary rehabilitation in chronic pulmonary interstitial disease. In *Pulmonary rehabilitation*, edited by A.P. Fishman, 683-700. New York: Marcel Dekker.

8. Bach, J.R. 1996. Pulmonary rehabilitation in musculoskeletal disorders. In *Pulmonary rehabilitation*, edited by A.P. Fishman, 701-23. New York: Marcel Dekker.

Acknowledgments

Pulmonary rehabilitation deals with an interdisciplinary team of specialists who use their skills and expertise to work with patients who have lung disease. The writers and reviewers of the second edition of these Guidelines represent a truly interdisciplinary team who volunteered their knowledge and time to this project. We would like to thank the following individuals:

Editors

Gerilynn Connors, BS, RCP, RRT, FAACVPR,
  Co-Chair
Director, Cardiopulmonary Rehabilitation
Clinical Coordinator, Nicotine Intervention Program
St. Helena Hospital
Deer Park, CA

Lana Hilling, RCP, FAACVPR,
  Co-Chair
Coordinator, Pulmonary Rehabilitation
Mt. Diablo Medical Center
Concord, CA

Writing Committee Members

Rebecca Crouch, MS, PT, FAACVPR
Coordinator, Pulmonary Rehabilitation
Duke University Medical Center
Durham, NC

Mary Ellen Dorko, MS, FAACVPR
Program Coordinator, Pulmonary Rehabilitation
Temple University Hospital
Philadelphia, PA

Bonnie Fahy, RN, MN, FAACVPR
Pulmonary Clinical Nurse Specialist
Pulmonary Rehabilitation Coordinator
St. Joseph's Hospital and Medical Center
Phoenix, AZ

Donna Lopes, BSN, MPA
Supervisor of Cardiology Services, Cardiac and
  Pulmonary Rehabilitation
St. Rose Hospital
Hayward, CA

Jamie Sheldon-Villalobos, PT, FAACVPR
Pulmonary and Transplant Rehabilitation
UCSD Medical Center
San Diego, CA

Douglas R. Southard, PhD, MPH, PA-C, FAACVPR
Director, Physician Assistant Program
College of Health Sciences
Roanoke, VA

Kenneth Tolep, MD
Associates in Pulmonary Medicine
Fort Myers, FL

Richard L. ZuWallack, MD
Assistant Chief, Section of Pulmonary and
  Critical Care Medicine
St. Francis Hospital and Medical Center
Hartford, CT

Special thanks to the AACVPR representatives of the American College of Chest Physicians/AACVPR Evidence-Based Pulmonary Rehabilitation Guidelines Committee who thoroughly reviewed the document:

Brian W. Carlin, MD, FAACVPR
Medical Director, Pulmonary Rehabilitation
Allegheny General Hospital
Pittsburgh, PA

Charles F. Emery, PhD, FAACVPR
Associate Professor, Department of Psychology
Ohio State University
Columbus, OH

John E. Hodgkin, MD, FAACVPR
Clinical Professor of Medicine, University of
    California, Davis
Medical Director, Respiratory Care and
    Pulmonary Rehabilitation
St. Helena Hospital
Deer Park, CA

Virginia Carrieri-Kohlman, DNSc, RN
Professor, University of California
School of Nursing
San Francisco, CA

Sincere appreciation to the following reviewers of the document from throughout the United States who represent the pulmonary rehabilitation community with their wealth of knowledge and dedication to the profession:

Rhonda N. Barr, PT, MA, CCS
University of Iowa Hospitals and Clinics
Department of Physical Therapy
Iowa City, IA

William Bell, PhD, RN, MBA, FAACVPR
Colorado Lung Center Research
Englewood, CO

Richard Casaburi, PhD, MD
Professor of Medicine and Associate Chief of the
    Division of Pulmonary Critical Care Medicine
Harbor-UCLA Medical Center
Torrance, CA

Anne M. Gavic
Highland Park Hospital
Highland Park, IL

Linda Koch, RRT, MEd
West Country Sports Fitness and
    Rehabilitation Center
Creve Coeur, MO

Trina Limberg, BS, RRT
Program Director, Pulmonary Rehabilitation
UCSD Medical Center
San Diego, CA

Barry Make, MD, FAACVPR
Director, Pulmonary Rehabilitation and
    Respiratory Care
National Jewish Center for Immunology
Denver, CO

Michael G. Moran, MD
Director of Adult Psychiatry
National Jewish Medical and Research Center
Associate Professor of Psychiatry
University of Colorado
Denver, CO

Jane Reardon, MSN, CS, FAACVPR
Hartford Hospital
Department of Medicine
Hartford, CT

Andy L. Ries, MD, MPH, FAACVPR
Professor of Medicine
UCSD Medical Center
San Diego, CA

Susan L. Ruppel, RD
Duke University Medical Center
Durham, NC

Rebecca Schein, PhD
Duke/FAHEC, Coordinator,
    Psychological Services
Fayetteville, NC

Dennis Sobush, MA, PT
Associate Professor
College of Health Sciences
Marquette University
Milwaukee, WI

Wayne Sotile, PhD, FAACVPR
Sotile Psychological Associates
Winston-Salem, NC

Susan L. Swails, RN, C, BSN
Holy Spirit Hospital
Camp Hill, PA

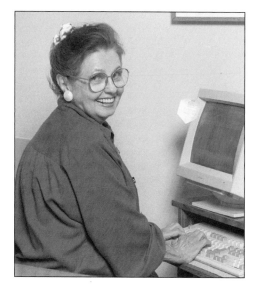

A key figure in the interdisciplinary team is our patient. We would like to thank Beverly Striplin, a Mt. Diablo Medical Center Pulmonary Rehabilitation Program graduate and volunteer who unselfishly spent hundreds of hours assisting us with her word processing skills to complete this manuscript. Thank you Beverly, we love you dearly.

We thank our editor at Human Kinetics, Julie Marx, for her encouragement and patience as this book has been in development and production. And our AACVPR staff liaison, Jane Shepard, for her words of encouragement.

The AACVPR expresses its gratitude to all of those that contributed ideas, authored sections, reviewed chapters and provided editorial comments.

And lastly, we thank our patients for their inspiration and our colleagues for "hanging in there" in these challenging times.

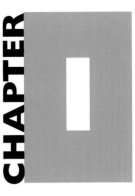

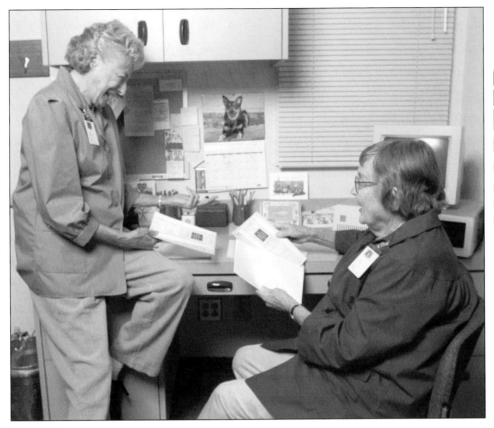

CHAPTER 1

Definition and Overview of Pulmonary Rehabilitation

Pulmonary rehabilitation has evolved over the past eight decades[1] in response to the continued increase in patients with chronic pulmonary diseases and the need to optimize their care. The strategies and techniques used in comprehensive pulmonary rehabilitation have been well established.[2-6] The documented benefits are substantial and include decreased symptoms, improved quality of life, increased exercise tolerance, independence in activities of daily living, and decreased utilization of medical resources. See the *Pulmonary Rehabilitation: Evidence-Based Guidelines* in appendix A, which review the current state of evidence for the scientific basis of pulmonary rehabilitation.

Pulmonary rehabilitation has traditionally focused on patients with chronic obstructive pulmonary disease (COPD), defined as chronic bronchitis and/or emphysema with obstruction to airflow demonstrated on a spirogram. Pulmonary rehabilitation, however, can also benefit patients with other conditions including asthma, alpha 1 antitrypsin deficiency, cystic fibrosis, interstitial lung disease, neuromuscular and neurological disorders, primary pulmonary hypertension, lung cancer, before and after volume reduction surgery or lung transplantation, patients who require ventilatory support, and pediatric patients with pulmonary disease (see chapter 7).

Pulmonary rehabilitation can benefit patients with conditions other than COPD.

This chapter covers a variety of issues: the definition and outcomes of pulmonary rehabilitation, how the *Guidelines* may be utilized, the epidemiology of lung disease, the prevention of disease, the philosophy of pulmonary rehabilitation, the importance of setting appropriate and individualized patient and program goals, and the essential components of a comprehensive pulmonary rehabilitation program. Pulmonary rehabilitation includes assessment, patient training, exercise, psychosocial intervention, and follow-up, with prevention incorporated into every component of rehabilitation. Each of these issues is critical to understanding the need for pulmonary rehabilitation and developing a successful pulmonary rehabilitation program. The definition and outcomes of pulmonary rehabilitation will set the foundation for pulmonary rehabilitation programs. An understanding of the epidemiological data of lung disease supports the need for pulmonary rehabilitation in patients with lung disease. To succeed in pulmonary rehabilitation, the patient, significant others, and the interdisciplinary team members need to understand and believe in the philosophy of pulmonary rehabilitation. Setting patient and program goals allows for the program to be individualized to meet the patients' needs. Finally, it is essential that the interdisciplinary team providing pulmonary rehabilitation understands the essential components of pulmonary rehabilitation since it is not just an exercise or education program.

Pulmonary rehabilitation is not just an exercise or education program—it includes assessment, patient training, exercise, psychosocial intervention, and follow up, with prevention incorporated into every component of rehabilitation.

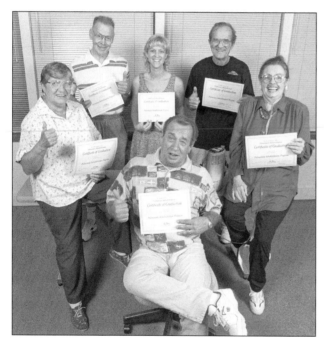

DEFINITION AND OUTCOMES

Pulmonary rehabilitation was defined in 1974 by a committee of the American College of Chest Physicians.[7] That same definition was included in the official American Thoracic Society statement on pulmonary rehabilitation in 1981:

Pulmonary rehabilitation may be defined as an art of medical practice wherein an individually tailored, multidisciplinary program is formulated which through accurate diagnosis, therapy, emotional support, and education, stabilizes or reverses both the physio- and psychopathology of pulmonary diseases and attempts to return the patient to the highest possible functional capacity allowed by his pulmonary handicap and overall life situation. (p. 663)[8]

In 1994, the National Institutes of Health Consensus Conference on Pulmonary Rehabilitation developed the following definition to describe the process:

A multidimensional continuum of services directed to persons with pulmonary disease and their families, usually by an interdisciplinary team of specialists, with the goal of achieving and maintaining the individual's maximum level of independence and functioning in the community. (p. 826)[9]

The following definition summarizes the views of a graduating class of the pulmonary rehabilitation program at Mt. Diablo Medical Center in Concord, California:

> *"Pulmonary rehabilitation has been a life-saving pathway between inactivity and activity, isolation and socialization, depression and hope, and from being an observer of life to an active participant." (p. 445)*[10]

Pulmonary rehabilitation programs are adjuncts to standard medical care and assist to control and alleviate symptoms, optimize functional capacity, and improve the quality of life for patients with chronic pulmonary diseases. These programs have been studied most extensively for patients with COPD[11] but have also been shown to be beneficial for patients with other conditions as detailed in chapter 7. The benefits[12, 13] and outcomes of pulmonary rehabilitation have been demonstrated by randomized clinical trials and scientific studies,[6, 14-19] empirical studies, and patient testimonials such as the following:

> *"The program has given me more control of my life; I am very grateful as living is so wonderful now."*

> *"Pulmonary rehabilitation has allowed me to return to the mainstream of life, both emotionally and physically."*

See table 1.1 for the demonstrated outcomes of pulmonary rehabilitation.

Table 1.1 Demonstrated Outcomes of Pulmonary Rehabilitation
Reduced hospitalizations and use of medical resources
Improved quality of life
Reduced respiratory symptoms (e.g., dyspnea)
Improved psychosocial symptoms (e.g., reversal of anxiety and depression and improved self-efficacy)
Increased knowledge about pulmonary disease and its management
Increased exercise tolerance and performance
Enhanced ability to perform activities of daily living
Increased survival in some patients (e.g., use of continuous oxygen in patients with severe hypoxemia)
Return to work for some patients

Adapted, by permission, from A.L. Ries, 1990, "Position paper of the American Association of Cardiovascular and Pulmonary Rehabilitation: Scientific basis of pulmonary rehabilitation," *Journal of Cardiopulmonary Rehabilitation* 10:418-441. ©AACVPR.

In the utilization of pulmonary rehabilitation by the general medical community, however, there is room for improvement.[20, 21] According to Corsello,

> *Although the medical literature is filled with reports attesting to the benefits of pulmonary rehabilitation, skepticism and a lack of enthusiasm for it persist among many physicians, including pulmonologists, more than 20 years after the seminal studies of Drs. Petty and Cherniack. (p. 197)*[21]

To have a positive impact on the pulmonary patient's quality of life, this skepticism and lack of enthusiasm for pulmonary rehabilitation must change. For many years the standard of care for pulmonary patients included inactivity and rest. Pulmonary rehabilitation programs encourage the exact opposite. Patients need to be active participants in their health care. In fact, Hippocrates stated in 460-377 B.C. that "use strengthens, disuse debilitates."

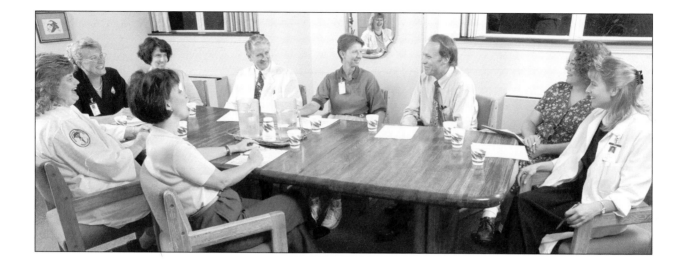

APPLICATION OF THE *GUIDELINES*

This second edition of the American Association of Cardiovascular and Pulmonary Rehabilitation's (AACVPR) *Guidelines for Pulmonary Rehabilitation Programs* expands on each of the components of pulmonary rehabilitation in addition to addressing the importance of earlier detection and prevention of lung disease and the role of pulmonary rehabilitation for patients with special conditions. This book is not intended as a detailed step-by-step process of rehabilitation or as a thorough explanation of the scientific basis of pulmonary rehabilitation; instead this book is intended as a guideline to emphasize the following:

- Essential components of pulmonary rehabilitation, including assessment, patient training, exercise, psychosocial intervention, and follow-up
- Integration of prevention into pulmonary rehabilitation
- Earlier screening and detection of lung disease to make pulmonary rehabilitation more accessible to patients
- Patient selection criteria beyond those for patients with COPD
- Programs tailored to the patient's individual needs
- Documentation of outcomes

These guidelines are intended for the following people:

- Professionals (interdisciplinary team members) developing and updating pulmonary rehabilitation programs
- Physicians and other allied health care professionals referring patients for pulmonary rehabilitation
- Patients and significant others interested in knowing what a pulmonary rehabilitation program should consist of prior to selecting a program to attend
- Third-party payers evaluating pulmonary rehabilitation programs
- Educators training health care professionals (e.g., respiratory therapists, nurses, physicians, physical and occupational therapists, etc.) about pulmonary rehabilitation

This book is not intended as a detailed step-by-step process of rehabilitation or as a thorough explanation of the scientific basis of pulmonary rehabilitation; instead this book is intended as a guideline.

▌ Individuals involved in educating the media and public about pulmonary rehabilitation

EPIDEMIOLOGY

According to a 1996 publication, over 30 million Americans are living with chronic lung disease.[22] They include 14.6 million with asthma, of which 4.8 million are under the age of 18; and 16 million with COPD, of which 14 million have chronic bronchitis and 2 million have emphysema.[22] The impact of morbidity is not just a statistic. Its affect on the patients' and their families' quality of life is immense. In 1996 the American Lung Association stated, "Lung disease is not only a killer. Lung disease is usually chronic, making each breath barely possible—a constant struggle to stay alive from moment to moment" (p. 1).[22]

The cost of lung disease in terms of lives affected and dollars utilized is enormous. Lung disease is the leading cause of disability in the United States according to the American Lung Association's 1996 publication on lung disease data.[22] It costs the American economy approximately $33.4 billion in direct health care expenditures every year and $51 billion in indirect costs—a total of $84.4 billion.[22] The economic cost of caring for patients with COPD was approximately $23.5 billion, which included $14.7 billion in direct health care expenditures and $8.8 billion in indirect costs.[22] COPD is the third ranking condition (after congestive heart failure and stroke) necessitating at-home care. The cost of caring for patients with asthma[23] was an estimated $12.4 billion, of which $9.8 billion was for direct medical expenditures and $2.6 billion made up indirect costs.[22] The impact of chronic lung disease on morbidity and mortality has increased dramatically in recent decades. In the United States, COPD and allied conditions rank as the fourth leading cause of death as shown in table 1.2.[24]

Table 1.2 Ten Leading Causes of Death in the United States	
All causes	**2,312,203**
1. Heart disease	738,781
2. Cancer	537,969
3. Stroke	158,061
4. Chronic obstructive pulmonary diseases and allied conditions	104,756
5. Accidents and adverse effects	89,703
6. Pneumonia and influenza	83,528
7. Diabetes mellitus	59,085
8. Human immunodeficiency virus (HIV) infection	42,506
9. Suicide	30,893
10. Chronic liver disease and cirrhosis	24,848

Note: Data are provisional, estimated from a 10% sample of deaths. Figures may not add to totals because of rounding. Rates have been recomputed based on revised population estimates.

Source: National Center for Health Statistics, U.S. Dept. of Health and Human Services, 1995.

Adapted from *The World Almanac and Book of Facts 1997.* Copyright 1996 by K-111 Reference corporation.

PREVENTION

The traditional standard of care for patients with COPD is often medication therapy, including oxygen. As stated by Kaplan and Ries, however, "it is widely recognized that these measures cannot cure COPD and that much of the effort in the management of this condition must be directed toward preventive treatment strategies, improving symptoms, patient functioning and quality of life"[25] (p. 383). Because the onset of COPD is insidious, developing over 20 to 30 years with a long asymptomatic period, the early detection and rehabilitation of these patients is critical. Early detection may prevent the progression of COPD to a chronic and disabling state. The symptoms of lung disease such as breathlessness, cough, sputum production, and wheezing often cause the patient to be anxious, apprehensive, fatigued, and fearful that the next breath will not come. Patients with COPD tend to live in "emotional straightjackets," as all expressions of emotion lead to distressing or disabling symptoms, as stated by Dudley et al.[26] Through pulmonary rehabilitation, however, these issues and symptoms can be addressed and often improved.

> *Because the onset of COPD is insidious, developing over 20 to 30 years with a long asymptomatic period, the early detection and rehabilitation of these patients is critical.*

The goal of earlier detection is not just for the COPD population but for any patient with pulmonary disease. Anyone with a history of smoking, family history of lung disease, occupational or environmental exposures, and symptoms of cough and mucus production should automatically be considered for a spirometry test,[27] which is considered the best assessment tool to determine whether an individual has lung abnormalities.[28] In 1979, Macklem and Permutt stated,

> *In considering the simplicity of determination of FEV$_1$ and its potential use in detecting individuals who are headed toward serious trouble at a time when intervention might have prevented a disastrous outcome, it is interesting to explore the reasons why the spirometer has not achieved a position comparable to the clinical thermometer, the sphygmomanometer, the ophthalmoscope, the chest x-ray and the electrocardiogram.* [29]

> *The goal of earlier detection is not just for the COPD population but for any patient with pulmonary disease.*

Pulmonary rehabilitation should address health promotion and disease prevention; this can be accomplished when prevention is integrated into pulmonary rehabilitation.[30] Prevention is defined in three ways: primary, secondary, and tertiary.[31] Primary prevention involves health promotion and addressing risk factors. Intervention is accomplished through behavioral change that decreases the risk of disease before any evidence of disease appears (e.g., smoking cessation/nicotine addiction programs). Secondary prevention occurs after a disease is present without apparent symptoms. According to Coultas and Samet, "Clinicians need to understand the natural history of COPD and the associated opportunity for intervention at a time before smoking-caused decline of lung function has resulted in overt disease."[32] Tertiary prevention is applied to a patient with symptomatic disease; the prevention is directed toward slowing the deterioration and complications of the disease to avoid or lessen disability. These preventive strategies include teaching the patients about the need for immunizations, how to identify their asthma triggers, what the early warning signs of an infection are, and when to notify their physician or implement their medication self-management plan. These preventive strategies are critical to promoting better health.

> *Pulmonary rehabilitation should address health promotion and disease prevention; this can be accomplished when prevention is integrated into pulmonary rehabilitation.*

PHILOSOPHY

Successful pulmonary rehabilitation requires that the patient, significant other, and the interdisciplinary team members believe in the philosophy of pulmonary rehabilitation. This philosophy should include a rehabilitation process that is directed toward the patient but occurs with the patient's cooperation. As described in the Code of Ethics, pulmonary rehabilitation team members should serve as role models in attitude, communication style, and professionalism for the patient, significant other, and the general and medical community.

Code of Ethics for Pulmonary Rehabilitation Team Members

As pulmonary rehabilitation specialists involved in the care of patients with pulmonary disease, we must strive, both individually and as a team, to maintain the highest ethical standards.

The principles set forth in this document outline the ethical and moral standards to which each pulmonary rehabilitation team member should conform.

The pulmonary rehabilitation specialist shall practice medically acceptable methods of pulmonary rehabilitation and shall not extend his or her practice beyond the competence and authority vested in him or her by the pulmonary rehabilitation medical director.

The pulmonary rehabilitation specialist shall always strive to increase and improve his or her knowledge and expertise and render to each pulmonary rehabilitation patient/significant other the full measure of his or her ability. All treatment modalities and training sessions shall be provided with respect for the dignity of the patient/significant other, unrestricted by considerations of social, economic, personal, or religious beliefs.

The pulmonary rehabilitation specialist shall be responsible for the competent, efficient, and thorough performance of his or her designated duties.

The pulmonary rehabilitation specialist shall hold in strict confidence all patient information.

The pulmonary rehabilitation specialist, as a vital member of the interdisciplinary health care team, shall strive for the prevention and early detection, not just the treatment, of pulmonary disease.

Adapted, by permission, from the American Association for Respiratory Care, 1986, *Code of Ethics.* 11030 Ables Lane, Dallas, TX 75229.

PATIENT GOALS AND PROGRAM GOALS

Pulmonary rehabilitation staff should be consistent in their understanding of the goals of pulmonary rehabilitation as they pertain to the individual patient and to the overall program. Patient goals need to be established and reviewed with the patient/significant other at the beginning of the program. Goals should be realistic and readily achievable to improve patient motivation, adherence, and outcomes. Patient goals may include (but are not limited to) the following:

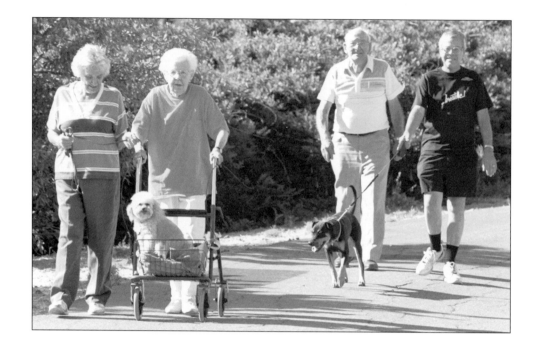

Patient goals should be realistic and readily achievable to improve patient motivation, adherence, and outcomes.

▌ Breathe better

▌ Be more active

▌ Have a better quality of life

▌ Increase strength and endurance

▌ Be able to perform activities of daily living including hobbies

▌ Travel

▌ Decrease anxiety and/or depression

▌ Prevent exacerbations and hospitalizations

▌ Be independent and self-reliant

▌ Return to work

The program goals should be based upon the interdisciplinary team's assessments, which may include (but are not limited to) the following:

▌ Integrate prevention into the patient's treatment plan

▌ Design and implement an individualized treatment plan (e.g., smoking cessation, weight loss/gain, etc.)

▌ Improve the patient's/significant other's quality of life

▌ Control and alleviate, as much as possible, the symptoms and pathophysiological complications of respiratory impairment

▌ Increase exercise tolerance

▌ Decrease psychological symptoms such as anxiety or depression

▌ Increase patient compliance with the medical regime

▌ Train, motivate, and rehabilitate the patient to his or her maximum potential in self-care

▌ Train, motivate, and involve the patient's significant other in the patient's treatment plan

▌ Reduce the economic burden of pulmonary disease on society through reduction of acute exacerbations, frequency of hospitalizations and length of stay, emergency room visits, long-term duration of convalescence, etc.

▌ Return the patient to gainful employment or active retirement

▌ Educate the general public and health care professionals about pulmonary health and rehabilitation

▌ Increase the medical community's awareness regarding the importance of early detection of pulmonary disease through screenings (e.g., spirometry, etc.)

▌ Increase the community's awareness of the harmful effects of smoking, nicotine addiction, secondhand smoke, and available treatment for nicotine addiction/smoking cessation and so on

ESSENTIAL COMPONENTS

The essential components of pulmonary rehabilitation are assessment, patient training, exercise, psychosocial intervention, and follow-up.[2] Prevention strategies should be integrated into every aspect of the program.[30] As shown in figure 1.1, pulmonary rehabilitation is not simply an exercise or education program. Instead, it is an individualized program that meets the specific needs of the pulmonary patient through all of the essential components listed above. The pulmonary rehabilitation interdisciplinary team must understand this concept when developing a complete and individualized plan for the patient. The composition of the interdisciplinary team will depend on the facility resources and patient needs (see chapter 8). Not every patient requires all of the interdisciplinary services mentioned in figure 1.1, but these services should be available if needed.

> The essential components of pulmonary rehabilitation are assessment, patient training, exercise, psychosocial intervention, and follow-up. Prevention strategies should be integrated into every aspect of the program.

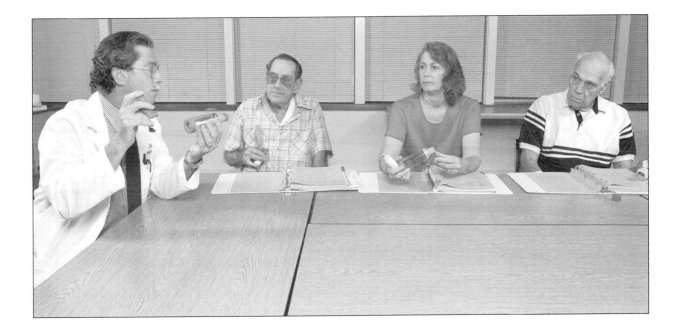

ESSENTIAL COMPONENTS

Team Assessment*

Patient selection

Medical history

Diagnostic tests

Symptom assessment

Physical assessment

Nutritional assessment

Activities of daily living assessment

Educational assessment

Exercise assessment

Psychosocial assessment

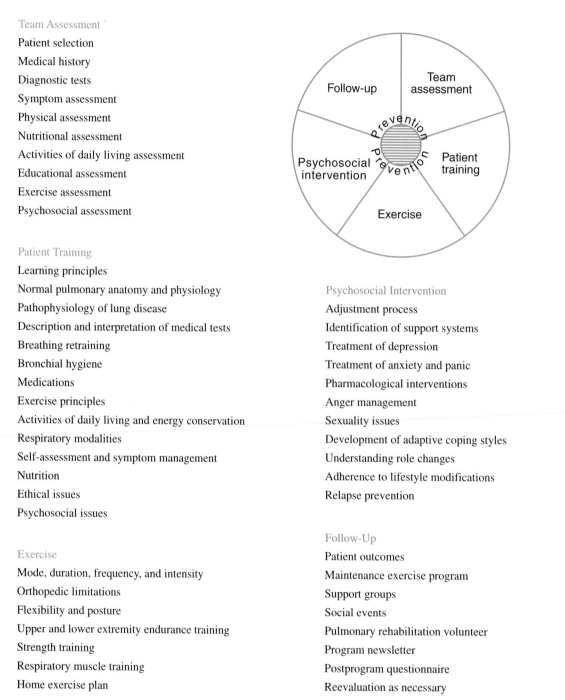

Patient Training

Learning principles

Normal pulmonary anatomy and physiology

Pathophysiology of lung disease

Description and interpretation of medical tests

Breathing retraining

Bronchial hygiene

Medications

Exercise principles

Activities of daily living and energy conservation

Respiratory modalities

Self-assessment and symptom management

Nutrition

Ethical issues

Psychosocial issues

Psychosocial Intervention

Adjustment process

Identification of support systems

Treatment of depression

Treatment of anxiety and panic

Pharmacological interventions

Anger management

Sexuality issues

Development of adaptive coping styles

Understanding role changes

Adherence to lifestyle modifications

Relapse prevention

Exercise

Mode, duration, frequency, and intensity

Orthopedic limitations

Flexibility and posture

Upper and lower extremity endurance training

Strength training

Respiratory muscle training

Home exercise plan

Follow-Up

Patient outcomes

Maintenance exercise program

Support groups

Social events

Pulmonary rehabilitation volunteer

Program newsletter

Postprogram questionnaire

Reevaluation as necessary

* An individualized pulmonary rehabilitation program meets the specific needs of the patient. Not every member of the pulmonary rehabilitation interdisciplinary team may be involved with the patient.

Figure 1.1   Essential components of a pulmonary rehabilitation program.

Note: Pulmonary rehabilitation should address health promotion and disease prevention, which can be accomplished when prevention is integrated into every component. Training or exercise alone does not constitute a pulmonary rehabilitation program.

Reprinted, by permission, from L. Beytas and G.L. Connors, 1993, Organization and management of a pulmonary rehabilitation program. In *Pulmonary rehabilitation: Guidelines to success,* 2ed., edited by J.E. Hodgkin, G.L. Connors, and C.W. Bell. Copyright 1993 by J.B. Lippincott.

CONCLUSION

Pulmonary rehabilitation is a comprehensive preventive and therapeutic treatment program individualized to the patient's needs. The essential components of pulmonary rehabilitation are assessment, patient training, exercise, psychosocial intervention, and follow-up. Prevention should be integrated into every aspect of the comprehensive program. The interdisciplinary team's understanding of the program goals and the patients'/significant others' goals for pulmonary rehabilitation will allow optimum care for the patient with pulmonary disease. Hodgkin stated nearly ten years ago that "an effective pulmonary rehabilitation program is no longer a luxury but a necessity for patients with pulmonary disease."[33] This is even more true today as lung disease continues to steadily increase in terms of lives affected, morbidity, mortality, and health care cost. As pulmonary rehabilitation specialists, we must be proactive not reactive in this changing health care environment.

REFERENCES

1. Woodhead, G.S., and P.C. Varrier-Jones. 1917. Experiences in colony treatment and after-care. *Lancet* 2:779-85.

2. American Association of Cardiovascular and Pulmonary Rehabilitation. 1993. *Guidelines for pulmonary rehabilitation programs*. Champaign, IL: Human Kinetics.

3. Hodgkin, J.E., G.L. Connors, and C.W. Bell, eds. 1993. *Pulmonary rehabilitation: Guidelines to success*. 2d ed. Philadelphia: Lippincott.

4. Casaburi, R., and T.L. Petty. 1993. *Principles and practice of pulmonary rehabilitation*. Philadelphia: W.B. Saunders.

5. Hass, F., and K. Axen, eds. 1991. *Pulmonary therapy and rehabilitation*. Baltimore: Williams & Wilkins.

6. American Thoracic Society. 1995. Standards for the diagnosis and care of patients with chronic obstructive pulmonary disease. *Am J Respir Crit Care Med* 152 (Suppl):77-120.

7. Petty, T.L. 1975. *Pulmonary rehabilitation*. In *Basics of RD*. Vol. 4. New York: American Thoracic Society, pg. 1.

8. Hodgkin, J.E. et al. 1981. Pulmonary rehabilitation: Official ATS statement. *Am Rev Respir Dis* 124:663-66.

9. Fishman, A.P. 1994. NIH workshop summary: Pulmonary rehabilitation research. *Am J Respir Crit Care Med* 149:825-33.

10. Hilling, L., and J. Smith. 1995. Pulmonary rehabilitation. In *Cardiopulmonary physical therapy*. 3d ed. Edited by S. Irwin and J.S. Tecklin, 445-470. St. Louis: Mosby.

11. Celli, B.R. 1995. Pulmonary rehabilitation in patients with COPD. *Am J Respir Crit Care Med* 152:861-64.

12. Hodgkin, J.E. 1993. Benefits and the future of pulmonary rehabilitation. In *Pulmonary rehabilitation: Guidelines to success*. 2d ed. Edited by J.E. Hodgkin, G.L. Connors, and C.W. Bell, 587-604. Philadelphia: Lippincott.

13. Hodgkin, J.E. 1996. Benefits of pulmonary rehabilitation. In *Pulmonary rehabilitation, Lung biology in health and disease*, edited by A.P. Fishman. Vol. 91, 33-46. New York: Marcel Dekker, Inc.

14. Ries, A.L. 1990. Position paper of the American Association of Cardiovascular and Pulmonary Rehabilitation: Scientific basis of pulmonary rehabilitation. *J Cardiopulm Rehabil* 10:418-41.

15. Goldstein, R.S. et al. 1994. Randomized controlled trial of respiratory rehabilitation. *Lancet* 344:1394-97.

16. Reardon, J. et al. 1994. The effect of comprehensive outpatient pulmonary rehabilitation on dyspnea. *Chest* 105 (4):1046-52.

17. O'Donnell, E.D. et al. 1995. The impact of exercise reconditioning on breathlessness in severe chronic airflow limitation. *Am J Respir Crit Care Med* 152:2005-13.

18. Strijbos, J.H. et al. 1996. A comparison between an outpatient hospital-based pulmonary rehabilitation program and a home-care pulmonary rehabilitation program in patients with COPD. *Chest* 109:366-72.

19. Ries, A.L. et al. 1995. Effects of pulmonary rehabilitation on physiologic and psychosocial outcomes in patients with chronic obstructive pulmonary disease. *Ann Intern Med* 122:823-32.

20. Fishman, A.P., ed. 1996. Pulmonary rehabilitation: From empiricism to science. In *Pulmonary rehabilitation, Lung biology in health and disease.* Vol. 91, 15-16. New York: Marcel Dekker, Inc.

21. Corsello, P.R. 1991. Rehabilitation of the chronic obstructive pulmonary disease patients: General principles. In *Pulmonary therapy and rehabilitation,* edited by F. Haas and K. Axen, 197-212. Baltimore: Williams & Wilkins.

22. American Lung Association. 1996. *Lung disease data.* New York: American Lung Association.

23. Weiss D.B., P.J. Gergen, and T.A. Hodgson. 1992. An economic evaluation of asthma in the United States. *N Engl J Med* 326:862.

24. Famighetti, R. et al. 1996. *The world almanac and book of facts.* Mahwah, NJ: Funk & Wagnalls.

25. Kaplan, R.M., and A.L. Ries. 1996. Cost-effectiveness of pulmonary rehabilitation. In *Pulmonary rehabilitation, Lung biology in health and disease,* edited by A.P. Fishman. Vol. 91, 383. New York: Marcel Dekker, Inc.

26. Dudley, D.L. et al. 1980. Psychosocial concomitants to rehabilitation in chronic obstructive pulmonary disease. *Chest* 77:413-544, 677.

27. Petty, T.L. 1994. Pulmonary rehabilitation: Where we've been and where we should be going. Paper presented at the Ninth Annual Meeting of the American Association of Cardiovascular and Pulmonary Rehabilitation (October). Included in Meeting Syllabus published by AACVPR, Portland, OR.

28. Enright, P.L., and J.E. Hodgkin. 1991. Pulmonary function tests. In *Respiratory care: A guide to clinical practice.* 3d ed. Edited by G.G. Burton, J.E. Hodgkin, and J.J. Ward, 157-79. Philadelphia: Lippincott.

29. Macklem, P.R., and S. Permutt. 1979. *The lung in transition between health and disease.* New York: Marcel Dekker.

30. Connors, G.L. 1995. A primary role in secondary prevention. *J Respir Care Prac* (February/March):31-34.

31. Peters, J.A. 1993. Preventive care in pulmonary rehabilitation. In *Pulmonary rehabilitation: Guidelines to success.* 2d ed. Edited by J.E. Hodgkin, G.L. Connors, and C.W. Bell, 102-18. Philadelphia: Lippincott.

32. Coultas, D.B., and J.M. Samet. 1996. Smoking cessation and pulmonary rehabilitation. In *Pulmonary rehabilitation, Lung biology in health and disease,* edited by A.P. Fishman. Vol. 91, 401. New York: Marcel Dekker, Inc.

33. Bunch, D. 1988. Pulmonary rehabilitation: The next ten years. *AARC Times* 12 (3):54.

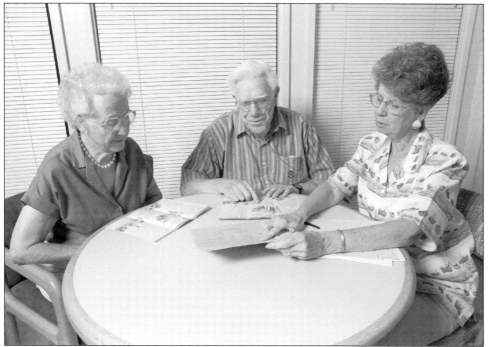

CHAPTER 2

Selection and Assessment of the Pulmonary Rehabilitation Candidate

A comprehensive pulmonary rehabilitation program may be adapted for any individual with pulmonary disease, which expands the patient selection criteria. The practice of reserving pulmonary rehabilitation for patients with end-stage lung disease or severe limitation of function results in many individuals being denied the opportunity to benefit from pulmonary rehabilitation. Therefore, as pulmonary rehabilitation specialists we need to educate the public and the medical community about the importance of prevention, early detection, and rehabilitation of patients with lung disease.

The first component of a pulmonary rehabilitation program is the interdisciplinary team assessment. This assessment sets the foundation for tailoring the program to meet the patient's individual needs. The components of patient training, exercise, or psychosocial interventions alone or together do not constitute pulmonary rehabilitation unless an initial and ongoing assessment is included.

> The practice of reserving pulmonary rehabilitation for patients with end-stage lung disease or severe limitation of function results in many individuals being denied the opportunity to benefit from pulmonary rehabilitation.

PATIENT SELECTION

A list of conditions considered appropriate for pulmonary rehabilitation is shown in table 2.1. The degree of impairment in pulmonary function testing is commonly used as the primary selection criteria in establishing patient eligibility for pulmonary rehabilitation. Although helpful in patient evaluation, pulmonary function tests are not sufficient as selection criteria alone. Symptoms, especially dyspnea, correlate better with functional ability than FEV_1 or other measures of pulmonary function.[1] In addition to the presence of disease, an important selection criterion should be an impairment in health-related quality of life resulting from the disease or its comorbidity. Reductions in physical activity, occupational performance, activities of daily living, and increases in medical resource consumption should be evaluated and used in the

---

Table 2.1   Conditions Appropriate for Pulmonary Rehabilitation

Obstructive Diseases

- Chronic obstructive pulmonary disease (COPD)
  - Chronic bronchitis
  - Emphysema
- Alpha 1 Antitrypsin Deficiency (a1AT)
- Asthma and asthmatic bronchitis
- Bronchiectasis
- Cystic fibrosis
- Bronchiolitis obliterans

Restrictive Diseases

- *Interstitial diseases*
  - Interstitial fibrosis, including rheumatoid lung and other disorders secondary to collagen-vascular disease
  - Occupational or environmental lung disease
  - Sarcoidosis
- *Chest wall diseases*
  - Kyphoscoliosis
  - Spondylitis
- *Neuromuscular diseases*
  - Parkinson's disease
  - Postpolio syndrome
  - Amyotrophic lateral sclerosis
  - Diaphragm dysfunction
  - Multiple sclerosis

Other Conditions

- Lung cancer
- Primary pulmonary hypertension
- Post-thoracic surgery
- Before and after lung transplantation
- Before and after volume reduction surgery
- Ventilator dependency
- Pediatric patients with pulmonary disease
- Morbid obesity
- Sleep apnea

---

selection process.[2] The criteria used for selecting a patient for pulmonary rehabilitation are listed in table 2.2.

Concurrent diseases or conditions that may interfere with the rehabilitation process or place the patient at substantial risk during exercise should be corrected or stabilized before the patient enters the program. Permanent or temporary conditions that may be considered contraindications to pulmonary rehabilitation include, but are not limited to, the conditions listed in table 2.3.

Current smoking status has been used by some programs as a consideration in accepting or denying patients' participation. Some programs exclude active cigarette smokers from participating in pulmonary rehabilitation, believing they are less motivated and committed than the non- or ex-smoker. If active smokers are accepted, smoking cessation is a major goal of the rehabilitation process.

Patient motivation is also a necessary consideration in patient selection, although difficult to assess. Patients must agree to commit to complete the program and be an

Pulmonary function tests are not sufficient as selection criteria alone; another important selection criterion should be an impairment in health-related quality of life resulting from the disease or its comorbidity.

Table 2.2 Patient Selection Criteria for Pulmonary Rehabilitation

Impaired quality of life

Reduction in physical activity

Decreased occupational performance

Dependence in activities of daily living

Noncompliance with medication regime (e.g., oxygen, aerosolized medications)

Psychosocial problems (e.g., anxiety, depression, etc.)

Increased use of medical resources (e.g., hospitalizations, urgent care/emergency room visits, physician visits)

Comorbidity

Pulmonary function abnormalities

Arterial oxygenation

Smoking history

Motivation for rehabilitation, including time commitment and active program participation

Transportation needs

Financial resources

Reprinted, by permission, from L. Beytas and G.L. Connors, 1993, Organization and management of a pulmonary rehabilitation program. In *Pulmonary rehabilitation: Guidelines to success,* 2ed., edited by J.E. Hodgkin, G.L. Connors, and C.W. Bell. Copyright 1993 by J.B. Lippincott.

Table 2.3 Possible Contraindications to Pulmonary Rehabilitation

Ischemic cardiac disease	Metastatic cancer
Congestive heart failure	Disabling stroke
Acute cor pulmonale	Active substance abuse
Severe pulmonary hypertension	Severe cognitive deficit
Significant hepatic dysfunction	Severe psychiatric disease

Reprinted, by permission, from L. Beytas and G.L. Connors, 1993, Organization and management of a pulmonary rehabilitation program. In *Pulmonary rehabilitation: Guidelines to success,* 2ed., edited by J.E. Hodgkin, G.L. Connors, and C.W. Bell. Copyright 1993 by J.B. Lippincott.

active participant. Patients who initially appear resistant to rehabilitation, however, often show dramatic improvement and become advocates of the program. Therefore, patient motivation shouldn't be considered too strongly in the evaluation criteria.

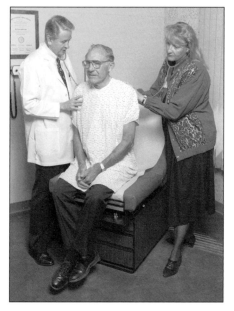

Discussing the patient's financial ability to meet the anticipated expenses of pulmonary rehabilitation is necessary. Third-party payers should be contacted to determine if the rehabilitation program is a covered benefit and, if so, to what extent. Patients are then able to determine if they can afford the out-of-pocket expenses. Verbal and written information regarding program fees and coverage must be given to the patient prior to admission.

Patients being considered must also have a means of transportation to and from the program. This may be provided by family members, friends, or public transit. Local and regional telephone books have transportation assistance information available from state and federal agencies. It is often listed under "disabled," "handicapped," or "aging" headings. Patients too ill to regularly attend outpatient pulmonary rehabilitation may be candidates for admission to an inpatient rehabilitation facility or home care. If the pulmonary rehabilitation facility has a social services department, their staff may assist patients with financial issues, transportation, and access to community support networks.

PATIENT ASSESSMENT

The initial assessment may be performed by members of the interdisciplinary team, as determined by the patient's individualized needs.

The initial assessment should include a patient interview and the components listed in table 2.4. These assessments may be performed by various members of the interdisciplinary team, as determined by the patient's individualized needs. An in-depth interview with the patient and family or significant other is necessary to help assess the patient and to establish appropriate individual goals.[3] Figure 2.1 illustrates a sample form that may be filled out by the pulmonary rehabilitation specialist during the initial interview. Another approach to obtain patient information is to request that the patient complete a questionnaire prior to the interview. A sample questionnaire is shown in figure 2.2.

The importance of the initial interview cannot be overstated. Not only are assessments made and goals formulated, but also the foundations of trust and credibility are generated at this time. The interview allows the patient to interact on a personal level with the rehabilitation staff, see where the program is located, and possibly meet rehabilitation graduates.

Table 2.4 Components of the Initial Patient Assessment	
Patient interview	Activities of daily living assessment
Medical history	Educational assessment
Diagnostic test	Exercise assessment
Symptoms assessment	Psychosocial assessment
Physical assessment	Goal development
Nutritional assessment	

INITIAL INTERVIEW FORM

Name: _____ Date: _____

Address: _____ Phone: _____

Emergency contact: _____ Phone: _____

Age: _____ Sex: _____ Occupation: _____

Height: _____ Weight: _____ Highest Level of Education: _____

Marital Status: _____ Advance Directives: _____

Diagnosis: _____ Insurance Provider: _____

Referring Physician: _____

Primary Care Physician: _____

Referral Source: _____

Chief Complaint: _____

History

How many times have you been hospitalized in the last year due to lung problems? _____

days in the hospital in the last year due to lung disease? _____

How many E.R. visits have you had in the past year as a result of breathing difficulty? _____

Last hospital admission: _____ Release: _____

Previous hospitalizations: _____

Have you ever attended a pulmonary rehabilitation program? _____

Have you ever had any chest injuries or surgeries? Yes / No

  Type _____

Do you have any upcoming surgeries? Yes / No _____

Do you have any physical limitations that may affect your ability to exercise (sensory loss, amputation, stroke, surgeries,

  fractures, etc.)? _____

Do you have any other medical problems?

Cardiovascular disease _____

Hypertension _____

Diabetes _____

G-I problems _____

Reflux/hiatal hernia _____

Osteoporosis _____

Sinusitis _____

Vision or hearing problems _____

Other _____

Have you ever had or do you have:

Emphysema	_____	Valley fever	_____
Asthma	_____	Tuberculosis	_____
Bronchitis	_____	Pleurisy	_____
Pneumonia	_____	Lung cancer	_____
Bronchiectasis	_____	Sinus trouble	_____
Blood clot in lung	_____	Other	_____
High pressure in lungs	_____		

(continued)

Figure 2.1 Pulmonary rehabilitation initial interview form.

Reprinted courtesy of the Pulmonary Rehabilitation Program at St. Joseph's Hospital and Medical Center, Phoenix, AZ.

Do you have a family history of respiratory disease? _____

Have you ever used tobacco? _____ What form? Chew/Smoke _____

Do you chew/smoke now? _____ How long did/have you used tobacco? _____

When did you stop chewing/smoking? _____

If you are still smoking, do you plan to quit? _____

Do you live with any smokers? _____

Other substance abuse? _____

Have you ever been exposed to:

Asbestos dust	Yes/No		Paint fumes	Yes/No
Cotton dust	Yes/No		Plastic fumes	Yes/No
Mining dust	Yes/No		Solvent fumes	Yes/No
Other dusts	Yes/No		Other fumes	Yes/No

Do you consume alcohol? _____ How much? _____

Do you have any allergies (food, pollen, drugs, etc.)? _____

How many colds do you get per year? _____

Vaccines: Flu Yes/No   Pneumonia Yes/No

Do you ever have chest pain? _____ Location _____

  Type of pain _____ Frequency _____

Have you ever had a heart attack? _____ When? _____

Major Symptomatology

What are your symptoms today? _____

What were your symptoms last year? _____

What were your symptoms five years ago? _____

When did you realize that you had lung problems? _____

Disease Impact

Do you sleep flat or with your head elevated? _____

  If elevated, how high? _____

Do you awaken during the night? _____ How often? _____

  Why? _____

Do your ankles ever swell up? _____ When? _____

Do you cough? _____ What part of the day? _____

Do you cough up sputum? _____ When? _____

  Describe _____

  Have you ever coughed up blood? _____

Dyspnea Index

_____ Class 1:   If SOB, consistent with activity

_____ Class 2:   SOB climbing hills or stairs

_____ Class 3:   Can walk at own pace but not at normal pace without SOB

_____ Class 4:   SOB walking 100 yards on level ground, dressing, or talking

Do you use oxygen? _____ How often? _____ LPM: _____

Type of oxygen delivery system _____ Supplier _____

Are you on any home respiratory therapy? _____ Type _____

Do you use any respiratory equipment? _____ Type _____

  How do you clean the equipment? _____

(continued)

Figure 2.1 *(continued)*

18

Do you have trouble eating? _____ Why? _____

Do you have trouble gaining or losing weight? _____

Have you experienced a recent weight change? _____

Do you have a special diet? _____

Are you able to care for yourself? _____

Are you able to take care of your home? _____

Do you exercise? _____ If yes, how? _____ How often? _____

Do you have exercise equipment? _____ Type _____

Has your physician limited your activities? _____

Any special interests or hobbies? _____

What activities does your breathing difficulty prevent you from doing that you would like to do? _____

Does your breathing interfere with your ability to have sexual relations? _____

Are others close to you affected by your health? _____

   If yes, how? _____

Are you affected by trying to live up to others' expectations? _____

   How? _____

Do you find yourself worrying daily? _____ occasionally? _____ almost never? _____

Does your income cover your expenses and needs? _____

Do you live alone? _____

Do you have transportation? _____ How? _____

How do you heat and cool your home? _____

Do you have any pets? _____

Medications

Type	Amount	Frequency

Medication compliance: Yes/No

M.D.I. technique:

Spacer: Yes/No   Type:_____   Needs training: Yes/No

Observations

   Color _____   Skin turgor _____

   Mentation _____   Energy level _____

   Nutritional status _____

   B/P_____   Pulse _____   Edema _____

(continued)

Figure 2.1 *(continued)*

Respirations (rate, rhythm, depth) _____

Accessory breather? _____   Pursed lips? _____

Abdominal breathing? _____   Other _____

Auscultation _____

Data From Patient's Records

FEV$_1$ _____   FEV$_1$/FVC _____   ABGs _____   Hb/Hct _____

Alb _____   EKG _____   Other _____

Client's Stated Goals

Please state your goals or what you expect to achieve from this rehabilitation program.

_____

_____

Patient's signature _____

Estimated Learning Ability

_____ No baseline, slow learner   _____ Some baseline, slow learner

_____ No baseline, good learner   _____ Some baseline, good learner

_____ Needs only comprehensive review and reinforcement

Degree of motivation _____

Candidacy: Accept _____   Reject _____

Evaluator's signature _____

Figure 2.1   (continued)

Medical History

The medical history is important in highlighting comorbid conditions that may have a direct bearing on the patient's health, well-being, and progress in the pulmonary rehabilitation program.

A thorough review of the patient's medical status is essential for the initial assessment. Much of this information can be obtained from patient records in the physician's office or the hospital. The medical history is important in highlighting comorbid conditions that may have a direct bearing on the patient's health, well-being, and progress in the pulmonary rehabilitation program. One example is a patient with a hip or knee disorder who may need to have the frequency, intensity, and mode of exercise adjusted. A listing of the medical history information to be gathered is summarized below.

Medical History

▌ Respiratory history

▌ Family history of respiratory disease

▌ Active medical problems

▌ Other medical and surgical history

▌ Utilization of medical resources (e.g., hospitalizations, urgent care/emergency room visits, physician visits)

▌ All current medications including over-the-counter drugs

▌ Allergies and drug intolerance

▌ Smoking history

(continued on page 26)

PARTICIPANT QUESTIONNAIRE

Date: _____ Physician: _____

Name: _____

Address: _____

City/State: _____ Zip: _____ Phone: _____

Age: _____ Birth date: _____ Marital status: M S W D

Spouse's name: _____

Social Security #: _____ Medicare #: _____

Insurance: _____
_____

Diagnosis: _____

Living Situation: ____ House   ____ Apartment   ____ Mobile home   ____ Condo

Level: _____ Single ____ Multi

Entrance: ____ Incline   ____ Stair(s) # ____

Household members: _____

(Relationship & name) _____

Household pets: _____

(Type & name) _____

Usual household duties I perform: ___ Cooking ___ Cleaning ___ Finances ___ Laundry ___ Transportation

___ Yard work ___ Grocery shopping

My major source(s) of support: (names and relationships) _____

Transportation: ____ Currently drive   ____ Rely on family   ____ Rely on friends

____ Use public transportation ____ Is a real problem for me

Occupational History:

Current or former occupation: _____

Retirement/disability date: _____

Occupational exposure: ____ Welding ____ Pottery ____ Asbestos ____ Mines/foundry ____ Gas/fumes

____ Quarry ____ Sandblasting ____ Chemicals ____ Dust

Educational History:

The last grade I completed was: _____

I learn information best by: ___ Explanation ___ Reading ___ Video/TV ___ Computer ___ Demonstration

Medical History:

(Please check those that apply; mark with F if family history exists)

___ Asthma	___ High blood pressure
___ Chronic bronchitis	___ Arthritis
___ Emphysema	___ Pulmonary fibrosis
___ Bronchiectasis	___ Fractures (specify) _____
___ Osteoporosis	___ Cancer
___ Cystic fibrosis	___ Pneumonia
___ Tuberculosis	___ Heart disease
___ Diabetes	___ Sarcoidosis
___ Sinus problems	___ Collapsed lung

(continued)

Figure 2.2 Pulmonary rehabilitation participant questionnaire.

Adapted from Pulmonary Rehabilitation Programs at Long Beach Memorial Medical Center, Long Beach, CA, Mt. Diablo Medical Center, Concord, CA, and Union Hospital, Dover, OH.

Allergy History:

I have seen an allergist. ___ Yes ___ No

Skin testing performed. ___ Yes ___ No

I am allergic to the following:

    Food(s): _____

    Medications: _____

    Environmental: ___ Dust ___ Mold ___ Pollens ___ Grass Other: _____

I have difficulty when exposed to the following environmental irritants:

    ___ Dust ___ Smog ___ Solvents ___ Humidity ___ Perfumes/colognes

    ___ Rapid changes in temperature ___ Tobacco smoke ___ Wind ___ Other: _____

Vaccine History:

I receive the flu vaccine annually. ___ Yes ___ No

    If no, why? _____

I have received the pneumonia vaccine. ___ Yes ___ No

    Year received: _____

Smoking History:

___ I have never smoked.

___ I have smoked in the past but do not smoke now.

    Year started _____ Year quit _____

    Number of packs smoked per day _____

___ I am currently a smoker.

    Number of packs smoked per day _____

Exposure to secondhand smoke: ___ None ___ Home

                                                    ___ Social situations ___ Work

Pulmonary Health History:

Cough: ___ No ___ Yes ___ A.M. ___ P.M.

                                                                  ___ Nighttime ___ Around the clock

Mucus: Normal color: _____

                     ___ Thick ___ Thin ___ Moderate

          Amount/day: ___ 1 tsp. ___ 1-2 tsp. ___ 1 Tbsp. ___ 1/4 cup ___ 1/2 cup ___ 1 cup ___ >1 cup

          When: ___ A.M. ___ P.M. ___ Around clock

I use the following to help me raise my mucus:

    ___ Drink warm liquids ___ Inhalers

    ___ Aerosol treatments ___ Chest percussion

    ___ Postural drainage ___ Increase my fluids

I have coughed up blood. ___ Yes ___ No

                            When: _____

I have taken steroid pills (e.g., Prednisone). ___ Yes ___ No

Length of time: _____ Last date: _____

Highest dose: _____

I experience the following:

    ___ Chest pain ___ Dizziness/unsteadiness ___ Hoarseness

    ___ Fatigue ___ Ankle swelling ___ Weight change

    ___ Wheezing ___ A.M. ___ P.M.

    Known trigger factors: _____

(continued)

Figure 2.2 *(continued)*

I have been on a ventilator (respirator) in an intensive care unit. ___ Yes ___ No Last date: _____

What I remember most about that experience is: _____

_____

I see my lung doctor every (please give a time frame): _____

Pulmonary Infections:

Number/year: _____

Antibiotic usually taken: _____

I know I have an infection when: _____

Pulmonary Hospitalizations:

Number in past year: _____

Number in previous year: _____

Emergency Room Visits for Pulmonary Reasons:

Number in past year: _____

Number in previous year: _____

Shortness of Breath:

I have experienced shortness of breath since: _____

My breathing is most difficult: ___ Early A.M. ___ A.M. ___ P.M. ___ Bedtime

I use the following to decrease or avoid being short of breath:

___ Stop and rest	___ Use aerosol machine
___ Use inhalers	___ Use belly/diaphragm breathing
___ Use a fan/air conditioner	___ Open windows
___ Remove myself from the irritant	___ Limit my activity
___ Practice a relaxation technique	___ Avoid exposure to irritants
___ Check the air pollution forecast	___ Check my peak flow
___ Use pursed lip breathing	___ Avoid tobacco smoke exposure

Dietary History:

Current height: _____ Current weight: _____

I have recently had a change in my weight. ___ Yes ___ No

Gained _____ lbs.

Lost _____ lbs.

Over this period of time _____

I can attribute this weight change to: _____

I would like to weigh _____ lbs.

I follow the following type of diet:

___ No special diet	___ Diabetic
___ Low sodium (salt)	___ Ulcer
___ Low cholesterol	___ Hiatal hernia
___ Low saturated fat	___ Other_____
___ Caloric restriction	

My appetite is: ___ Good ___ Fair ___ Poor

I drink this amount of each of these a day:

Water _____	Sodas _____	Coffee _____
Tea _____	Wine _____	Hard liquor _____
Milk _____	Juice _____	Beer _____

(continued)

Figure 2.2 *(continued)*

I have difficulty with: chewing   ___ Yes   ___ No

swallowing   ___ Yes   ___ No

digestion   ___ Yes   ___ No

I take vitamins.   ___ Yes   ___ No

If yes, please list: _____

Sleeping History:

Usual bedtime _____   Usual time of waking up _____

Naps taken during the day: Number _____   Length _____

Number of pillows used when sleeping _____

Medications/strategies used to help me sleep _____

Medication Name/Strength	Amount & Frequency on a Daily Basis	Time(s) of the Day Medication Taken	Purpose of Medication	Comments That You Have
Example: 1. Albuterol	2 puffs 4 times a day	6 A.M., 2 P.M., 6 P.M., 11 P.M.	improve breathing	works well
Example: 2. Lasix 40 mg.	1 tablet once a day	in the morning usually 6 A.M.	blood pressure	

Activities of Daily Living:

Use this SHORTNESS OF BREATH SCALE to answer the following questions:

SCALE: 0 = NONE 1 = MINIMAL 2 = MODERATE 3 = GREAT 4 = UNABLE

To what degree do you get short of breath at rest?_____

To what degree do you get short of breath when climbing stairs? _____

How many stairs? _____

To what degree do you get short of breath during the following activities:

___ Eating?

___ Simple personal care? (washing face, combing hair, etc.)

___ Taking full bath/shower?

___ Dressing?

___ Picking up/straightening up?

___ Sweeping/vacuuming?

___ Shopping?

___ Laundry?

___ Cooking/doing dishes?

___ Walking around your house?

___ Walking your own pace on level surface?

___ Walking one block?

___ Walking with others your age?

___ Walking up a slight hill?

(continued)

Figure 2.2 *(continued)*

Activity/Exercise History:

Yes   No   I currently do purposeful walking ____ days a week for ____ minutes.

Yes   No   I do calisthenics ____ days/week.

Yes   No   I do no purposeful exercise program.

The following things limit my ability to remain active:

    ___ Shortness of breath   ___ Lightheadedness

    ___ Fatigue   ___ Joint problems (specify): _____

    Other: _____

I have the following exercise equipment available:

    ___ None

    ___ Stationary bike   ___ Treadmill   ___ Stair-stepper

    ___ Pool   ___ Weights   ___ Other: _____

Equipment/Assistive Device History:

I use the following items:

    ___ Walker   ___ Eyeglasses

    ___ Wheelchair   ___ Electric cart

    ___ Cane   ___ Hearing aid

    ___ 4-point/quad cane   ___ Other: _____

Respiratory Home Care Equipment History:

I use the following items: Frequency used:

    ___ Peak flow meter   _____

    ___ Aerosol machine (e.g., Pulmoaide)   _____

    ___ Suction machine   _____

    ___ Ventilator   _____

    ___ Mechanical chest percussor   _____

    ___ PEP valve   _____

    ___ Oxygen: ___ Flowrate   System: ___ Concentrator

                                           ___ Tank

                                         ___ Liquid

                                         ___ Pulse

Oxygen used: ___ Continuously   ___ Only when I need it   ___ With sleep only   ___ With exercise only

    ___ With sleep and exercise

I change my oxygen tubing every:

    ___ Week   ___ 2 weeks   ___ 3-4 weeks   ___ 1-2 months

    ___ Oops! I didn't know I need to change it.

My home care equipment vendor is: _____

Day to Day Living:

I am sexually active   ___ Yes   ___ No

My present interests and hobbies are: _____

Former interests and hobbies in which I can no longer participate are: _____

This is what I do for fun: _____

I would describe my present temperament (mood) as: _____
(examples: worried, sad, impatient, frustrated, depressed, anxious, contented, cheerful, etc.)

(continued)

Figure 2.2 *(continued)*

This is what makes me feel this way: _____

I use the following to relax:

    ___ Read   ___ Alcohol   ___ Other: _____

    ___ Deep breathing   ___ Yoga

    ___ Smoke   ___ Pursed lip breathing

    ___ TV   ___ Tranquilizer

This has been the most difficult adjustment for me because of my lung disease:

_____

This is how my lung disease has affected how I feel about myself: _____

_____

My goals for completing pulmonary rehabilitation are: _____

_____

Figure 2.2 *(continued)*

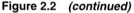

- Occupational, environmental, and recreational exposures

- Alcohol and other substance abuse history

- Comorbid conditions, especially osteoporosis, cardiovascular disease, peripheral vascular disease, cancer, acid-peptic disease including gastroesophageal reflux, dysphasia, diabetes, sinusitis, rhinitis, sleep disturbances including sleep apnea, and neuromuscular or orthopedic impairment

Diagnostic Tests

Baseline diagnostic studies assist in proper diagnosis of the rehabilitation candidate and the development of an appropriate plan of care.

The baseline diagnostic studies listed in table 2.5 assist in proper diagnosis of the rehabilitation candidate and the development of an appropriate plan of care.[4] These diagnostic tests identify the patient's disease(s) and establish a baseline of the patient's current clinical status and may be used postprogram to evaluate outcomes. Additional laboratory tests listed in table 2.6 may also be helpful for selected patients as determined by the initial and ongoing assessments.

Table 2.5 Diagnostic Tests for Initial Evaluation of the Pulmonary Rehabilitation Candidate
Spirometry pre- and postbronchodilator
Lung volumes
Diffusing capacity
Resting arterial blood gas
Arterial oxygen saturation by pulse oximetry
Chest radiograph
Resting electrocardiogram
Exercise test with cutaneous oximetry and/or arterial blood gas (e.g., simple or modified test such as 6- or 12-minute walk, calibrated cycle ergometer, or motorized treadmill)
Complete blood count
Basic blood chemistry panel

Note: It is acceptable not to repeat these tests if done within the three months prior to entering the pulmonary rehabilitation program or as determined by the pulmonary rehabilitation medical director.

Table 2.6   Diagnostic Tests to Consider for Selected Patients
Maximal voluntary ventilation
Maximal inspiratory and expiratory pressures
Theophylline level
Pulmonary exercise stress test (metabolic study) with continuous ECG monitoring
Postexercise spirometry
Bronchial challenge
Cardiovascular tests (e.g., holter monitor, echocardiogram, thallium exercise stress test)
Polysomnography
Sinus x-rays
Upper gastrointestinal series
Skin tests
Risk for falling (Tinetti score)
Anxiety and depression inventory (e.g., Beck Depression Inventory, see also appendix C)

Symptom Assessment

Dyspnea, cough, sputum production, and fatigue are common symptoms in patients with respiratory disease and should be documented if present. Onset, location, quality, quantity, frequency, and duration are often used to describe symptoms. In addition, identifying and alleviating irritating factors is important. Information from symptom assessment may be used to document outcomes and is often used by third-party payers to determine medical necessity for payment authorization. A listing of items to include in the symptom assessment is summarized below.

Symptom Assessment

- Dyspnea: on exertion, paraoxysmal, at rest, nocturnal
- Cough
- Sputum volume, color, consistency, smell
- Fatigue
- Wheeze
- Hemoptysis
- Chest pain
- Postnasal drainage
- Reflux, heartburn
- Edema: pedal, pretibial
- Dysphagia, swallowing problems

An objective rating of dyspnea is especially valuable in the assessment because it is usually the overriding symptom in lung disease and is reduced by pulmonary rehabilitation.[1] See appendix A for further information on the reduction of dyspnea through rehabilitation. Dyspnea during exercise is commonly rated with a 10-point Borg Scale

Information from symptom assessment may be used to document outcomes and is often used by third-party payers to determine medical necessity for payment authorization.

An objective rating of dyspnea is especially valuable in the assessment because it is usually the overriding symptom in lung disease and is reduced by pulmonary rehabilitation.

or a Visual Analog Scale. These two methods of rating dyspnea are explained in chapter 4. The impact of dyspnea on physical function can be measured with the Baseline Dyspnea Index, and changes in dyspnea with rehabilitation can be rated with the Transitional Dyspnea Index described in appendix C.

Physical Assessment

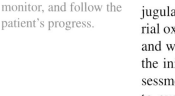

The physical assessment represents a simple and noninvasive way to evaluate, monitor, and follow the patient's progress.

Physical assessment includes measuring and evaluating vital signs, use of accessory muscles of respiration, chest examination, finger clubbing, edema, and other signs of heart failure such as jugular venous distention.[5] Measurement of arterial oxygen saturation with pulse oximetry at rest and with activity is frequently performed during the initial physical assessment. The physical assessment represents a simple and noninvasive way to evaluate, monitor, and follow the patient's progress. A listing of the physical assessment is summarized below.

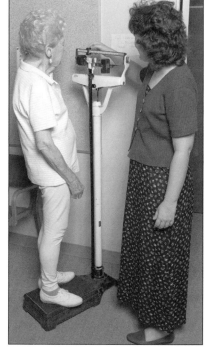

Physical Assessment

▌ Vital signs: height, weight, blood pressure, heart rate, respiratory rate, temperature

▌ Breathing pattern

▌ Use of accessory muscles of respiration

▌ Chest examination: inspection, palpation, percussion, symmetry, diaphragm position, breath sounds, duration of expiratory phase, forced expiratory time, adventitious sounds

▌ Signs of congestive heart failure: S3 gallop, crackles, peripheral edema, jugular venous distention

▌ Presence of finger clubbing

▌ Arterial oxygen saturation measured with pulse oximetry at rest and with activity

Nutritional Assessment

Patients with pulmonary disease often have significant alterations in nutritional status.

Patients with pulmonary disease often have significant alterations in nutritional status.[6] Chronic lung disease causes an increased energy expenditure during breathing, which results in increased caloric needs.[7] Problems of maintaining adequate nutrition are present in 40% to 60% of patients with COPD,[8] and poor nutritional status is a significant predictor of mortality.[9] Weight gain is indicated for the underweight patient. Patients who are overweight possibly due to inactivity or medications require a weight loss program. These patients experience an increase in their work of breathing and shortness of breath as a result of being overweight.

Minimal nutritional assessment includes measurement of height and weight and documentation of recent weight change; in addition, fluid intake and alcohol consumption should be recorded. See figure 2.3 for a sample assessment tool. Other assessments should be based on the needs of the patient. A listing of items included in the nutritional assessment is summarized on page 30.

NUTRITIONAL ASSESSMENT

Name: _____ Date: _____

Height: _____ Weight: _____

What is your "usual" adult weight? _____

Have you gained or lost any weight recently?   No   Yes   How much? _____

Over what period of time? _____

What do you attribute it to? _____

Have you noticed any changes in your eating habits since your pulmonary problems began?

If so, describe them: _____

Do you follow any of these dietary restrictions?

   Low salt   Diabetic   Gout   Ulcer   Low fat/cholesterol   Hiatal hernia   Other: _____

Caloric intake: _____

How would you describe your appetite? _____

Is this usual for you?   No   Yes

Do you take vitamin or mineral supplements?   No   Yes   Specify name, strength, and frequency.

_____

_____

Do you have any food allergies?   No   Yes   What are they?

_____

_____

Describe any problems you have with:

  Dental: _____

  Chewing: _____

  Swallowing: _____

  Digestion: _____

  Constipation/diarrhea: _____

  Bloating: _____

  Nausea: _____

  Fatigue: _____

  Shortness of breath: _____

How many ounces of the following fluids do you drink:

	Daily	Weekly	Rarely
Water	_____	_____	_____
Soft drinks*	_____	_____	_____
Juice	_____	_____	_____
Milk	_____	_____	_____
Coffee*	_____	_____	_____
Tea*	_____	_____	_____
Beer	_____	_____	_____
Wine	_____	_____	_____
Hard liquor	_____	_____	_____
*Caffeine/decaffeinated			

(continued)

Figure 2.3   Nutritional assessment form.

Reprinted courtesy of the Pulmonary Rehabilitation Program at Mt. Diablo Medical Center, Concord, CA.

FOR STAFF USE ONLY:

%IBW: _____   BMI: _____

Weight change: Mild   Moderate   Severe

Supplements? _____

Available Labs: Albumin _____   Cholesterol _____   Other _____

Possible drug/nutrient interactions?

_____

_____

Comments:

_____

_____

Assessment and recommendations:

_____

_____

_____

_____

Date: _____   Dietitian: _____ , RD

Figure 2.3   *(continued)*

Nutritional Assessment

▌ Height and weight

▌ Weight change

▌ Dietary history, diet recall (3 to 7 days)

▌ Person responsible for shopping and food preparation

▌ Fluid intake

▌ Alcohol consumption

▌ Laboratory tests of nutritional status: serum albumin, pre-albumin

▌ Body mass index (weight in kilograms divided by height in meters squared)

▌ Drug/nutrient interactions

▌ Lean body mass determination, when indicated

▌ Need for nutritional supplements

Activities of Daily Living Assessment

Dyspnea often leads to a decreased ability and willingness to perform activities of daily living (ADLs) independently; therefore, the patient's ability to function independently in ADLs and leisure activities should be assessed. The ADLs assessment should include energy conservation techniques, upper extremity strength, proper breathing techniques with daily activities, and need for adaptive equipment.[10] If appropriate, functional task performance and the work environment's demands should be assessed to establish a baseline for planning treatment and measuring outcomes. Table 2.7 lists levels of energy expenditure for common household and leisure activities (in METs) that may be used as a tool to assess ADLs. An interview with a significant other frequently adds complementary information to the patient's self-report. Two recently developed questionnaires, the Pulmonary Functional Status Scale (PFSS),[11] and the Pulmonary Functional Status and Dyspnea Questionnaire (PFSDQ),[12] emphasize functional activities assessment and are described in appendix C.

Dyspnea often leads to a decreased ability and willingness to perform ADLs independently.

Table 2.7 Representative Levels of Energy Expenditure (in METs)[16, 17, 18]

1.5–2 METs	**4–5 METs**
Walking 1 mph	Calisthenics
Standing	Cycling outdoors 6 mph
Driving automobile	Painting
Sitting at desk or typing	Golfing (carrying clubs)
2–3 METs	Playing tennis (doubles)
Walking 2.5–3 mph	**5–6 METs**
Dusting furniture, light housework	Walking 4 mph
Preparing a meal	Digging in garden
3–4 METs	Ice or roller skating 9 mph
Sweeping	Doing carpentry
Vacuuming	**6–7 METs**
Ironing	Stationary cycling (vigorous)
Walking 3 mph	Playing tennis (singles)
Golfing (power cart)	Shoveling snow
Pushing light lawnmower	Mowing lawn (nonpowered)

Note: One MET is the level of energy expenditure at rest, or approximately 3.5 ml/kg/min of oxygen consumption.

Sexual dysfunction resulting from chronic pulmonary disease is another important area to be assessed.[13] See chapter 5 for additional information on sexuality. Understanding the patient's concerns and previous patterns of sexual activity will help in the plan for counseling, if necessary. The reaction of the significant other to the disease and its effect on mutual sexual function is important to determine. A listing of the Activities of Daily Living assessment is summarized below.

Sexual dysfunction resulting from chronic pulmonary disease is another important area to be assessed.

Activities of Daily Living Assessment

- Functional task performance
- Breathing techniques with ADLs
- Upper extremity function
- Energy conservation
- Need for adaptive equipment
- Food procurement and preparation
- Leisure impairment

    ▍ Sexual function

    ▍ Work environment demands

Educational Assessment

Patients' knowledge of the level of their individual disease process and strategies used to cope with their illness can be measured during the initial assessment. This can provide a baseline for evaluation of change in knowledge during and after the program and is a method of documenting outcomes. An example of a pretest used for assessing the patient's knowledge is shown in figure 2.4. A number of areas in addition to patients' knowledge of their disease should be evaluated,[14] including the ability to read or write, hearing or vision impairment, cognitive impairment, language barriers, and cultural diversity (ethnicity, cultural beliefs, and customs). This information can be ascertained during the initial interview session. See chapter 3 for further information on how to develop an educational plan. A listing of items included in the educational assessment is summarized on the next page.

		True	False	Not Sure
1.	The diaphragm is a muscle that does most of the work of breathing.	1	2	3
2.	Emphysema is a disease that primarily affects air sacs (alveoli).	1	2	3
3.	"Pursed-lip breathing" helps prevent small airways from collapsing.	1	2	3
4.	People with chronic lung disease can abruptly stop taking a steroid medication such as prednisone at any time without ill effects	1	2	3
5.	Changing the flow rate on oxygen equipment can be dangerous for a person with chronic lung disease.	1	2	3
6.	For a person with chronic lung disease, eating six small meals a day rather than three large meals can help to reduce shortness of breath during and after meals.	1	2	3
7.	For a person with chronic lung disease, foods that are high in protein, such as fish, are an important part of the diet.	1	2	3
8.	Drinking water has no effect on the mucus in the lungs.	1	2	3
9.	A person with chronic lung disease should rinse out the mouth after using a steroid metered-dose inhaler.	1	2	3
10.	When climbing stairs, a person with chronic lung disease should hold his or her breath briefly while taking a step.	1	2	3
11.	For people with chronic lung disease, the most efficient method of completing a task is to work quickly in short bursts and to take frequent rests.	1	2	3
12.	During activity, people with chronic lung disease should exhale when they exert themselves.	1	2	3
13.	If someone with chronic lung disease is taking antibiotics, it is fine for that person to stop taking them when he or she feels better.	1	2	3
14.	During diaphragmatic breathing, it is important for a person with chronic lung disease to pull in the abdomen during inhalation.	1	2	3
15.	It is important for a person with chronic lung disease to keep the shoulder muscles relaxed to decrease the amount of oxygen used for breathing.	1	2	3
16.	A bronchodilator, such as Theodur, gets rid of infection.	1	2	3

Figure 2.4 Sample quiz for patients with chronic lung disease.

Adapted, by permission, from Y. Scherer, L. Schmeider, and S. Shimmell, 1995, "Outpatient instruction for individuals with COPD," *Perspectives in Respiratory Nursing* 6 (3):3.

Educational Assessment

▮ Knowledge of disease, treatment, and so forth

▮ Hearing

▮ Vision

▮ Cognitive ability

▮ Language

▮ Literacy

▮ Cultural diversity

Exercise Assessment

The safety of an exercise training program and the appropriateness of the exercise prescription are determined by the thoroughness of the initial exercise assessment. This assessment includes evaluation of the patient's exercise tolerance, physical limitations, and requirements for supplemental oxygen. An evaluation of cardiac function and physical limitation should also be included in the assessment.

Exercise assessment includes evaluation of the patient's exercise tolerance, physical limitations, and requirements for supplemental oxygen.

The assessment of physical limitations serves to establish a baseline of strength, range of motion, posture, functional abilities, and activities.[15] The evaluation should also address orthopedic limitations, any restrictions to activity requiring exercise modification, and transferring abilities such as from chair to standing or floor to standing. See chapter 4 for a detailed description of an exercise assessment. A list of the information to be obtained in the exercise assessment is summarized below.

Exercise Assessment

▮ Physical limitations (e.g., strength, range of motion, posture, functional abilities, and activities)

▮ Orthopedic limitations

▮ Transferring abilities

▮ Exercise tolerance

▮ Exercise hypoxemia including the need for supplemental oxygen therapy

▮ Cardiac function

▮ Exercise modification

Psychosocial Assessment

The psychosocial assessment should address several areas: motivation level, emotional distress, substance abuse, cognitive impairment, interpersonal conflict, other psychopathology (e.g., depression, anxiety), significant neuropsychological impairment (e.g., memory, attention/concentration, problem-solving abilities during daily activities), coping style, and sexual dysfunction. Failure to detect the presence of significant psychosocial pathology may result in poor progress with rehabilitation. The findings from the psychosocial assessment are most useful if they lead to specific and

Failure to detect the presence of significant psychosocial pathology may result in poor progress with rehabilitation.

individually tailored treatment goals and are integrated into the overall interdisciplinary treatment plan.

In general, psychosocial evaluation and treatment should be integrated into every
component of pulmonary rehabilitation from assessment through follow-up. Psychosocial assessment is covered in detail in chapter 5. A listing of items included in the
psychosocial assessment is summarized below.

Psychosocial Assessment

▌ Perception of quality of life and ability to adjust to the disease

▌ Interpersonal conflict

▌ Psychopathology (e.g., depression, anxiety, etc.)

▌ Substance abuse

▌ Neuropsychological impairment

▌ Sexual dysfunction

▌ Motivation for pulmonary rehabilitation

GOAL DEVELOPMENT

Setting realistic goals
that are compatible
with the patient's
underlying disease, the
patient's needs and
expectations, and the
program's objectives is
important.

Measurable, patient-specific goals are formulated from data collected during the initial patient assessment. Setting realistic goals that are compatible with the patient's
underlying disease, the patient's needs and expectations, and the program's objectives
is important. Goals should be formulated with the patient and must be objectives the
patient is eager to achieve. Examples of such goals include the ability to walk to the
mailbox, bowl, play golf, perform proper breathing techniques, and better understand
the disease and its therapy. The patient must have a clear understanding of the goals
and should agree to work toward their attainment. Involving significant others in the

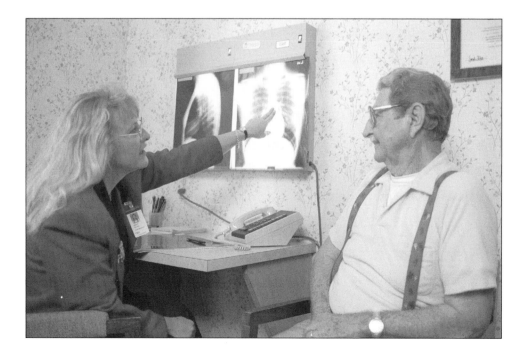

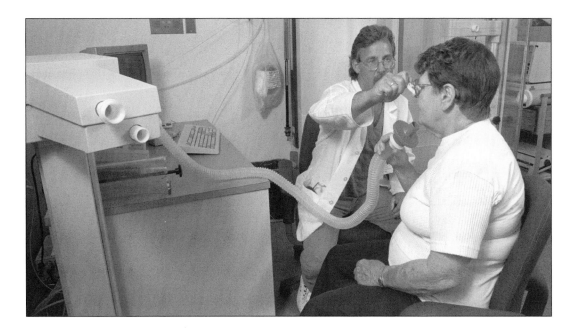

goal-setting process at the beginning of the program helps to ensure that everyone understands what can and cannot be expected as a result of the program.

CONCLUSION

In the patient selection process, we need to remember that pulmonary rehabilitation is not just for the COPD population but for any patients impaired in their ADLs as a result of their lung disease. Assessment of the pulmonary rehabilitation patient by an interdisciplinary team sets the foundation for an individualized and comprehensive pulmonary rehabilitation program. Assessment is one of the most critical components of a program, a precursor to patient training, psychosocial intervention, exercise, and follow-up. Realistic patient goals are determined during the assessment and reevaluated during the program as necessary. Assessment is the key to prevention and early detection of lung disease when intervention may prevent a disastrous outcome.

Assessment is the key to prevention and early detection of lung disease when intervention may prevent a disastrous outcome.

REFERENCES

1. Mahler, D.A., and A. Harver. 1990. Clinical measurement of dyspnea. In *Dyspnea,* edited by D.A. Mahler, 75-100. Mount Kesco, NY: Futura.

2. American Thoracic Society. 1995. Standards for the diagnosis and care of patients with chronic obstructive pulmonary disease. *Am J Respir Crit Care Med* 152 (Suppl): 93-94.

3. Ries, A.L. 1995. What pulmonary rehab can do for your patients. *J Respir Dis* 16 (8): 685-704.

4. Connors, G.L., L.R. Hilling, and K.V. Morris. 1993. Assessment of the pulmonary rehabilitation candidate. In *Pulmonary rehabilitation: Guidelines to success.* 2d ed. Edited by J.E. Hodgkin, G.L. Connors, and C.W. Bell, 64-68. Philadelphia: Lippincott.

5. Pierson, D.J., and R.L. Wilkins. 1992. Clinical skills in respiratory care. In *Foundations of Respiratory Care,* edited by D.J. Pierson and R.M. Kacmarek, 431-45. New York: Churchill Livingstone.

6. Schols, A., P. Soeters, A. Dingemans, et al. 1993. Prevalence and characteristics of nutritional depletion in patients with stable COPD eligible for pulmonary rehabilitation. *Am Rev Respir Dis* 147:1151-56.

7. Schols, A., P. Soeters, A. Dingemans, et al. 1991. Energy balance in chronic obstructive pulmonary disease. *Am Rev Respir Dis* 143:1248-52.

8. Wilson, D.O., R.M. Rogers, and D. Openbrier. 1986. Nutritional aspects of chronic obstructive pulmonary disease. *Clin Chest Med* 7:643-56.

9. Gray-Donald, K. et al. 1996. Nutritional status and mortality in chronic obstructive pulmonary disease. *Am J Respir Crit Care Med* 153:961-66.

10. Reed, K.L. 1991. Cardiopulmonary disorders. In *Quick reference to occupational therapy,* 195-209. Gaithersberg, MD: Aspen.

11. Weaver, T., and G. Narsavage. 1992. Physiological and psychological variables related to functional status in chronic obstructive pulmonary disease. *Nurs Res* 41:286-91.

12. Lareau, S. et al. 1994. Development and testing of the Pulmonary Functional Status and Dyspnea Questionnaire (PFSDQ). *Heart Lung* 23:242-50.

13. Selecky, P.A. 1993. Sexuality and the patient with lung disease. In *Principles and practice of pulmonary rehabilitation,* edited by R. Casaburi and T.L. Petty, 382-91. Philadelphia: Saunders.

14. Gilmartin, M.E. 1986. Patient and family education. *Clin Chest Med* 7 (4): 619-27.

15. Hilling, L., and J. Smith. 1995. Pulmonary rehabilitation. In *Cardiopulmonary physical therapy,* edited by S. Irwin and J.S. Teckin, 450-56. St. Louis: Mosby.

16. Fo, S.M., J.P. Naughton, and P.A. Gorman. 1972. Physical activity and cardiovascular health. The exercise prescription: Frequency and type of activity. *Mod Concepts Cardiovas Dis* 41:25-30.

17. Scanlan, M., L. Kishbaugh, and D. Horne. 1993. Life management skill in pulmonary rehabilitation. In *Pulmonary rehabilitation: Guidelines to success.* 2d ed. Edited by J.E. Hodgkin, G.L. Connors, and C.W. Bell, 246-67. Philadelphia: Lippincott.

18. Blair, S.N. et al. 1986. *Guidelines for exercise testing and prescription.* 3d ed. Philadelphia: Lea & Febiger.

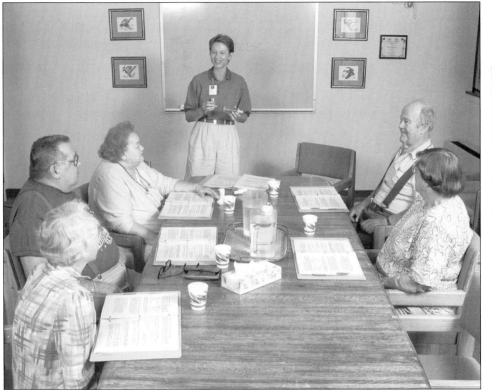

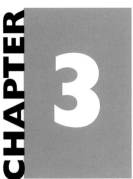

Patient Training

Upon completing a thorough assessment the interdisciplinary team can begin to develop the necessary training sessions for the pulmonary rehabilitation patient. Achieving the goals of pulmonary rehabilitation requires that the patient and the significant other understand the patient's underlying pulmonary disorder and the principles of collaborative self-management.[1, 2] The patient training objectives should therefore encourage patients to make behavioral changes that lead to improved health and enable them to become active participants in their own health care.[3, 4] The process of behavioral change is ongoing. It is achieved through providing a strong educational foundation that allows patients to build on their knowledge. This chapter discusses the basic principles of patient training that should be included in the content of a pulmonary rehabilitation program.

Achieving the goals of pulmonary rehabilitation requires that the patient and the significant other understand the patient's underlying pulmonary disorder and the principles of collaborative self-management.

TRAINING PROCESS

Key steps in the training process include the following:

▌ Assess the patient's educational needs (see chapter 2).

▌ Determine how the patient learns best.

▌ Select the training approach or style that most benefits the patient.

Each patient will have an individualized approach to accepting the information based on his or her life experiences.[5, 6] No single approach or style of learning is best; but repetition, straight forwardness, and mutual respect are key aspects in achieving successful learning. Present the material in an organized sequence using appropriate terminology, document the training sessions, and determine the reinforcement and follow-up needed.

The development of pulmonary disease is often a long-term process resulting in middle-age or older patients entering pulmonary rehabilitation. Therefore, these patients may not have been in a structured educational setting for many years. As educators we need to create a comfortable and relaxed educational environment for these patients, which will allow them to become at ease with the setting and the material taught. Everyone learns differently, but patients' retention of material can be improved by the way we present the information.

Patients acquire new information through the following processes: visual, auditory, or tactile/psychomotor.[7] In developing the training program, team members should use each of these processes to improve patients' ability to retain newly learned material.

Figure 3.1 depicts a scale of learning that demonstrates the ability to increase retention through the use of the senses (hearing, seeing, touching, doing). To help prevent or reduce communication barriers using the auditory and visual senses the interdisciplinary team should carefully address speaker communication behavior, environmental barriers, and listener/patient variables. Interdisciplinary team members can improve their communication style by making sure they face the patient(s), get the patient's attention, leave their faces or mouths uncovered when talking, do not face away from the patient to speak (especially when writing on a board or flipchart), speak in a volume that is neither too loud nor too soft, speak slowly, and articulate as clearly as possible. The setting/environment used may also present barriers that need to be avoided such as background noise, inadequate lighting, distractions, sound reverberation, poor seating arrangement, lack of assistive technology, and too great a distance between the speaker and listener. The last variable to have an impact on good communication is the patient/listener. When patient training is done by the interdisciplinary team the patient/listener variables that should be evaluated are emotional status, attention span, fatigue level, general health, type and severity of hearing loss, and knowledge and acceptance of the hearing loss and how to cope with it.

Providing written material such as a patient education manual helps improve comprehension and retention of the vast amount of information presented during the pulmonary rehabilitation program. This manual is an important resource for the patient and significant other(s) throughout the program and post graduation (see figure 3.2 for a sample table of contents). In developing the training sessions and written materials, consider the following: reading level of the patient, visual or hearing impairments, language barriers, and other comorbid conditions (e.g., hypoxemia).

PROGRAM CONTENT

A primary objective of pulmonary rehabilitation is to assist the patient in achieving his or her optimum level of function.[8] The patient's and family's educational needs are determined during the initial evaluation and may need to be reassessed during the program. Professionals from any of the disciplines represented by the rehabilitation team who have expertise in a particular content area may present the relevant training

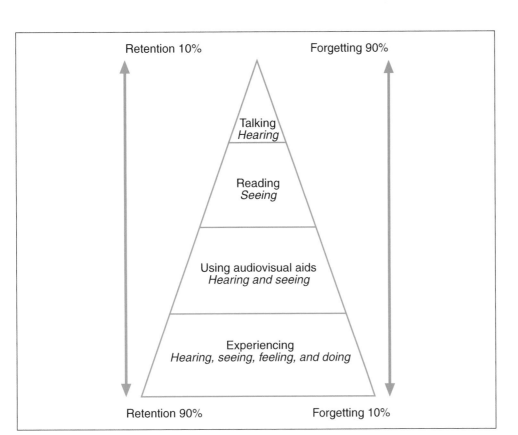

Figure 3.1 The scale of learning.

Reprinted with permission from "Education of Patients and Their Families" by J.W. Hopp and S.E. Maddox. In *Pulmonary Rehabilitation: Guidelines to Success* (p. 55) by J.E. Hodgkin, E.G. Zorn, and G.L. Connors (Eds.). Copyright 1984 by J.E. Hodgkin.

sessions. Many excellent educational resources are available for content development (e.g., the internet, the AACVPR Educational Resource Guide, medical textbooks).[9-14] Refer to appendix B for additional patient training information. Depending on the patient's individual needs, any or all of the following topics may be included in the training component of the pulmonary rehabilitation program:

The patient's and family's educational needs are determined during the initial evaluation and may need to be reassessed during the program.

▌ Normal pulmonary anatomy and physiology

▌ Pathophysiology of lung disease

▌ Description and interpretation of medical tests

▌ Breathing retraining

▌ Bronchial hygiene

▌ Medications

▌ Exercise principles

▌ Activities of daily living (ADLs) and energy conservation

▌ Respiratory modalities

▌ Self-assessment and symptom management

▌ Nutrition

▌ Psychosocial issues

▌ Ethical issues

TABLE OF CONTENTS

I. Chronic Lung Disease
- A. The Respiratory System: Structure and Function
- B. Disease Process
  - 1) Asthma
  - 2) Chronic Bronchitis
  - 3) Emphysema
  - 4) Bronchiectasis
  - 5) Restrictive Diseases
  - 6) Other Conditions
- C. Oxygen as a Drug
- D. Preventing Infection
- E. Controlled Coughing Technique
- F. Postural Drainage Therapy
- G. Patient Testing

II. Time and Energy Conservation
- A. Activities of Daily Living
- B. My Daily Routine Activity Sheet for Planning My Day
- C. Leisure Time Techniques
- D. Travel

III. Exercise
- A. Exercise Log Form
- B. Exercise Principles
- C. Taking Your Pulse
- D. Strengthening Exercises (Arms, Legs)
- E. Aerobic Exercise
- F. Breathing Retraining
- G. Home Exercise Prescription

IV. Coping With Illness
- A. Stress Management
- B. Relaxation Exercise
- C. Panic Control
- D. Coping With Chronic Disease: Sexuality
- E. Sleeping Less

V. Medications
- A. Inhalers
- B. General Information
- C. Bronchodilators
- D. Bronchodilators by Mouth
- E. Bronchodilators by Inhalation
- F. Steroids by Mouth
- G. Steroids by Oral Inhalation
- H. Antibiotics
- I. Tranquilizers and Sedatives
- J. Diuretics (Water Pills)

VI. Nutrition
- A. An Important Part of Better Breathing
- B. Weight Management
- C. Calcium-Rich Foods
- D. Food Pyramid
- E. Vitamin and Mineral Supplements
- F. What Is Sodium?
- G. Seasoning With Herbs and Spices
- H. Problems With Eating
- I. Antireflux Diet Suggestions
- J. Fluid Intake

VII. Smoking
- A. Facts
- B. Physiological Effects
- C. Nicotine Addiction
- D. Secondhand Smoke (Passive Smoking)
- E. Strategies for Quitting
- F. Weight Gain
- G. Stop Smoking Benefits
- H. Listing of Smoking Cessation Programs in Your Area

VIII. Miscellaneous
- A. Aerosol Treatments
- B. Oxygen (Cleaning Equipment)
- C. Medical Consumer Magazine Subscriptions
- D. Commonly Used Terms

Figure 3.2 Sample table of contents from a patient manual.

Figure 3.3 is a sample form for the documentation of training sessions. The form can be individualized to reflect a patient's progress and the specific content of the training topic.

Normal Pulmonary Anatomy and Physiology

Presenting basic anatomy and physiology of the respiratory system is sufficient for most participants in the program. It is particularly useful to use demonstration models and other teaching aides when discussing this material, as it is frequently difficult for the layperson to envision the pulmonary anatomy.

Patient name: _____

Medical record #: _____

DIAPHRAGMATIC AND PURSED LIP BREATHING (DB/PLB)

	Goals	Objectives	Assessment	Outcome
Session I	Instruct on anatomy and physiology of normal lung, disease process, and the effect of bronchial collapse.	Identify the effects of bronchial collapse, increase O_2 sat during technique.	Written or verbal review. Participant able to identify effects of bronchial collapse, O_2 sat pre- and post-PLB.	Met Not met Date ____ _____ _____ Comments: _____ _____ Sig: _____
Session II	Instruct and demonstrate proper techniques of DB/PLB.	Will be able to demonstrate the proper techniques of DB/PLB while using a __ lb. wt. on abdomen while lying, if there are no contraindications.	Pt. demonstrated proper DB/PLB technique with __ lb. wt. on abdomen.	Met Not met Date ____ _____ _____ Comments: _____ _____ Sig: _____
Session III	Instruct and demonstrate use of DB/PLB with activities of daily living.	Will be able to demonstrate proper use of DB/PLB while performing activities of daily living.	Pt. demonstrated proper DB/PLB technique with activities of daily living.	Met Not met Date ____ _____ _____ Comments: _____ _____ Sig: _____
Session IV	Instruct on the benefits of using DB/PLB for panic control.	Will be able to verbally explain/identify the importance and purpose of DB/PLB for panic control.	Given written or verbal review questions. Will be able to give correct response on the purpose of using DB/PLB for panic control.	Met Not met Date ____ _____ _____ Comments: _____ _____ Sig: _____

Figure 3.3   Example of pulmonary rehabilitation progress notes for diaphragmatic and pursed lip breathing.

Adapted from Missouri Baptist Medical Center Pulmonary Rehabilitation Program, St. Louis, Missouri.

Pathophysiology of Lung Disease

Content discussed regarding the pathophysiology of the patient's disease should be tailored to mirror the diagnosis that the patient has received from his or her physician. With a basic understanding of their specific lung disease, most patients are more willing to comply with their prescribed therapeutic interventions. Numerous anatomy and physiology texts addressing pathophysiology are available from different disciplines.[11-17]

Medical Tests

The description and interpretation/results of medical tests can be very confusing to the patient, and instruction should be kept simple. Many times patients have never seen their test results, nor have they understood how their results compare to the normal range. The more the patient understands—including why the tests are done, what the results mean, and how his or her treatment program is individualized based upon these results—the more the patient will desire to follow the treatment recommendations. An example is the difficulty that patients often have in understanding the poor correlation between shortness of breath and oxyhemoglobin saturation. Some of the topics that you might discuss with patients to explain their medical tests are listed next:

- Timed distance walk (6- or 12-minute)[18]
- Pulmonary function tests [19]
- Cardiopulmonary stress test [20]
- Arterial blood gases [21]
- Pulse oximetry [22, 23]
- Chest x-ray
- ECG
- CBC/electrolytes
- Sleep study

Breathing Retraining

It is important to teach every patient proper breathing techniques. Diaphragmatic and pursed-lip breathing may help patients control and relieve breathlessness and panic, improve their ventilatory pattern (slow respiratory rate and increase tidal volume), prevent dynamic airway compression, improve respiratory synchrony of abdominal and thoracic musculature, and improve gas exchange.[24-26] Teaching paced breathing is useful to enhance the patient's ability to perform activities of daily living.[27] Utilizing a pulse oximeter to demonstrate an increase in oxygen saturation while performing pursed-lip breathing may increase patient understanding of proper breathing techniques.[28]

Bronchial Hygiene

Bronchial hygiene ensures that the pulmonary patient is receiving optimal air flow. These techniques are appropriate for those patients who have difficulty clearing excessive sputum on a continuous or intermittent basis. Bronchial hygiene may include the following: [29-33]

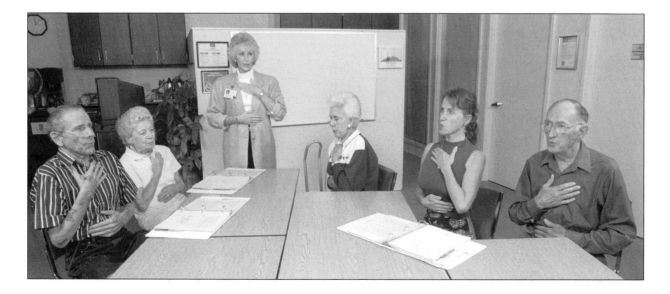

▮ Cough techniques

▮ Percussion

▮ Postural drainage

▮ Vibration

▮ Positive airway pressure

▮ Positive expiratory pressure (PEP or flutter valves)

▮ Autogenic drainage

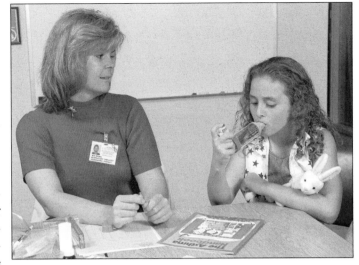

Having a thorough knowledge of these various techniques, and the specific needs of your patient, will enable you to match the most effective technique to your patient's needs. Patients using inhaled bronchodilators should be instructed in the importance of their use prior to performing their bronchial hygiene techniques. Patient demonstration of bronchial hygiene techniques is encouraged, and repeat instruction is frequently necessary.

Medications

Training in the prescribed dosage, frequency, side effects, interactions, and role of medications, including oxygen, in the treatment and prevention of lung impairment is of utmost importance for all patients with lung disease.[26, 34-37] The primary emphasis in pulmonary rehabilitation may be on the respiratory medications, including oxygen, but it is equally important that patients understand the proper use of *all* of their medications. They also should understand the importance of telling *all* of their physicians and pharmacists what prescribed and over-the-counter medications they are currently taking. This practice, and encouraging the patient to utilize just one pharmacy for acquiring all medications, should reduce the possibility of harmful drug interactions. Instruction in these matters should be individualized and include return demonstration of inhaler/spacer use. A major outcome measure of patient responsibility in self-care is adherence to and compliance with their medication regimen.

A major outcome measure of patient responsibility in self-care is adherence to and compliance with their medication regimen.

Exercise Principles

The benefits of exercise for improving patients' functional capacity and activities of daily living are well established (see chapter 4).[38, 39] Teaching this information to patients improves their understanding about the importance of their individualized exercise program. To facilitate compliance, it is important that a home exercise program is developed for each patient prior to completion of the rehabilitation program. An exercise log or diary may be developed for patients to self-record their home exercise. The benefits of lifelong exercise should be stressed and patients encouraged to continue in a maintenance exercise program, if available.

Activities of Daily Living

Independence in activities of daily living is a primary goal for the pulmonary patient.[40, 41] The patient's individualized treatment plan is established based on the initial

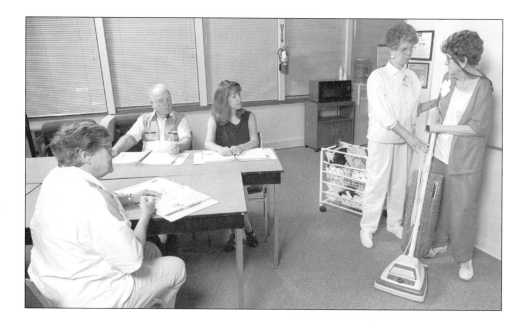

The goal of the treatment plan is to provide patients with the tools necessary to adapt to their limitations and improve their quality of life.

assessment. The goal of the treatment plan is to provide patients with the tools necessary to adapt to their limitations and improve their quality of life. The training sessions may include but are not limited to the areas listed here:

▮ Energy conservation

▮ Work simplification

▮ Time management techniques

▮ Panic control

▮ Relaxation techniques

▮ Pacing techniques

▮ Food procurement and preparation

▮ Leisure activities

▮ Adaptive equipment

▮ Sexuality

▮ Travel considerations [42]

▮ Community resources

▮ Vocational retraining

Respiratory Modalities

Patients with pulmonary disease frequently use various types of respiratory therapy modalities and equipment to aid their breathing. The use of specific modalities is based upon the patient's disease and individual needs. Reinforcement and additional training may be necessary to ensure that patients are correctly using their modalities and are compliant with their physician's prescription. Respiratory therapy modalities for patients with pulmonary disease may include those listed next:

▮ Metered-dose inhalers/spacers [34, 35]

▮ Nebulizers/compressors [43]

■ Peak flow meters[44]

■ Oxygen delivery systems (concentrators, liquid, compressed gas)[45]

■ Oxygen-conserving devices[46]

■ Transtracheal oxygen (TTO)[47]

■ Inspiratory muscle training[48]

■ Positive expiratory pressure[32]

■ Sleep assessment equipment (oximetry, apnea monitors)

■ CPAP and BiPAP

■ Suctioning in the home

■ Tracheostomy care

■ Ventilator management in the home

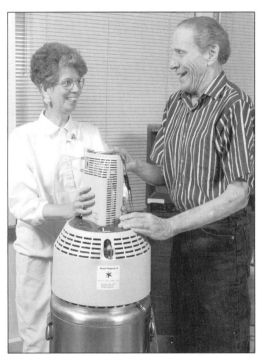

Instruction should include proper use, care, and cleaning of home respiratory equipment.

Self-Assessment and Symptom Management

In patients with lung disease, treatment is geared toward slowing the progression and complications of their disease to minimize disability. This is considered tertiary prevention in pulmonary rehabilitation. Patients must learn to avoid occupational and environmental irritants, especially first- and secondhand cigarette smoke. It is critical that this is emphasized. Indications for when to call the doctor and signs and symptoms of a respiratory exacerbation should be included in patient training.[26] Simple techniques such as hand washing and covering the mouth when coughing are often overlooked in instructional sessions. Dyspnea management is an area that is often found to be most advantageous to patients and their families. Next is a list of specific topics to be discussed with pulmonary rehabilitation program participants:

In patients with lung disease, treatment is geared toward slowing the progression and complications of their disease to minimize disability.

■ Nicotine dependency intervention [49, 50, 51]

■ Hazards of secondhand smoke

■ Environmental and occupational irritant avoidance

■ When to call the doctor

■ Signs and symptoms of a respiratory infection

■ Management strategies for symptoms, including dyspnea and medication changes

Nutrition

General nutritional principles apply to all patients who have lung disease (see chapter 2).[52-54] The pulmonary patient can fall anywhere along the weight spectrum. On the one hand, the metabolic cost of breathing can increase caloric expenditure with resultant weight loss. On the other hand, a sedentary lifestyle and steroid use can lead to obesity. Instruction should be geared to the individual needs of your patient as indicated on initial and follow-up assessments. It may be beneficial to refer the patient for dietary counseling should this area need to be emphasized. Examples of nutritional topics to cover with your patients include the following:

▍ Need for weight loss or gain

▍ Adequate fluid intake

▍ Sodium restriction

▍ Food allergies

▍ Low-fat, complex carbohydrate diet

▍ Cholesterol reduction

▍ Reflux diet

▍ Diabetic training

▍ Treatment of osteoporosis

▍ Alcohol consumption/restriction

Ethical Issues

Advance directives help to improve communication among the patient, family, and physician.

Advance directives, living wills, and durable powers of attorney for health care are underutilized in the general population, especially with geriatric patients. These topics are particularly important to discuss with patients with lung disease because of the frequency of respiratory failure and need for mechanical ventilation in this population.[55-57] Advance directives help to improve communication among the patient, family, and physician. The development of a treatment plan that includes mutual goals is most practical. This plan may be derived from patients' understanding of their disease, the ramifications of dialing 9-1-1, the implications of resuscitation in the home, their values and life goals, and the physician's estimation of mortality and morbidity outcomes in certain clinical situations.

If the decision is made to limit medical intervention given by emergency medical services (EMS) providers in nonacute care hospital settings (e.g., home, long-term care facility, or during transport to or from a health care facility), specific rules or laws may apply. Information and sample forms addressing these areas as well as advance directives are available from a county medical society, hospital association, or local EMS provider. Examples of ethical issues to cover with patients include the following:

▍ Ramifications of dialing 9-1-1

▍ Community EMS (specific rules or laws may apply to limit medical intervention outside the acute care setting)

▍ Advance directives

▍ Living wills

▍ Durable power of attorney for health care

Psychosocial Issues

Some patients cope better than others with the emotional aspects of lung disease.[58] Group interaction is often successful in helping patients share their coping mechanisms. The staff should provide assistance, where appropriate, on an individual basis. See chapter 5 for additional information about psychosocial intervention issues. If severe psychosocial issues arise, the patient may warrant a referral for counseling. Areas of psychosocial intervention are listed:

- Strategies for coping with lung disease
- Depression management
- Panic control
- Stress reduction
- Relaxation techniques
- Anger control
- Support systems
- Patient/caregiver relationships
- Well spouse issues
- Sexuality
- Modifying addictive behaviors (e.g., nicotine, alcohol, prescribed medication, illegal drugs, etc.)
- Memory improvement skills

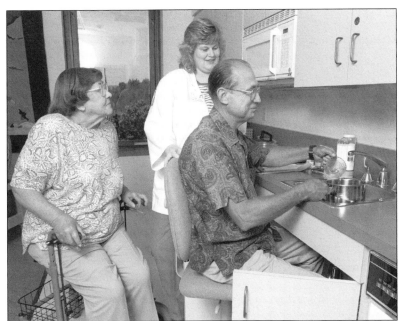

CONCLUSION

An effective pulmonary rehabilitation training program helps the patient and significant others to develop a working knowledge of the patient's disease process and an appropriate, effective treatment program of collaborative self-management.[3] It is important that patients become aware of the nature of their disease and its resultant disturbances of function, as well as the purpose and value of each aspect of care. Rehabilitation team members should be sensitive to patient expectations and work together with them to set realistic goals. This will allow patients to take control of their disease, improve their compliance with treatment recommendations, and lessen their fears and anxiety.[59]

Rehabilitation team members should be sensitive to patient expectations and work together with them to set realistic goals.

REFERENCES

1. Hopp, J.W., and C.M. Neish. 1993. Patient and family education. In *Pulmonary rehabilitation: Guidelines to success*. 2d ed. Edited by J.E. Hodgkin , G.L. Connors, and C.W. Bell, 72-85. Philadelphia: Lippincott.

2. Make, B. 1994. Collaborative self-management strategies for patients with respiratory disease. *Respir Care* 39:566-79.

3. Neish, C.M., and J.W. Hopp. 1988. The role of education in pulmonary rehabilitation. *J Cardiopulm Rehabil* 8 (11): 439-41.

4. Gilmartin, M.E. 1986. Patient and family education. *Clin Chest Med* 7 (4): 619-27.

5. Mast, M.E., and M.J. VanAtta. 1986. Applying adult learning principles in instructional module design. *Nurse Educ* 11 (1): 35.

6. Babcock, D.E., and M.A. Miller. 1994. The adult learner. In *Client education: Theory and practice,* 19-25. St. Louis: Mosby.

7. AARC. 1996. Clinical Practice Guideline: Providing patient and caregiver training. *Respir Care* 41 (7): 658-63.

8. American Thoracic Society. 1981. Pulmonary rehabilitation. *Am Rev Respir Dis* 24:661-63.

9. Pierson, D.J., and R.M. Kacmarek, eds. 1992. *Foundations of respiratory care*. New York: Churchill Livingstone.

10. West, J. 1995. *Respiratory physiology: The essentials.* 5th ed. Baltimore: Williams & Wilkins.

11. Lung disease care and education staff. 1991. *COPD resource guide*. New York: American Lung Association.

12. Dettenmeier, P. 1992. *Pulmonary nursing care*. St. Louis: Mosby

13. Kersten, L.D. 1989. *Comprehensive respiratory nursing*. Philadelphia: Saunders.

14. Lipson, J., S. Dibble, and P. Minarik. 1996. *Culture and nursing care: A pocket guide*. San Francisco: UCSF Nursing Press.

15. National Heart, Lung and Blood Institute. 1992. *Expert panel report 2: Guidelines for the diagnosis and management of asthma.* NIH Publication No. 97-4051. Bethesda, MD.

16. National Heart, Lung and Blood Institute. 1993. *Chronic obstructive pulmonary disease.* NIH Publication No. 93-2020. Bethesda, MD.

17. Parsons, P., and J.E. Heffner, eds. 1997. *Pulmonary/respiratory therapy secrets*. Philadelphia: Hanley & Belfus.

18. Steele, B. 1996. Timed walking tests of exercise capacity in chronic cardiopulmonary illness. *J Cardiopulm Rehabil* 16:25-33.

19. Snow, M., and R. Beauchamp. 1992. Assessment of airflow. In *Foundations of respiratory care*, edited by D.J. Pierson and R.M. Kacmarek, 457-75. New York: Churchill Livingstone.

20. American College of Sports Medicine. 1991. *Guidelines for exercise testing and prescription*. Philadelphia: Lea & Febiger.

21. Kacmarek, R. 1992. Assessment of gas exchange and acid-base balance. In *Foundations of respiratory care*, edited by D.J. Pierson and R.M. Kacmarek, 477-512. New York: Churchill Livingstone.

22. Sonnersso, G. 1991. Are you ready for pulse oximetry? *Nursing91* 21 (8): 61-64.

23. AARC. 1991. Clinical Practice Guideline: Pulse oximetry. *Respir Care* 36 (12):1406-09.

24. Faling, L.J. 1993. Controlled breathing techniques and chest physical therapy in chronic obstructive pulmonary disease and allied conditions. In *Principles and practice of pulmonary rehabilitation*, edited by R. Casaburi and T.L. Petty, 167-74. Philadelphia: W.B. Saunders.

25. Rochester, D.F., and S.K. Goldberg. 1980. Techniques of respiratory physical therapy. *Am Rev Respir Dis* 122 (Suppl): 133-46.

26. Moser, K.M. et al. 1991. *Shortness of breath: A guide to better living and breathing.* St. Louis: Mosby Year Book.

27. Hillegass, E.H., and H.S. Sadowsky. 1994. *Essentials of cardiopulmonary physical therapy*. Philadelphia: W.B. Saunders.

28. Tiep, B. et al. 1986. Pursed lip breathing training using ear oximetry. *Chest* (August): 5-29.

29. AARC. 1991. Clinical Practice Guideline: Postural drainage therapy. *Respir Care* 36 (12): 1418-26.

30. AARC Clinical Practice Guideline. 1993. Directed cough. *Respir Care* 38 (5): 495-99.

31. AARC Clinical Practice Guideline. 1993. Use of positive airway pressure adjuncts to bronchial hygiene therapy. *Respir Care* 38 (5): 516-21.

32. Mahlmeister, M.J. et al. 1991. Positive-expiratory-pressure mask therapy: Theoretical and practical considerations and review of the literature. *Respir Care* 36 (11): 1218-29.

33. Hardy, K.A. 1994. A review of airway clearance: New techniques, indications and recommendations. *Respir Care* 39 (5): 440-55.

34. American Lung Association. 1993. *Understanding lung medications.* New York: American Lung Association.

35. Jenne, J.W. 1993. Pharmacology in the respiratory patient. In *Pulmonary rehabilitation: Guidelines to success.* 2d ed. Edited by J.E. Hodgkin, G.L. Connors, and C.W. Bell, 135-99. Philadelphia: Lippincott.

36. Cooper, C.B. 1993. Long term oxygen therapy. In *Principles and practice of pulmonary rehabilitation*, edited by R. Casaburi and T.L. Petty, 183-203. Philadelphia: W.B. Saunders.

37. Nocturnal Oxygen Trial Group. 1980. Continuous or nocturnal oxygen therapy in hypoxemic chronic lung disease: A clinical trial. *Ann Intern Med* 93:391-98.

38. Celli, B. 1994. Physical reconditioning of patients with respiratory diseases: Legs, arms and breathing retraining. *Respir Care* 39 (5): 482-95.

39. Casaburi, R. 1993. Exercise training in chronic obstructive lung disease. In *Principles and practice of pulmonary rehabilitation*, edited by R. Casaburi and T.L. Petty, 204-24. Philadelphia: W.B. Saunders.

40. Ogden, L.S., and C. deRenne. 1985. *Chronic obstructive pulmonary disease: Program guidelines for occupational therapists and other health professionals.* Laurel, MD: RAMSCO.

41. Reed, K.L. 1991. Cardiopulmonary disorders. In *Quick reference to occupational therapy,* 195-209. Gaithersberg, MD: Aspen.

42. Stoller, J.K. 1994. Travel for the technology-dependent individual. *Respir Care* 39 (4): 347-62.

43. AARC. 1992. Clinical Practice Guideline: Selection of aerosol delivery device. *Respir Care* 37 (8): 891-97.

44. National Heart, Lung and Blood Institute. 1992. Peak expiratory flow monitoring. In *International consensus report on diagnosis and treatment of asthma.* NIH Publication No. 92-3091. Bethesda, MD.

45. McDonald, G. 1994. Home oxygen therapy. In *Handbook of adult and pediatric respiratory home care,* edited by J. Turner, G. McDonald, and N. Larter, 247-72. St. Louis: Mosby.

46. Tiep, B.L, and M.L. Lewis. 1987. Oxygen conservation and oxygen-conserving devices in chronic lung disease: A review. *Chest* 92:263-72.

47. Hoffman, L. et al. 1991. Transtracheal delivery of oxygen: Efficacy and safety for long term continuous therapy. *Ann Otolaryngol* 100:108.

48. Pardy, R.L. et al. 1981. The effects of inspiratory muscle training on exercise performance in chronic airflow limitation. *Am Rev Respir Dis* 123:426-33.

49. Fisher, E.B. et al. 1990. Smoking and smoking cessation: State of the art. *Am Rev Respir Dis* 142:702-20.

50. Agency for Health Care Policy and Research. 1996. *Clinical practice guideline: Smoking cessation.* AHCPR Publication No. 96-0692. Washington, DC.

51. Nett, L. 1993. Nicotine addiction treatment. In *Principles and practice of pulmonary rehabilitation*, edited by R. Casaburi and T.L. Petty, 289-99. Philadelphia: W.B. Saunders.

52. Mancino, J.M., M. Donahoe, and R. Rogers. 1992. Nutritional assessment and therapy. In *Foundations of respiratory care*, edited by D.J. Pierson and R.M. Kacmarek, 336-50. New York: Churchill Livingstone.

53. Angillo, V.A. 1993. Nutrition and the pulmonary patient. In *Pulmonary rehabilitation: Guidelines to success.* 2d ed. Edited by J.E. Hodgkin, G.L. Connors, and C.W. Bell, 311-21. Philadelphia: Lippincott.

54. Rogers, R.M., and M. Donahoe. 1996. Nutrition in pulmonary rehabilitation. In *Pulmonary rehabilitation, Lung biology in health and disease,* edited by A.P. Fishman. Vol. 91, 544-64. New York: Marcel Dekker, Inc.

55. Heffner, J.E., B. Fahy, and C. Barbieri. 1996. Advance directive education during pulmonary rehabilitation. *Chest* 109:373-79.

56. Heffner, J.E. et al. 1996. Attitudes regarding advance directives among patients in pulmonary rehabilitation. *Am J Respir Crit Care Med* 154:1735-40.

57. Heffner, J.E. et al. 1997. Outcomes of advance directive education of pulmonary rehabilitation patients. *Am J Respir Crit Care Med.* 155:1055-59.

58. Petty, T.L., and L.M. Nett. 1984. *Enjoying life with emphysema.* Philadelphia: Lea & Febiger.

59. Ferguson, G.T., and R.M. Cherniack. 1993. Management of chronic obstructive lung disease. *N Engl J Med* 328:1017-22.

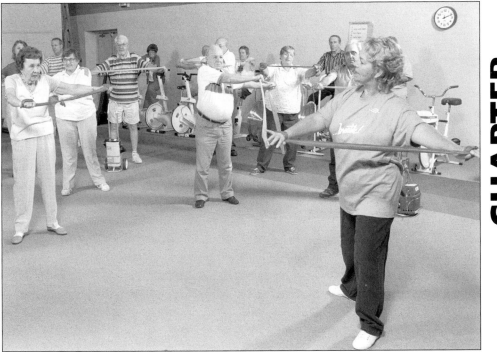

Exercise Assessment
and Training

Exercise assessment, testing, and training are essential components of comprehensive pulmonary rehabilitation programs. Each program should have appropriate facilities for testing and training patients. Facilities and equipment will vary, depending upon resources available and patient needs. The benefits of exercise training (see appendix A) for improving dyspnea,[1] functional capacity,[2, 3] performance of activities of daily living,[4] and quality of life[5, 6] have been well established. Exercise training, therefore, should be incorporated into the rehabilitation program for the majority of the pulmonary patients, unless contraindicated. The role of exercise in prevention is to optimize an individual's general well-being. Exercise increases endurance, promotes a higher level of functioning, decreases blood pressure, counteracts depression, promotes relaxation, improves high-density lipoprotein cholesterol levels, helps with blood sugar regulation, improves performance of activities of daily living, and facilitates sleep. Exercise is an important component in pulmonary rehabilitation and improves wellness regardless of one's health status.

The benefits of exercise training have been well established; therefore, exercise training should be incorporated into the rehabilitation program for the majority of pulmonary patients, unless contraindicated.

EXERCISE ASSESSMENT

Exercise assessment of the patient with chronic pulmonary disease may be used to

▎ evaluate exercise capacity prior to beginning a program,[7]

▎ establish a baseline for outcome documentation,

▌ assist in formulating an exercise prescription for training,[8, 9]

▌ detect exercise hypoxemia and aid with supplemental oxygen therapy,[10]

▌ evaluate nonpulmonary limitations to exercise[11] (e.g., musculoskeletal),

▌ help detect underlying cardiac abnormalities,[11] and

▌ screen for exercise-induced bronchospasm.

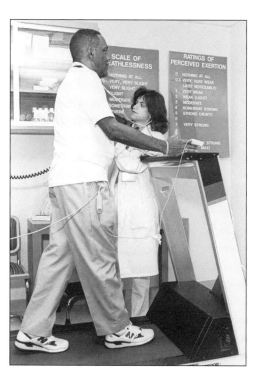

Contraindications to exercise testing for patients with pulmonary disease are relatively few. Standard lists of absolute and relative contraindications (see table 4.1 from the American College of Sports Medicine[12]) are concerned primarily with patients with known or suspected cardiovascular abnormalities. For many pulmonary patients without known or suspected cardiac problems, exercise testing, even to maximum levels, is relatively safe. One exception may be the individual with primary pulmonary vascular disease with pulmonary hypertension (i.e., primary pulmonary hypertension or chronic thromboembolic pulmonary embolism). In such individuals, some experts advise caution because of the risk of serious cardiac arrhythmias or even sudden death.

A variety of exercise testing procedures and protocols have been used to evaluate patients in pulmonary rehabilitation programs. Testing methods range from simple, noninvasive procedures to those that are more complex, invasive, and technically sophisticated. No single testing protocol is clearly established as the most appropriate for all patients and programs. Selection of an appropriate exercise test may depend on:

▌ individual patient status and goals,

▌ program objectives,

▌ questions identified in the initial patient assessment (see chapter 2),

▌ type of exercise training program,

▌ available laboratory resources, and

▌ cost

Equipment and Personnel Recommendations

The recommendations for exercise testing of the pulmonary patient are listed next:

Minimum Recommendations

▌ A measured walking distance used for timed distance walk tests (at least 100 feet in length with minimal traffic)

▌ Manual blood pressure measurement equipment

Contraindications to exercise testing for patients with pulmonary disease are relatively few.

Testing methods range from simple, noninvasive procedures to those that are more complex, invasive, and technically sophisticated. No single testing protocol is clearly established as the most appropriate for all patients and programs.

Table 4.1   Contraindications to Exercise Testing

Absolute Contraindications

1. A recent significant change in the resting ECG suggesting infarction or other acute cardiac events
2. Recent complicated myocardial infarction
3. Unstable angina
4. Uncontrolled ventricular dysrhythmia
5. Uncontrolled atrial dysrhythmia that compromises cardiac function
6. Third-degree A-V block
7. Acute congestive heart failure
8. Severe aortic stenosis
9. Suspected or known dissecting aneurysm
10. Active or suspected myocarditis or pericarditis
11. Thrombophlebitis or intracardiac thrombi
12. Recent systemic or pulmonary embolus
13. Acute infection
14. Significant emotional distress (psychosis)

Relative Contraindications

1. Resting diastolic blood pressure > 120 mmHg or resting systolic blood pressure > 200 mmHg
2. Moderate valvular heart disease
3. Known electrolyte abnormalities (hypokalemia, hypomagnesemia)
4. Fixed-rate pacemaker (rarely used)
5. Frequent or complex ventricular ectopy
6. Ventricular aneurysm
7. Cardiomyopathy, including hypertrophied cardiomyopathy
8. Uncontrolled metabolic disease (e.g., diabetes, thyrotoxicosis, or myxedema)
9. Chronic infectious disease (e.g., mononucleosis, hepatitis, AIDS)
10. Neuromuscular, musculoskeletal, or rheumatoid disorders that are exacerbated by exercise
11. Advanced or complicated pregnancy

Reprinted, by permission, from Guidelines for Exercise Test Administration, 1995. In *ACSM Guidelines for exercise testing and prescription,* 5th ed. (Philadelphia: Lea & Febiger), 42.

- Stethoscope
- Cutaneous pulse oximeter
- Supplemental oxygen source
- Stopwatch
- Walker, cart, or wheelchair
- Emergency plan and supplies (refer to hospital/facility policy)
- Test-site personnel trained in basic life-support techniques

Additional Recommendations

▌ Calibrated cycle ergometer or motorized treadmill

▌ EKG monitoring during exercise testing

▌ Defibrillator and crash cart

▌ Access to a laboratory for arterial blood gas analysis

▌ Equipment for expired gas analysis to measure $\dot{V}O_2$ (oxygen uptake), $\dot{V}CO_2$ (carbon dioxide elimination), minute ventilation, and derived variables[5] (see table 4.2)

▌ ACLS certification for test-site personnel.

▌ Spirometry equipment for use in screening for exercise-induced bronchospasm

Table 4.2   Exercise Response Interpretation

Measurement	Deconditioning	Cardiac	COPD	Fibrosis	Pulmonary vascular
$\dot{V}O_2$max	Low	Low	Low	Low	Low
HR/workload	High	High			High
MVV–$\dot{V}_E$max	High	High	Low	Low	
O_2sat			Low	Low	Extra low
O_2 pulse		Low			Low
V_D/V_T			High	High	Extra high

Reprinted, by permission, from P.L. Enright and J.E. Hodgkin, 1997, Pulmonary function tests. In *Respiratory care: a guide to clinical practice,* 4ed., edited by G.G. Burton, J.E. Hodgkin, and J.J. Ward (Philadelphia: Lippincott-Raven Publishers), 244.

Functional Performance Assessment

The functional performance assessment in pulmonary rehabilitation is used to evaluate the problems that influence the patient's ability to perform functional activities.

Musculoskeletal problems can be especially prominent in the older pulmonary rehabilitation population.

The functional performance assessment in pulmonary rehabilitation is used to evaluate the problems that influence the patient's ability to perform functional activities; table 4.3 outlines some of these limitations.[13] The performance assessment should also evaluate the function of the respiratory muscles (e.g., diaphragmatic excursion, thoraco-abdominal synchrony) as well as any orthopedic limitations or other musculoskeletal contraindications to exercise.

Musculoskeletal problems can be especially prominent in the older pulmonary rehabilitation population. It is important to make a thorough assessment of the patient's baseline levels of strength, range of motion, posture, orthopedic limitations, and simple activities of daily living (ADLs) movements (e.g., transfers such as sitting to standing and lying to standing).[13, 14] Following the assessment an individualized treatment plan can be included in the patient's exercise program. The team members involved in the evaluation may vary from program to program. (See figure 4.1 for a sample form of a Functional Performance Assessment.) As the rehabilitation program progresses, the patient's response to the treatment plan should be monitored in relation to the specific, individual goals and revised as necessary.

Nutritional Assessment

Because the nutritional status of the patient with pulmonary disease significantly influences his or her exercise performance, it is important to consider the dietary com-

Table 4.3 Problems Affecting Functional Activities

- Decreased muscle strength and endurance
- Joint pain, limited range of motion, or both
- Lack of understanding of fitness and exercise
- Decreased cardiopulmonary endurance
- Dyspnea with activity
- Reduction in leisure and recreational activities
- Poor stress management and coping skills
- Decreased ambulation affecting performance of ADLs
- Inability to manage self-care
- Vocational and work issues, including opportunities and skills evaluation
- Decreased work tolerance
- Fear of exertion
- Oxygen desaturation with activity

Adapted, by permission, from D. Horne and P. Corsello, 1993, "Physical and occupational therapy for patients with chronic lung disease," *Seminars in Respiratory Medicine* 14 (6):466-481. Copyright 1993 by Thieme Medical Publishers.

ponent when assessing and planning an exercise training program. Often, appropriate loss or gain of total body weight may enhance both specific exercise performance and the ability to carry out ADLs. See chapter 2 for additional information on nutritional assessment.

Because the nutritional status of the patient with pulmonary disease significantly influences his or her exercise performance, it is important to consider the dietary component when assessing and planning an exercise training program.

Timed Distance Walk Test

The 6- or 12-minute walk test is commonly used to measure exercise ability in pulmonary rehabilitation. This test is relatively easy to administer, is relevant to activities of daily living, and requires minimal resources. Its simplicity makes it a valuable outcome measure for pulmonary rehabilitation. To obtain valid and reliable results, however, it is essential to standardize the test procedure (e.g., number of tests at baseline, patient instructions, reinforcement during testing, use of supplemental oxygen, etc.).[8] Because the 6- and 12-minute timed distance walk tests correlate well, it is more common to perform the 6-minute walk test to decrease patient fatigue and testing time if multiple tests are administered. During the timed distance walk test, patients typically improve performance with repeat testing as they learn to do the test more efficiently. Therefore, in order to establish a true baseline, it is important to allow patients to perform the timed distance walk test more than once. Although it would be ideal to perform repeat testing on separate days, many programs perform repeat tests on the same day with at least a 10- to 15-minute rest period between testing.

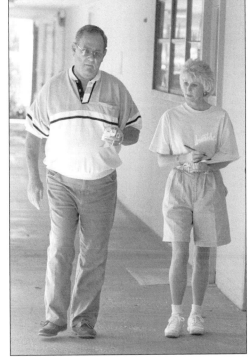

The timed distance walk test is performed in a premeasured walking distance (e.g, hallway, track, etc.) not on a treadmill. The patient is instructed to walk as far as possible during the 6- or 12-minute time interval. The distance walked (in feet or meters) is recorded as well as the number of times the patient stopped to rest

FUNCTIONAL PERFORMANCE ASSESSMENT

Name: _____ Age: _____ Date: _____
_____ (Initial)

Diagnosis (chief complaint):_____ Date: _____
_____ (Follow-up)

Onset: _____ Other information: _____
_____

Medical history: _____
_____

Orthopedic history: _____
_____

Body type: Lithe _____   Medium _____   Stout _____
Average daily activity: _____

Range of Motion	Initial	Follow-up
Cervical		
Forward flexion		
Extension		
Rotation R/L		
Lateral flexion R/L		
Trunk mobility		
Forward flexion		
Extension		
Side-bending R/L		
Rotation R/L		
Upper extremities		
Shoulders		
Scapula		
Elbows		
Wrists and hands		
Lower extremities		
Hips		
Knees		
Ankles and feet		
Rib mobility		
Opposite elbow to knee		
Hands behind head		
Hands behind back		
Chest excursion (inches)		
Inspiration-exhalation		
Strength	**Initial**	**Follow-up**
Upper extremities		
Distal		
Proximal		

(continued)

Figure 4.1   Sample pulmonary rehabilitation functional performance assessment.

"Functional Peformance Assessment" form is reprinted courtesy of the Pulmonary Rehabilitation Program at Mt. Diablo Medical Center, Concord, CA.

Lower extremities		
Distal		
Proximal		
Posture	**Initial**	**Follow-up**
A/P balance		
Head		
Scapula		
Thoracic curve		
Lumbar curve		
Abdomen		
Lateral balance		
Head tilt		
Shoulder level		
Chest (convex/concave)		
Pelvic level		
Functional Grading	**Initial**	**Final**
Dyspnea		
At rest		
With slight action		
With level walking		
With light activity		
With unlimited walking		

Functional mobility

Up and down from floor: _____

Breathing pattern: _____

_____

Patient's goals: _____

_____

Physical therapist's goals: _____

_____

Initial assessment: _____

_____

Follow-up assessment: _____

Physical therapist: _____ Date: _____

Physical therapist: _____ Date: _____

Figure 4.1 *(continued)*

and the total time spent resting. Figure 4.2 explains the procedure for performing the timed distance walk test (6- or 12-minute). Figure 4.3 shows a sample evaluation form for use in the 6-minute walk test. One can calculate speed (mph) and MET level using the distance and time walked, which may be useful information in formulating an initial exercise prescription. MET levels correlate with the patient's level of physical exertion; one MET is the amount of energy required while the body is at rest. Activities are expressed as requiring a multiple of this resting requirement; therefore, the MET level is helpful in setting up a patient's initial exercise prescription. Miles per hour and MET level may be calculated by using the following formulas:

The 6- or 12-minute walk test is commonly used to measure exercise ability in pulmonary rehabilitation.

$$\text{To calculate speed:} \quad \frac{\text{number of feet walked in one hour}}{\text{number of feet in one mile}}$$

Example: 6-minute walk

$$\text{MPH} = \frac{(300 \text{ feet walked in 6 minutes}) (10)}{5,280 \text{ feet in one mile}} \quad \text{MPH} = .56$$

Example: 12-minute walk

$$\text{MPH} = \frac{(2,000 \text{ feet walked in 12 minutes}) (5)}{5,280 \text{ feet in one mile}} \quad \text{MPH} = 1.9$$

Equipment:

Method to measure walking distance (e.g., rolling distance marker); ideal walking distance at least 100 feet in length with minimal traffic; stopwatch; cutaneous pulse oximeter; copy of the 10-point Borg scale in large print; sphygmomanometer; stethoscope; a walker, cart, or wheelchair for patients who require supported walking (e.g., patients with severe dyspnea or orthopedic conditions, etc.); chairs to be positioned along the walking course to be used if needed

Procedure:

1. Prior to the walk test the following information may be documented: blood pressure, pulse, oxyhemoglobin saturation, dyspnea level (show patient 10-point Borg Scale), medications, oxygen, and assistive devices. Patients who use prescribed medications prior to exercise/activity (e.g., inhaled beta agonist, nitroglycerin) should do so before performing the test. Also patients who use oxygen with exercise/activity should do so during the test at their prescribed liter flow. The portable oxygen equipment may be carried by the staff, or it may be placed in a cart or wheelchair for the patient to push as determined by the patient's individual needs. The walker, cart, or wheelchair may also be used for patients who require supported walking.

2. If a team member accompanies the patient during the test, that member should walk behind the patient so that she does not influence the patient's pace. During the test the team member may provide words of encouragement (e.g., "you're doing great," "keep up the good work," "hang in there").

3. Oxyhemoglobin saturation should be assessed continuously during the test. Patients who desaturate to levels below 88% may be allowed to continue the test if severe symptoms are not present (e.g., increased dyspnea, chest pain). Realize that some patients may enter the pulmonary rehabilitation program with severe hypoxemia who have been functioning with these levels at home. The urgency to stop the test, therefore, may not be warranted unless the patient is experiencing significant symptoms. We want to document what is truly happening to the patient at home. If oxygen therapy is ordered and initiated these patients may then be retested.

4. Documentation during the walk test may include oxyhemoglobin saturation, heart rate, dyspnea level, patient symptoms and comments, and frequency and length of rest periods.

5. Documentation post walk test may include oxygenhomoglobin saturation; heart rate; blood pressure; dyspnea level; symptoms; patient and team member comments; if test was performed on room air or with oxygen (document liter flow); if patient required supported walking via a cart, walker, or wheelchair. The total time for the test is 6 or 12 minutes, which includes any rest stops. Example: Patient performed a 6-minute walk test and rested twice for 30 seconds each, for a total rest time of 1 minute. Patient walked 5 minutes of the 6-minute test and covered a total distance of 1,050 feet.

6. The following instructions should be given to the patients:

"The purpose of this test is to assess your exercise ability and to obtain a baseline of information (i.e., oxygen saturation, dyspnea level, blood pressure, heart rate, and distance walked). You will begin at the designated starting point and follow the walking course as directed, covering as much distance as possible or walking at your own pace in the 6- or 12-minute period. If you need to, you may stop and rest. You will be asked to rate your dyspnea level during the walk test and told to stop when the 6 or 12 minutes are up. To save your breath for the test do not carry on a conversation while walking." Patients should then be asked to repeat the instructions to verify that they understand them.

7. If two walk tests are performed, at least 10–15 minutes of rest between each test is advised.

Another option is to perform the tests on separate days.

Figure 4.2   Procedure for administering the timed distance walk test (6- or 12-minute).

One MET is the level of energy expenditure at rest or approximately 3.5 ml/kg/min of oxygen consumption.

To calculate METs: $$\frac{(mph)\ (26.83\ meters/min)\ (.1\ ml/kg/min)\ +\ (3.5\ ml/kg/min)}{3.5\ ml/kg/min\ the\ basal\ metabolic\ rate}$$

Example: 6-minute walk

$$METs\ =\ \frac{(.56\ mph)\ (26.83\ meters/min)\ (.1\ ml/kg/min)\ +\ (3.5\ ml/kg/min)}{3.5\ ml/kg/min}$$

METs = 1.4

Example: 12-minute walk

$$METs\ =\ \frac{(1.9\ mph)\ (26.83\ meters/min)\ (.1\ ml/kg/min)\ +\ (3.5\ ml/kg/min)}{3.5\ ml/kg/min}$$

METs = 2.45

TIMED DISTANCE WALK EVALUATION FORM

	Initial 6-minute walk		Discharge 6-minute walk	
	Walk: #1	*#2*	*Walk: #1*	*#2*
Total distance (ft)	_____	_____	_____	_____
Inside/outside	_____	_____	_____	_____
# rests	_____	_____	_____	_____
Time of rest(s)	_____	_____	_____	_____
Borg Scale	_____	_____	_____	_____
SO_2	_____	_____	_____	_____
F_IO_2	_____	_____	_____	_____
O_2L hr /m	_____	_____	_____	_____
BPmax	_____	_____	_____	_____
HRmax	_____	_____	_____	_____
MPH	_____	_____	_____	_____
METs	_____	_____	_____	_____
Patient symptoms *(see key)*	_____	_____	_____	_____
Supportive devices used *(see key)*	_____	_____	_____	_____
Other	_____	_____	_____	_____
comments:	_____	_____	_____	_____
	_____	_____	_____	_____
	_____	_____	_____	_____
Staff initials:	_____	_____	_____	_____
Date:	_____	_____	_____	_____

Key:
Patient symptoms: chest pain, dizziness, shortness of breath, leg pain, cramps, etc. Supportive walking devices used: walker, cart, wheelchair, cane, etc.

Staff signatures: _____

_____

Figure 4.3   Pulmonary rehabilitation timed distance walk evaluation form.

Incremental Maximal Exercise Test

Maximal exercise tolerance is typically measured with an incremental exercise test performed on a treadmill or stationary bicycle in a laboratory. Arm ergometry may be substituted for those patients unable to perform lower extremity exercise. Physiologic responses to graded exercise are commonly evaluated with ECG monitoring, blood pressure determinations, pulse oximetry, and ratings of perceived symptoms of breathlessness and muscle fatigue. Symptoms can be rated by using the Borg or visual analog scales.[15, 16] (See figures 4.4 and 4.5.)

0	Nothing at all	"No P"
0.3		
0.5	Extremely weak	Just noticeable
1	Very weak	
1.5		
2	Weak	Light
2.5		
3	Moderate	
4		
5	Strong	Heavy
6		
7	Very strong	
8		
9		
10	Extremely strong	"Max P"
11		
●	Absolute maximum	Highest possible

Borg CR10 scale
© Gunnar Borg, 1981, 1982, 1998

Figure 4.4   Category scale of breathlessness, a perceived symptom scale used to rate symptoms of breathlessness and fatigue during exercise testing.

Reprinted, by permission, from G. A. Borg, 1998, *Borg's perceived exertion and pain scales* (Champaign, IL: Human Kinetics), 50.

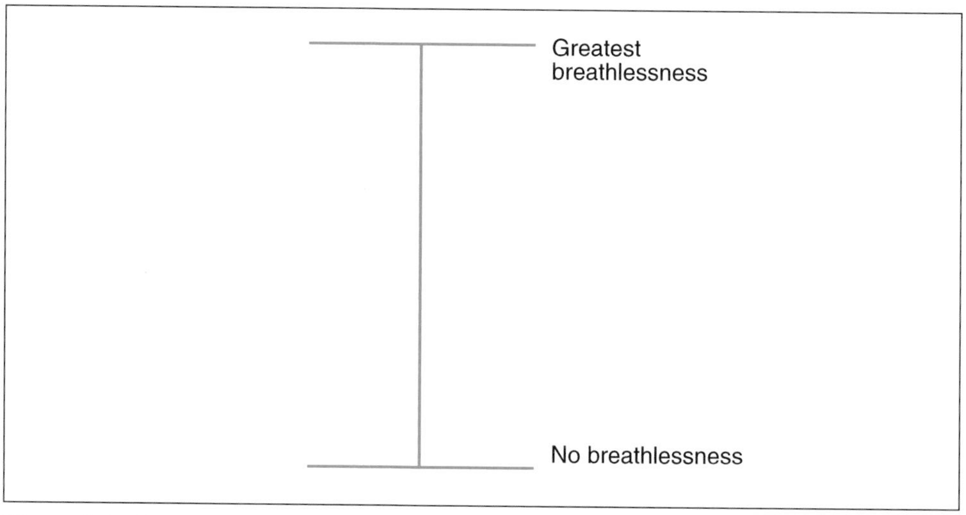

Greatest breathlessness

No breathlessness

Figure 4.5   Visual analog scale.

Adapted from R.C.B. Aitken, 1969, "Measurement of feelings using visual analogue scales," *Proc R Soc Med* 62:989-993.

In the absence of arterial and expired gas collection, the incremental exercise test may be used to measure maximal exercise capacity, detect exercise arterial oxyhemoglobin desaturation, develop an exercise prescription, and uncover potential coexisting cardiac abnormalities. With the addition of expired gas analysis, evaluation of ventilatory limitation, detection of nonpulmonary limitations to exercise, and measurement of the anaerobic threshold (when reached) can be performed.[3, 5] Addition of arterial blood gas analysis allows for the most accurate assessment of arterial oxygenation (i.e., alveolar-arterial oxygen gradient), carbon dioxide levels, and acid-base balance measurements.

Submaximal Exercise Test

Submaximal, steady-state exercise testing can be performed to assess supplemental oxygen requirements for ADLs. In this situation the test is conducted at a work rate that approximates those encountered during normal living conditions. A submaximal exercise test may also be conducted with patients with severe pulmonary hypertension or congestive heart failure, for whom maximal stress testing is contraindicated. Symptoms can be rated by using the Borg or visual analog scales.

Assessment of Exercise-Induced Bronchospasm

Patients with airway hyperresponsiveness, such as individuals with asthma or asthmatic bronchitis, commonly develop increased expiratory airflow obstruction after exercise (exercise-induced bronchospasm). This may occur even in the absence of clinically recognized lung disease. If such a condition is suspected, performing spirometry or other lung function tests before and after exercise may aid in its detection.

EXERCISE TRAINING

The exercise tolerance of patients with chronic lung disease is significantly decreased. As the severity of the underlying disease increases, the patient assumes a more sedentary lifestyle, avoiding the unpleasant sensation of dyspnea. This, in turn, leads to further deconditioning and increased exertional dyspnea. The "dyspnea spiral," which is depicted in figure 4.6, can be interrupted when the patient undergoes exercise reconditioning and breathing retraining as part of a pulmonary rehabilitation program.[17]

Most patients with severe chronic pulmonary disease have markedly reduced exercise capacity due to ventilatory rather than cardiovascular limitations to maximal exercise tolerance. Many of these individuals do not develop a significant lactic acidosis during maximum exercise testing, and they would not be expected to achieve the usual muscle and cardiovascular physiologic training responses seen in individuals with no disease or with less severe disease. Other pulmonary patients with less severe disease may develop significant lactic acidosis during maximum exercise testing associated with the added ventilatory response that may cause these individuals to reach a ventilatory limitation sooner. If such patients were to exercise above the lactate threshold, they would be expected to develop some of the usual physiologic benefits in addition to reducing their ventilatory demand at high exercise levels as their lactate threshold increases.[9]

Whether or not the anaerobic threshold is attained during incremental exercise testing and training, substantial increases in exercise ability (both endurance and

Most patients with severe chronic pulmonary disease have markedly reduced exercise capacity due to ventilatory rather than cardiovascular limitations to maximal exercise tolerance.

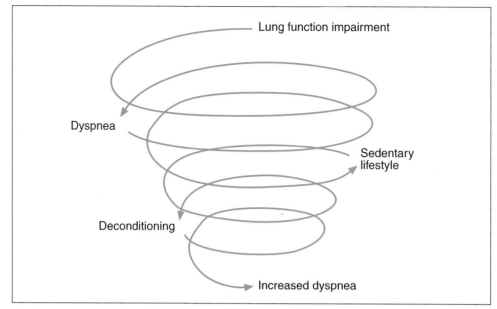

Figure 4.6 Dyspnea spiral.

Reprinted, by permission, from C. Prefaunt, A. Varray, and G. Vallet, 1995, "Pathophysiological basis of exercise training in patients with chronic obstructive lung disease," *European Respiratory Review*, 5(25): 27-32.

maximum level) are often observed after pulmonary rehabilitation in patients with chronic lung disease. Therefore, in the absence of contraindications, exercise training is recommended for rehabilitating virtually all patients with chronic lung disease, with the possible exception of patients with pulmonary hypertension due to primary pulmonary vascular diseases. (See chapter 7 for additional information concerning primary pulmonary hypertension).

Duration, Frequency, Mode, and Intensity

Exercise training in pulmonary rehabilitation can encompass both lower and upper extremity endurance training; strength training; and, possibly, respiratory muscle training. Duration, frequency, mode, and intensity of exercise should be included in the patient's individualized exercise prescription based on disease severity, degree of conditioning, and initial exercise test data. Various guidelines for exercise training have been suggested.[8, 12, 18]

The frequency and duration of the supervised exercise component during a pulmonary rehabilitation program may vary from three to five times per week, 30 to 90 minutes per session, over a period of 6 to12 weeks. Many different modes of exercise training have been used successfully with pulmonary patients, including walking (e.g., treadmill; track; supported walking via walker, cart, or wheel chair), cycling, stationary bicycling, arm ergometry, arm lifting exercises with or without weights, step exercise, rowing, water exercises, swimming, modified aerobic dance, and seated aerobics. Warm-up and cool-down periods must be included in each exercise session. Warm-up exercise allows for gradual increases in heart rate, blood pressure, ventilation, and blood flow to the exercising muscles. Cool-down reduces the risk of arrhythmias, orthostatic hypotension, syncopal episodes, and bronchospasm. For patients with chronic lung disease, exercise training is in many ways a tool to help them learn to cope with the frightening and disabling sensation of breathlessness that often limits their exercise capacity. Therefore, almost any type of exercise that the patient enjoys

For patients with chronic lung disease, exercise training is in many ways a tool to help them learn to cope with the frightening and disabling sensation of breathlessness that often limits their exercise capacity.

or is willing to do can be helpful in teaching patients to learn how to cope with their exertional symptoms.

Various methods have also been proposed for determining the appropriate exercise intensity during pulmonary rehabilitation for patients with chronic lung disease. No precise, well-established guidelines have been developed, however, for exercise training for patients with chronic lung disease.

For patients with chronic lung disease whose exercise tolerance is ventilatory limited (and who do not develop a significant lactic acidosis during exercise), the exercise training intensity can be set based on symptom limits. These patients are able to sustain exercise levels at or near the highest level reached on maximum exercise testing. Rating their perceived symptoms (using the Borg or visual analog scale) may help some patients target their exercise to a level of breathing discomfort, which may vary from time to time based on changes in the state of their underlying lung disease.[12, 19-21] For the purpose of training patients to build on increments of success, lower, submaximum intensity levels are often chosen to initiate exercise reconditioning. Then, duration and/or intensity of exercise can be increased as tolerated as the patient gains confidence with the training regimen.[8]

For patients with less severe lung disease who exceed the anaerobic (lactate) threshold during incremental maximum exercise testing, a target heart rate may be set at or above the anaerobic threshold (AT). This level may be set at a higher percentage of maximum than the typical 50 to 70% of maximum utilized in normal individuals.[8, 9, 12] In general, the standard heart rate ranges or targets used in normal populations have little application to ventilatory-limited individuals with disabling chronic lung disease. These patients usually stop exercise at low peak heart rates. Using any arbitrary submaximum percentage heart rate target often results in selecting target intensities that are too low for such individuals.

Regardless of the method used to select intensity training targets for patients with chronic lung disease, it is important to evaluate and periodically monitor the patients' oxyhemoglobin saturation (with cutaneous oximetry or arterial blood gas) with exercise to determine the need for supplemental oxygen. In particular, the arterial oxygen levels of patients with chronic lung disease change with exercise in an unpredictable fashion and cannot be determined by any measurement made at rest.[8] In general, it is

> No precise, well-established guidelines have been developed for exercise training for patients with chronic lung disease.

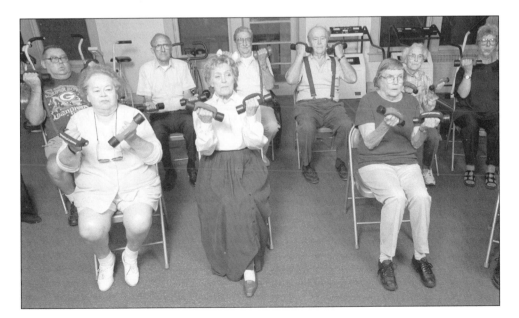

recommended that cutaneous oximetry estimates of oxyhemoglobin saturation be maintained at a level greater than 90% SaO_2 during exercise.[22-24] Cutaneous oximetry only estimates true arterial oxygen saturation within about $\pm$ 3 to 5% accuracy (and it tends to overestimate true saturation). Supplemental oxygen therapy, therefore, should be available in the rehabilitation setting for those patients who exhibit a hypoxemic response to exercise.

Upper and Lower Extremity Training

It is most beneficial to direct exercise training at those muscles involved in daily life activities. This typically includes training the muscles of both the upper and lower extremities. Upper extremity training improves performance for task-specific arm activities such as bathing, grooming, lifting, and so forth.[25] Types of upper extremity training may include the following:

- Arm ergometry
- Hand weights (e.g., wooden dowels, food cans)
- Elastic bands (Therabands)
- Wall pulleys
- Posture-specific exercises

Lower extremity training involves the large muscle groups and also improves performance in ADLs.[12] Types of lower extremity training may include the following:

- Walking
- Stationary bike
- Bicycling
- Rowing
- Stairs

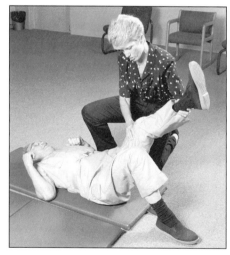 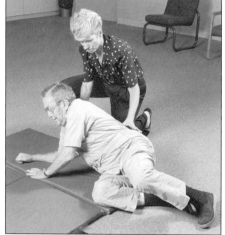

Along with strengthening the upper and lower extremities, various exercises to develop and maintain proper posture and good body symmetry should also be incorporated into a rehabilitation program. A lack of flexibility in particular muscle groups and imbalance in the muscular development of others can result in poor posture. A common postural deficit, such as rounded shoulders, may be due to a lack of muscular endurance in the scapular girdle abductors (i.e., middle trapezius and rhomboids), with a concomitant inflexibility in the pectoral muscles of the frontal chest area.[26] Focusing on strengthening the former muscle groups and increasing flexibility in the latter may aid in proper postural formation. Incorporating flexibility exercises with a goal to increase range of motion is also an integral component of the exercise program.

It is most beneficial to direct exercise training at those muscles involved in daily life activities.

Along with training the upper and lower extremities, various exercises to develop and maintain proper posture and good body symmetry should also be incorporated into a rehabilitation program.

Strength Training

In addition to endurance training, strength training may also be helpful to patients with chronic lung disease. Weight lifting may lead to improvement in muscle strength, exercise endurance, and fewer symptoms during ADLs.[7, 25] Examples of strength training modalities include

- hand and ankle weights,
- free weights, and
- circuit resistance.

Respiratory Muscle Training

Like their skeletal counterparts, the respiratory muscles of patients with chronic obstructive pulmonary disease can be trained. Respiratory muscle training can lead to an increase in respiratory muscle strength and endurance as well as a reduction in sensations of dyspnea.[27-30] Whether this results in an improved functional status or exercise capacity for the patient has not been clearly established.[31, 32]

Types of respiratory muscle training include flow resistive training (breathing through a progressively smaller orifice), threshold loading training (a preset inspiratory pressure, usually at some fraction of the maximal inspiratory pressure, is required) and isocapneic hyperventilation.[33] Suggested guidelines for employing resistive inspiratory muscle training include a frequency of four to five days a week; intensities of 25% to 35% of PImax (maximal inspiratory pressure measured at the mouth); and a duration of one 30-minute session per day, or two 15 minute sessions.[12, 34]

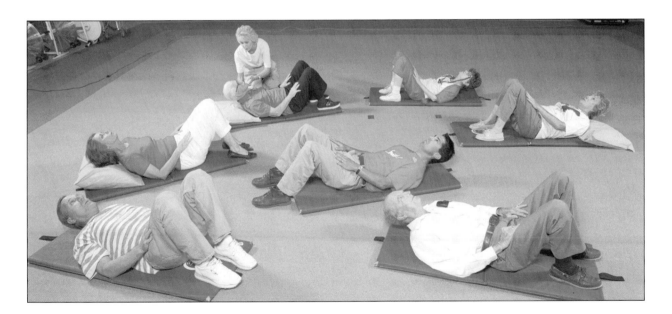

Home Exercise Training

Patients participating in rehabilitation should be provided with a home exercise prescription, which will allow them to engage in a continuum of physical activities outside the formal program setting. The home exercise prescription can be developed and begun early in the rehabilitation program, allowing the patient to gain confidence in independent exercise while in the program. Usually patients are expected to exercise

Patients participating in rehabilitation should be provided with a home exercise prescription.

regularly at home during the program. These unsupervised sessions may be monitored through exercise diaries, which can be reviewed during the supervised exercise sessions. Patient home exercise also aids the rehabilitation staff in adjusting the exercise prescription and addressing new problems that may arise. This exercise prescription can then be revised for a home maintenance program. Figure 4.7 is a sample form for a home exercise prescription.

EMERGENCY PROCEDURES

Personnel who work with pulmonary patients should be familiar with panic control techniques.

Appropriate emergency procedures and supplies must be available in the pulmonary rehabilitation exercise and patient training areas. All staff should be familiar with these emergency procedures. Minimum emergency equipment should include an oxygen source and delivery apparatus, resuscitation mask, first-aid supplies, and bronchodilator medications. In addition, personnel who work with pulmonary patients should be familiar with panic control techniques. In the patient with acute dyspnea, the following may be recommended:

- Have the patient stop the activity and assume a comfortable breathing position.
- Encourage the patient to use pursed-lip breathing and relaxation techniques.
- Use bronchodilator medication, if indicated.
- Monitor oxygen saturation, if equipment is available.

CONCLUSION

Exercise is one of the essential components of a comprehensive pulmonary rehabilitation program.

The importance of an exercise training program cannot be overemphasized. But before a safe program can be outlined, a thorough assessment needs to be done to evaluate exercise tolerance, formulate an appropriate exercise training prescription, detect exercise-induced hypoxemia, help determine the need for supplemental oxygen, and detect occult cardiac or other nonpulmonary limitations to exercise. The benefits of exercise training are well documented. They include increased tolerance for dyspnea, improved appetite, increased physical capability, and improved quality of life. Exercise is one of the essential components of a comprehensive pulmonary rehabilitation program.

REFERENCES

1. Reardon, J. et al. 1994. The effect of comprehensive outpatient pulmonary rehabilitation on dyspnea. *Chest* 105:1046-52.
2. Steele, B. 1996. Time walking tests of exercise capacity in chronic cardiopulmonary illness. *J Cardiopulm Rehabil* 16:25.
3. Ries, A.L. 1995. Effects of pulmonary rehabilitation on physiologic and psychosocial outcomes in patients with chronic obstructive pulmonary disease. *Ann Intern Med* 122:823-32.
4. Goldstein, R.S. et al.1994. Randomized controlled trial of respiratory rehabilitation. *Lancet* 1394-97.

PULMONARY REHABILITATION HOME EXERCISE PRESCRIPTION

Name: _____

The following instructions have been established based on your exercise performance in the pulmonary rehabilitation program. If there is a change in your condition, the instructions may need to be revised.

If you develop chest pain, severe shortness of breath (more than is usually associated with these exercises), light-headedness, or feel as if you are about to pass out—stop the exercise and consult your doctor.

If you are having a flare up of your lung condition, you should not exercise on that day and you should check with your doctor.

When exercising REMEMBER:

    A. Use your bronchodilator inhaler or aerosol treatment within two hours before you begin to exercise.

    B. Monitor your breathing level and heart rate.

    C. Do pursed-lip breathing.

During Exercise:

    A. On a scale of 0 to 10 (Borg scale), exercise at a maximum breathing level of _____ . If you are able to talk, you are okay.

    B. Your target heart rate (THR) is _____ beats/min. Try to stay within your THR. If you are above your THR, do not stop exercising abruptly. Slowly decrease the intensity of the exercise (e.g., walking, biking) until you bring your heart rate down.

    C. If oxygen is prescribed during exercise training, use at _____ liters/min.

Types of Exercise:

    1. Warm-ups

        Calisthenics: _____ minutes

        Stretching: _____ minutes

        Frequency: _____ daily, _____ x/week

    2. Walking/running

        May also try to walk/run _____ distance in _____ minutes

        Frequency: _____ x/week

    3. Supported walking: _____ minutes (pushing a cart or wheelchair) _____ distance

    4. Treadmill

        Speed: _____ miles/hour Duration: _____ minutes Grade of elevation: _____%

        Frequency: _____ x/week

    5. Stationary bicycle

        Speed: _____ miles/hour Duration: _____ minutes Work: _____ watts

        Frequency: _____ x/week

    6. Respiratory muscle training

        Threshold trainer set at _____ cmH_2O Should be done for _____ min/day

        Frequency: _____ daily, _____ x/week

    7. Strength training

        Hand weights: _____ sets of _____ repetitions _____ lbs. to be used as directed

        Leg weights: _____ sets of _____ repetitions _____ lbs. to be used as directed

        Frequency: _____ x/week

    8. Abdominal exercises:

        ___ sets of ___ repetitions Frequency:_____ daily, _____ x/week

    9. Back exercises

        ___ sets of ___ repetitions Frequency:_____ daily, _____ x/week

(continued)

Figure 4.7   Sample home pulmonary rehabilitation exercise prescription.

Adapted from Mt. Diablo Medical Center Pulmonary Rehabilitation Program Home Exercise Form, Mt. Diablo Medical Center, Concord, CA and Temple University Hospital Pulmonary Rehabilitation Program Home Exercise Form, Temple University Hospital, Philadelphia, PA.

10. Other
_____
_____
_____

11. Cool-down exercises

Lower extremity: _____ minutes

Upper extremity: _____ minutes

Calisthenics: _____ minutes

Stretching: _____ minutes

Frequency: _____ daily, _____ x/week

12. Diaphragmatic breathing

With a _____ lb. weight while lying down. Practice your relaxation exercises at this time, for 15 minutes, three to five times/week.

Comments: Do your exercises during the time of day that is best for you. Plan enough time for you to do the exercises without hurrying. Do what you are able to do.

_____
_____
_____

Pulmonary Rehabilitation Staff: _____   Date: _____

Figure 4.7 *(continued)*

5. Haggerty, M.C. et al. 1995. Connecticut Pulmonary Rehabilitation Consortium. The effects of pulmonary rehabilitation on functional status and exercise tolerance. (Abstract). *Am Rev Respir Crit Care Med* 151 (4): A683.

6. Vale, F., J.Z. Reardon, and R.L. ZuWallack. 1993. The long-term benefits of outpatient pulmonary rehabilitation on exercise endurance and quality of life. *Chest* 103:42-45.

7. Belman, M.J. Exercise in patients with chronic obstructive pulmonary disease. *Thorax* 48 (9): 936-46.

8. Ries, A.L. 1994. The importance of exercise in pulmonary rehabilitation. *Clin Chest Med* 15 (2): 327-37.

9. Casaburi, R. et al. 1991. Reductions in exercise lactic acidosis and ventilation as a result of exercise training in patients with obstructive lung disease. *Am Rev Respir Dis* 143:9-18.

10. Ries, A.L., J.T. Farrow, and J.L. Clausen. 1988. Pulmonary function tests cannot predict exercise-induced hypoxemia in chronic obstructive pulmonary disease. *Chest* 93 (3): 454-59.

11. Wasserman, K. et al. 1994. *Principles of exercise testing and interpretation.* Philadelphia: Lea & Febiger.

12. ACSM. 1995. *American College of Sports Medicine's guidelines for exercise testing and prescription.* 5th ed. Baltimore, MD: Williams & Wilkins.

13. Horne, D., and P. Corsello. 1993. Physical and occupational therapy for patients with chronic lung disease. *Sem Respir Med* 14 (6): 466-81.

14. Hillegass, E.A., and H.S. Sadowsky. 1994. *Essentials of cardiopulmonary physical therapy.* Philadelphia: W.B. Saunders.

15. Borg, G.A. 1998. *Borg's perceived exertion and pain scales.* Champaign: Human Kinetics.

16. Aitken, R.C.B. 1969. Measurement of feelings using visual analogue scales. *Proc Royal Soc Med* 62: 989-93.

17. Prefaut, C., A. Varray, and G. Vallet. 1995. Pathophysiological basis of exercise training in patients with chronic obstructive lung disease. *Eur Respir Rev* 5:25, 27-32.

18. Casaburi, R., and T.L. Petty, eds. 1993. *Principles and practice of pulmonary rehabilitation.* Philadelphia: W.B. Saunders.

19. Horowitz, M.B., and D.A. Mahler. 1993. The validity of using dyspnea ratings for exercise prescription in patients with COPD. *Am Rev Respir Dis* 147 (Suppl): A744.

20. Horowitz, M.B., B. Littenberg, and D.A. Mahler. 1996. Dyspnea ratings for prescribing exercise intensity in-patients with COPD. *Chest* 109:1169-75.

21. Faryniarz, K., and D.A. Mahler. 1990. Writing an exercise prescription for patients with COPD. *J Respir Dis* 11:638-44.

22. Nocturnal Oxygen Therapy Trial Group. 1980. Continuous or nocturnal oxygen therapy in hypoxemic chronic obstructive lung disease: A clinical trial. *Ann Intern Med* 93:391-98.

23. SEP Task Group. 1989. Recommendations for long term oxygen. *Eur Respir J* 2:160-64.

24. American Thoracic Society. 1995. Standards for the diagnosis and care of patients with chronic obstructive pulmonary disease (COPD). *Am J Respir Crit Care Med* 136:225-44.

25. Celli, B.R. 1994. Physical reconditioning of patients with respiratory disease: Legs, arms, and breathing retraining. *Respir Care* 39 (5): 482-501.

26. Alter, M.J. 1988. *Science of stretching.* Champaign, IL: Human Kinetics.

27. Harver, A., D.A. Mahler, and J.A. Daubenspeck. 1989. Targeted inspiratory muscle training improves respiratory muscle function and reduces dyspnea in patients with chronic obstructive pulmonary disease. *Ann Intern Med* 111:117-24.

28. Patessio, A. et al. 1989. Relationship between perception of breathlessness and inspiratory resistive loading: Report on a clinical trial. *Eur Respir J* 2:587-91s.

29. Leith, D.E., and M. Bradley. 1976. Ventilatory muscle strength and endurance training. *J Appl Physiol* 41 (4): 508-16.

30. Belman, M.J., and R. Shadmehr. 1988. Targeted resistive ventilatory muscle training in chronic obstructive pulmonary disease. *J Appl Physiol* 65 (6): 2726-35.

31. Goldstein, R.S. Ventilatory muscle training. *Thorax* 48:1025-33.

32. Smith, K. et al. 1992. Respiratory muscle training in chronic airflow limitation: A meta-analysis. *Am Rev Respir Dis* 145:533-39.

33. Belman, M.J. et al. 1994. Ventilatory load characteristics during ventilatory muscle training. *Am J Respir Crit Care Med* 149:925-29.

34. Larson, J.L. et al. 1988. Inspiratory muscle training with a pressure threshold breathing device in patients with chronic obstructive pulmonary disease. *Am Rev Respir Dis* 138 (3): 689-96.

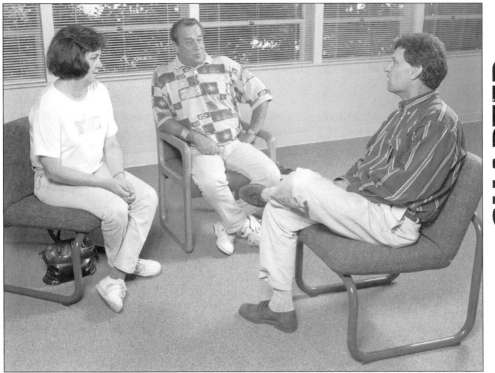

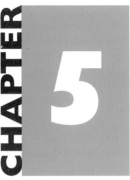

CHAPTER 5

Psychosocial Assessment and Intervention

The courage with which so many patients confront the enormous challenges associated with chronic lung disease is truly remarkable. Indeed, the capacity of patients to successfully adapt to these challenges is a major determinant of their quality of life. Although the ways that individuals cope with chronic lung disease vary considerably, there are some typical adjustment patterns as well as dysfunctional states of which practitioners should be aware. Psychosocial services provided within the pulmonary rehabilitation setting can facilitate the adjustment process by encouraging adaptive thoughts and behaviors, helping patients to reduce negative emotions, and providing a socially supportive environment.

The capacity of patients to successfully adapt to the enormous challenges associated with chronic lung disease is a major determinant of their quality of life.

ADJUSTMENT PROCESS

In the early stages of disease, patients and significant others are often unaware of, or deny, the existence and seriousness of the disease. Unlike the effects of other well-known diseases, the disabling effects and progression of chronic pulmonary disease are not well known to the public. This may make it easier to deny the relationship between pulmonary symptoms and the patient's past or present behavior (i.e., smoking history). Indeed, even as the disease progresses there appears to be some evidence

The presence of denial increases the risk of patient nonadherence with recommended medical interventions and changes in lifestyle.

An anxiety/dyspnea cycle is a frequent contributor to inactivity and overall disability in the patient with chronic lung disease.

that individuals with pulmonary disease are especially adept at suppressing emotions and concerns related to their illness.[1] Although suppressing one's emotions may be adaptive in reducing anxiety levels, the presence of denial also increases the risk of patient nonadherence with recommended medical interventions and changes in lifestyle.

As the disease progresses, most patients experience fear and anxiety[2] in anticipation of, and in association with, episodes of dyspnea.[3] Conversely, the heightened physiological arousal associated with anxiety can precipitate and exacerbate dyspnea. It is not, therefore, surprising that an anxiety/dyspnea cycle is a frequent contributor to inactivity and overall disability in the patient with chronic lung disease (see figure 5.1).

Patients' frustration with their poor health and inability to participate in many simple activities can also present in the form of irritability, pessimism, and a hostile attitude toward others. Overt expression of anger, however, may be suppressed to avoid an accentuation of dyspnea associated with acute physiological arousal.

In the later stages of disease, patients may develop a variety of psychosocial symptoms reflecting the progressive feelings of hopelessness and inability to cope with the disease process. Depression is common (51% to 74%)[4, 5] with signs and symptoms generally including[6]

▌ dysphoria (sadness);

▌ hopelessness;

▌ insomnia;

▌ loss of appetite;

▌ decreased interest in activities;

▌ decreased energy;

▌ loss of concentration leading to poor memory; and

▌ suicidal thoughts, particularly a sense of not caring to go on.

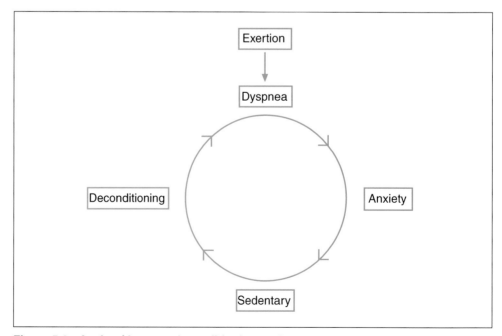

Figure 5.1   Anxiety/dyspnea deconditioning cycle.
Adapted, by permission, from L. Hilling and J. Smith, 1995, Pulmonary rehabilitation. In *Cardiopulmonary physical therapy,* 3d ed., edited by S. Irwin and J.S. Tecklin (St. Louis: Mosby).

As in the case of anxiety and dyspnea, a cycle of dysfunction may develop in which the loss of energy and desire to participate in physical activity may also contribute to deconditioning and progressive disability.

The tendency for depressed individuals to withdraw from social interactions with people outside of the immediate family can further serve to increase feelings of social isolation and depression for both the patient and primary caregivers. In contrast, patients may develop even greater dependency on one or more family members for their day-to-day care. This tendency to rely upon one or two caregivers often leads to considerable interpersonal conflict as the patient's needs, particularly when exacerbated by emotional distress, increase. In addition, sexual activity is often limited by depression, physical limitations, and the development of sustained sexual dysfunction.

Mild to moderate neuropsychological impairments may exist as a result of depression (as noted above) as well as hypoxemia. Such deficits generally involve difficulty in concentrating, poor memory, and some limitations in general cognitive processing. Patients experiencing such impairment may have difficulty in solving common problems involved in daily activities, miss office or clinic appointments, and fail to adhere to medical regimens.

> The tendency for depressed individuals to withdraw from social interactions with people outside of the immediate family can further serve to increase feelings of social isolation and depression for both the patient and primary caregivers.

Individuals with a history of preexisting mental health disorders can be expected to have the greatest difficulty adjusting to the chronic disease process. Particularly noteworthy is the presence of major depressive or anxiety disorders, previous adjustment disorder, personality disorder, alcohol or drug abuse, or history of psychosis.

As with other chronic illnesses, successful adaptation is often characterized by an active, engaging coping style with a positive, yet realistic, outlook on the future. Although some patients may find

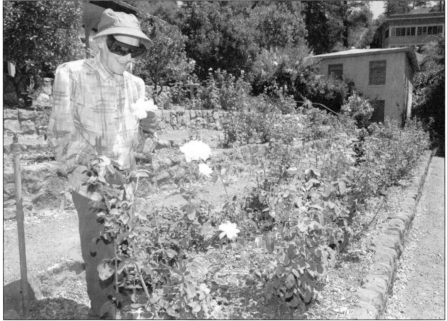

it helpful to deny some aspects of their illness, individuals coping through denial of their illness or treatment requirements, stoic denial of their feelings, or passive acceptance of their condition often experience a poor prognosis. A tendency to overly attend to somatic symptomatology (hypochondriasis) can also limit progress. It is also not surprising that in their efforts to cope, some patients may self-medicate with alcohol, overuse prescription medications, and maintain other self-destructive behaviors such as cigarette smoking.

> Successful adaptation is often characterized by an active, engaging coping style with a positive, yet realistic, outlook on the future.

An outline of medical and psychosocial stressors experienced by the patient with chronic pulmonary disease is presented in table 5.1. The clinician should also be aware that the patient's primary caregiver may also be under considerable stress. Though they may be deeply concerned about and dedicated to the patient's welfare, they are often emotionally and physically drained by the daily demands of their caregiving role. This may be particularly evident if caregivers perceive that the patient has become overly dependent on them.

Table 5.1. Medical and Psychosocial Stressors Associated With Chronic Pulmonary Disease

Medical

- Dyspnea
- Medication side effects
- Changes in physique due to disease process, medications, deconditioning, and aging
- Physical limitations imposed by disease (e.g., decreased ability to perform activities of daily living) and treatments (e.g., traveling with oxygen)
- Loss of cognitive functioning (concentration and memory)
- Comorbidity (e.g., CHD, arthritis, cataracts, CHF)
- Sleep deprivation (e.g., due to depression, hypoxemia)
- Surgical complications

Psychosocial

- Sense of impending mortality (both of self and with regard to other patients they have met in the program)
- Change in social roles
- Sexual dysfunction
- Family demands and reactions from others
- Public embarrassment (e.g., due to oxygen use)
- Loss of job/income
- Victim blaming
- Lack of visible signs of illness
- Major life events and other significant ongoing stressors (e.g., financial difficulties, comorbidity, legal concerns, role reversal)

PSYCHOSOCIAL ASSESSMENT

Programs are encouraged to develop a specific psychosocial screening protocol under the guidance of a mental health practitioner licensed to conduct such assessments.

Programs are encouraged to develop a specific psychosocial screening protocol (including instruments, procedures, and referral criteria) under the guidance of a mental health practitioner licensed to conduct such assessments. This practitioner may be a staff member or a consultant for protocol development only. If the latter, adequate mental health referral sites in the community should be identified. Several excellent references are also available that review relevant issues as well as the practice of conducting assessments appropriate to pulmonary rehabilitation settings.[7-11]

Practitioners are generally most effective in gathering quality assessment information through a combination of unstructured (open-ended questions) and structured (close-ended questions) interviewing formats. The practitioner can convey genuine empathy for the patient's welfare through the use of active listening skills, such as

- making appropriate eye contact;
- paraphrasing and summarizing patients' statements;
- asking questions to clarify important issues; and

▮ employing gentle, nonjudgmental confrontation regarding incongruencies between patient statements and behaviors.

It is also important that patients and practitioners have a mutual understanding of the nature and limitations of confidentiality in the professional relationship. For example, practitioners may convey medical information to other rehabilitation team members on a need-to-know basis. Interview questions should cover the following subjects:

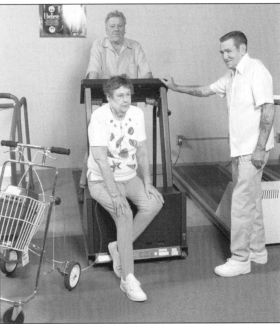

▮ Knowledge of the disease process and recommended treatments

▮ Perception of quality of life and ability to adjust to the disease

▮ Screening for psychopathology (i.e., depression, anxiety)

▮ Screening for significant neuropsychological impairment (e.g., memory, attention/concentration, and problem-solving abilities during daily activities)

As the patient's current level of sexual function may be a significant contributor to perceptions of quality of life, the practitioner should also assess the following:

▮ The patient's recent patterns of sexual activity

▮ Current fears and concerns (e.g., shortness of breath during sexual activity, development of impotence)

▮ Availability of a partner

▮ Partner's reaction to the disease and its effect on mutual sexual function

▮ Factors other than illness that may be affecting sexual functioning (e.g., age, medications, substance abuse, menopause, partner's health and emotional state)

Practitioners may wish to interview significant caregivers to gain a second perspective on the patient's medical history and to explore more fully issues related to dependency, interpersonal conflict, and intimacy. Such interviews should be conducted with the patient's consent and performed in a sensitive manner so as not to offend either patient or caregiver.

Clinician assessment of patients' verbal responses as well as direct observations of patients' affect and behavior should be supplemented by the use of questionnaires and/or psychometrically validated instruments. Although suitable for some screening purposes, it should be noted that unstandardized assessment tools may be less sensitive measures of pathology as compared to psychometrically validated instruments. Failure to detect the presence of significant psychosocial pathology may result in poor progress with rehabilitation. An outline of commonly used standardized instruments is presented in the *AACVPR Outcome Tools Resource Guide* in appendix C. Programs should seek the counsel of a licensed mental health provider in the administration and interpretation of these instruments.

Clinical interpretation and integration of findings from all assessment instruments is essential to avoid misdiagnosis or under-diagnosis. For example, many of the signs and symptoms of depression (insomnia, low energy, poor concentration) can be directly associated with hypoxemia secondary to pulmonary disease and may not be

Practitioners may wish to interview significant caregivers to gain a second perspective on the patient's medical history and to explore more fully issues related to dependency, interpersonal conflict, and intimacy.

Findings from the
psychosocial assess-
ment are most useful if
they lead to specific
and individually
tailored treatment goals
and are integrated into
the overall interdisci-
plinary treatment plan.

indicative of depression itself. In contrast, some patients with observable signs of
excessive anger may deny its existence on a written assessment.

Findings from the psychosocial assessment are most useful if they lead to specific
and individually tailored treatment goals and are integrated into the overall interdisciplinary treatment plan. Patients experiencing significant emotional distress, substance
abuse, cognitive impairment, or interpersonal conflict should be referred back to their
primary care physician or to a licensed mental health practitioner (psychologist, psy-
chiatrist, clinical social worker) for further evaluation.

PSYCHOSOCIAL INTERVENTIONS

All patients with chronic pulmonary disease are likely to benefit from some supportive counseling addressing one or more areas of concern (e.g., sexuality, anxiety, social
support). Interventions may be provided in a one-on-one or group format, depending
on the intensity of patient distress and the availability of therapeutic resources. Counseling can be delivered as a focused topic (e.g., stress management module) or during
the course of other rehabilitative activities (e.g., during breathing retraining). As noted
above, individuals experiencing significant emotional distress (e.g., depression) should
be referred for further evaluation. In such patients, subsequent treatment efforts within
pulmonary rehabilitation should be coordinated with the patient's primary care or mental
health provider.

Building Support Systems

Perhaps the psychoso-
cial intervention most
fundamental to pulmo-
nary rehabilitation is an
adequate support
system.

Perhaps the psychosocial intervention most fundamental to pulmonary rehabilitation
is an adequate support system.[7] Staff support, consisting of caring professionals dis-
playing good counseling skills, is key to successful programs. Such services often
entail good active listening and crisis management skills as well as patient advocacy
and facilitation of resource acquisition.

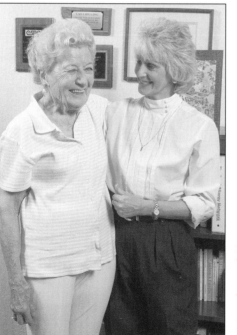

Additional support may be derived from family members, friends,
and other program participants. Such support can be enhanced
through patient involvement in support groups that encourage sharing of personal rehabilitation experiences as well as educational
presentations. The group environment is very conducive to partici-
pant-to-participant sharing of disease-related information and successful coping skills. It also provides an outlet for emotional release and elicitation of emotional support.

Additional opportunities for patient interaction can be developed
in waiting areas and during social events. To enhance their sense of
self-worth, some patients may also choose to serve as volunteers
for the rehabilitation program or other community activities.

Social support can also be fostered through involvement of significant others in the patient's rehabilitation program. Family members and significant others should be encouraged to participate in
support groups where family dynamics and interpersonal skills can
be observed, information can be shared, misperceptions clarified,
and fears and concerns addressed. Particularly important are dis-
cussions and skills development activities focusing on how family
members can provide support to the patient without promoting de-

pendency. For those patients having significant interpersonal or family conflict, referral to a clinical social worker or other counselor for family/relationship counseling may be necessary.

Addressing Issues of Sexuality

The sensitive topic of sexuality also needs to be addressed. Although general information may be provided during patient training in a small-group format, specific questions and concerns are generally best addressed in a one-on-one or couples format. An outline of topics that may be appropriate to discuss with patients is presented in table 5.2. The rehabilitation practitioner may be effective in facilitating discussion and resolution of sexual issues with many patients. Individuals experiencing significant emotional distress, however, or long-term difficulties with intimacy or sexual dysfunction should be referred to a licensed mental health provider.

Table 5.2 Issues to Address in Sexual Counseling With Heart and Lung Patients

Biological Issues

- Variations of sexual performance problems
- Effects of the aging process
- Sexual effects of organic factors related to the illness
- Is sexual activity safe?
- Effects of medications
- Evaluation and treatment options

Behavioral Factors

- Setting the appropriate sexual context
- Specific sexual technique

Emotional Factors

- Importance of relaxation and comfort
- Sexual effects of antierotic emotions

Cognitive Factors

- Anxiety-provoking beliefs
- Myths versus realities

Personality Factors

- Need for education, permission, or therapy

Relationship Factors

- Issues that relate to overall intimacy
- Sex versus sexuality in context

Sensory Factors

- Sensate focus as an antidote to anxiety
- Advisability of self-stimulation

Reprinted, by permission, from W.M. Sotile, 1996, *Psychosocial interventions for cardiopulmonary patients: a guide for health professionals* (Champaign, IL: Human Kinetics), 209.

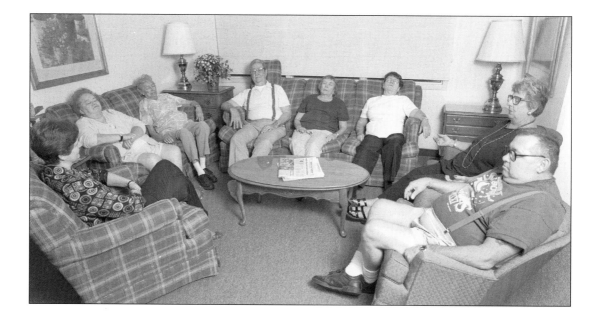

Managing Stress

Stress management training should include an easily understood, practical model for stress and its effects on the mind and body. Patients should be trained to recognize their own early warning signs and symptoms of stress (e.g., anxiety, dyspnea, muscle tension) and be capable of performing a variety of stress management techniques. Relaxation training for the mind and body can be accomplished via one or more methods. Examples include progressive muscle relaxation, imagery, autogenics, and yoga. To reinforce the training, relaxation tapes may be provided for home use. Relaxation practice may be supplemented through physiological monitoring (e.g., surface EMG, skin temperature) and auditory or visual feedback. In addition to in-class training, it is imperative that relaxation training be integrated into the patient's daily routine with specific application to dyspnea and panic attack control.

As patients with chronic pulmonary disease often experience medical or other life crises, the practitioner should be skilled in crisis management. Appropriate techniques include

▌ the ability to convey empathy through active listening skills,

▌ calming exercises (e.g., breathing retraining techniques),

▌ offering anticipatory guidance regarding upcoming stressors,

▌ assisting the patient with problem solving, and

▌ facilitating the identification of resources and support systems.[8]

The practitioner should be cautious to remain a concerned and supportive counselor, without behaving in a manner that would encourage patient dependency.

Treating Significant Emotional Distress

Cognitive-behavioral counseling techniques may be used for the treatment of depression. Cognitive interventions focus on gentle confrontation of irrational beliefs characteristic of depression. These include the tendency to selectively attend to, and overgeneralize from, negative events as well as the tendency to attribute negative events to personal inadequacies. Behavioral approaches generally include graduated activation and resumption of pleasurable activities.

Cognitive-behavioral counseling techniques may be used for the treatment of depression.

Patients experiencing anger control problems, a long-standing hostile attitude, or both, may benefit from individual and small-group counseling that addresses these issues.[8, 12] Management techniques for anger and hostility derive from general stress management training. These include early identification of anger-provoking stimuli ("hooks"), cognitive appraisal of the significance of these stimuli, and a cognitive decision regarding appropriate action. Assertiveness training is helpful to develop patient skills in expressing needs, fears, and concerns without putting the other individual on the defensive. Patients benefit from explicit instruction regarding how assertiveness differs from aggressive and passive behavior. In contrast, relaxation skills are useful for situations in which direct action is not likely to be effective. As in the management of depression, gentle confrontation of irrational beliefs may also be beneficial. Patients experiencing significant impairment of their quality of life due to anger and hostility may need referral to a mental health practitioner experienced in working with patients with chronic medical diseases.

Cognitive/behavioral interventions are also a critical component of therapeutic regimens (e.g., breathing retraining, medication use) used in the treatment of the anxiety/dyspnea cycle. Specific techniques include developing the patient's awareness of anxiety-promoting thoughts, enhancing the patient's ability to substitute more adaptive thinking, and initiating brief relaxation procedures. Antianxiety medications (anxiolytics; see table 5.3) such as benzodiazapenes can be used; however, long-term usage can result in psychological and/or physiological dependence. Evidence shows that anxiety levels in patients with COPD and comorbid depression can effectively be lowered with antidepressant medications.[13]

Pharmacological interventions for unipolar depression include the tricyclic antidepressants and the selective serotonin reuptake inhibitors (table 5.3). These medications are particularly helpful in restoring premorbid appetite and sleep patterns. Although often effective in the management of depression, significant side effects do occur. Particularly problematic may be tricyclic effects on secretions (dry mouth), the potential to exacerbate cardiac rhythm disturbances, and the development of sexual dysfunction (impotence, impaired ejaculation, and inhibited orgasm). As with other disorders, pharmacological interventions for depression are generally more effective when combined with psychological counseling than when either therapy is used alone.[14]

Modifying Lifestyles

Cognitive/behavioral interventions can also be useful in helping patients to adhere to recommended lifestyle modifications (e.g., diet, exercise, refraining from substance abuse).[15] Adherence to exercise is particularly important as it has been shown to enhance psychological adjustment in patients with COPD.[16-18] For smokers, nicotine replacement therapy in the form of gum, a transdermal patch, or a nasal spray may also be helpful. However, for optimum effectiveness, nicotine replacement therapy should be combined with a behavior modification program and social support.

Cognitive/behavioral interventions can also be useful in helping patients adhere to recommended lifestyle modifications.

Although the initial focus of cognitive/behavioral interventions is the development of new disease management skills, emphasis should also be placed on relapse prevention strategies that have been shown to facilitate long-term behavior change.[19] Therapeutic strategies that should be integrated into every aspect of the rehabilitation program are listed here:

Table 5.3   Tricyclic Antidepressants, Serotonin Reuptake Inhibitors, and Anxiolytic Agents

Tricyclic Antidepressants and Serotonin Reuptake Inhibitors

Generic	Brand
Amitriptyline	Elavil
Amoxapine	Asendin
Bupropion	Wellbutrin
Clomipramine	Anafranil
Desipramine	Norpramin
Fluoxetine	Prozac
Imipramine	Tofranil
Nortriptyline	Pamelor
Paroxetine	Paxil
Sertraline	Zoloft
Trazodone	Desyrel

Anxiolytic Agents

Generic	Brand
Alprazolam	Xanax
Buspirone	BuSpar
Chlordiazepoxide	Librium
Clonazepam	Klonopin
Diazepam	Valium
Hydroxyzine	Atarax
Lorazepam	Ativan
Oxazepam	Serax

> ▌ Enhance the patient's understanding and "ownership" of each component of the treatment regimen.

> ▌ Develop the patient's ability to identify situations (e.g., periods of emotional upset) in which the patient is likely to be at high risk of relapse (e.g., failing to maintain the exercise regimen, falling back into the anxiety/dyspnea attack cycle, misusing medications).

> ▌ Promote the patient's ability to solve problems independently as they arise during daily living.

> ▌ Encourage the patient and family's involvement in structured social support activities (e.g., clubs, exercise programs, volunteer activities).

Emphasis should also be placed on relapse prevention strategies that have been shown to facilitate long-term behavior change.

Reassessment of patients' adherence to the disease management regimen as well as their ability to implement relapse prevention strategies should be a major component of discharge planning.

CONCLUSION

The development of chronic pulmonary disease can have a marked impact on the overall quality of life for patients and their families. Screening for psychosocial disorders should be conducted during the initial assessment, with findings integrated into the comprehensive treatment plan. Individuals experiencing marked impairments in psychological functioning should be referred back to their primary care physician or a mental health provider for further evaluation and treatment. Psychosocial interventions, offered in either individual or group formats, can be effective in reducing distress and facilitating adaptive coping. Relaxation and stress management training can be beneficial in reducing the anxiety/dyspnea cycle and should be an integral part of the overall treatment plan. Reassessment of psychological status and refinement of interventions is an essential component of discharge planning.

REFERENCES

1. Dudley, D.L., C. Wermuth, and W. Hague. 1973. Psychosocial aspects of care in the chronic obstructive pulmonary disease patient. *Heart Lung* 2:289.

2. Prigatano, G.P, E.C. Wright, and D. Levin. 1984. Quality of life and its predictors in patients with mild hypoxemia and chronic obstructive pulmonary disease. *Arch Intern Med* 144:1613-19.

3. Heim, E., A. Blaser, and E. Waidelich. 1972. Dyspnea: Psychophysiologic relationships. *Psychosom Med* 34:405.

4. Agle, D.P., and G.L. Baum. 1977. Psychological aspects of chronic obstructive pulmonary disease. *Med Clin North Am* 61:749-58.

5. McSweeny, A.J. et al. 1982. Life quality of patients with chronic obstructive pulmonary disease. *Arch Intern Med* 142:473-78.

6. American Psychiatric Association. 1994. *Diagnostic and statistical manual of mental disorders*. 4th ed. Washington, DC: American Psychiatric Association.

7. Ries, A.L. 1990. Position paper of the American Association of Cardiovascular and Pulmonary Rehabilitation: Scientific basis of pulmonary rehabilitation. *J Cardiopulm Rehabil* 10:418-41.

8. Sotile, W.M. 1996. *Psychosocial interventions for cardiopulmonary patients*. Champaign, IL: Human Kinetics.

9. Hilling, L., and J. Smith. 1995. Pulmonary rehabilitation. In *Cardiopulmonary physical therapy*. 3rd ed. Edited by S. Irwin and J.S. Tecklin, 445-70. St. Louis: Mosby.

10. Prochaska, J.O., C.C. DiClemente, and J.C. Norcross. 1992. In search of how people change: Applications to addictive behaviors. *Am Psych* (September) 1102-14.

11. Emery, C.F. 1993. Psychosocial considerations among pulmonary patients. In *Pulmonary rehabilitation: Guidelines to success*. 2d ed. Edited by J.E. Hodgkin, G.L. Connors, and C.W. Bell, 279-92. Philadelphia: Lippincott.

12. Williams, R., and V. Williams. 1993. *Anger kills*. New York: Harper Collins.

13. Borson, S. et al. 1992. Improvement in mood, physical symptoms, and function with nortriptyline for depression in patients with chronic obstructive pulmonary disease. *Psychosom* 33:190-201.

14. Kahn, D. 1990. The dichotomy of drugs and psychotherapy. *Psych Clin North Am* 13:197-208.

15. Emery, C.F. 1995. Adherence in cardiac and pulmonary rehabilitation. *J Cardiopulm Rehabil* 15:420-23.

16. Emery, C.F. et al. 1994. Psychological functioning among middle-aged and older adult pulmonary patients in exercise rehabilitation. *Phys Occup Ther Geriatr* 12:13-26.

17. Emery, C.F. et al. 1991. Psychological outcomes of a pulmonary rehabilitation program. *Chest* 100:613-17.

18. Ries, A.L. et al. 1995. Effects of pulmonary rehabilitation on physiologic and psychosocial outcomes in patients with chronic obstructive pulmonary disease. *Ann Intern Med* 122:823-32.

19. Marlatt, G.A., and J.R. Gordon, eds. 1985. *Relapse prevention: Maintenance strategies in the treatment of addictive behaviors*. New York: Guilford.

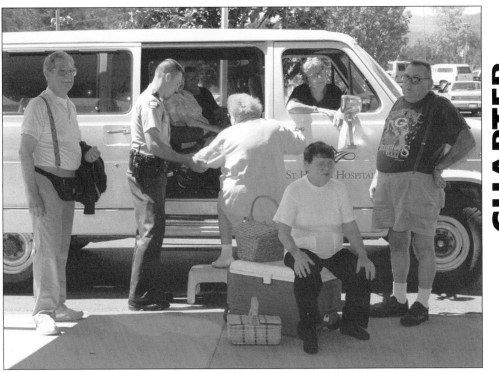

Continuous Quality Improvement and Follow-Up

Comprehensive pulmonary rehabilitation programs can enhance the quality of life and improve outcomes for patients with pulmonary disease.[1, 2, 3] With the health care atmosphere continually changing and the emphasis on quality, cost, and outcomes, it is increasingly important to incorporate outcome measurements into the rehabilitation program. In designing outcome measurements, a pulmonary rehabilitation program needs to incorporate a continuous plan for evaluating the quality of care provided in meeting their participants' and departmental goals and outcomes.[4] Before this can be done, the rehabilitation program personnel should understand more about continuous quality improvement (CQI). This knowledge will enable the staff to improve the quality of care of their participants.[5] In addition, to help maintain the benefits that the patients have achieved, the follow-up component is essential; numerous follow-up options are discussed in the later part of this chapter.

CONTINUOUS QUALITY IMPROVEMENT

A continuum of care, which begins at the start of a pulmonary rehabilitation program and continues through program discharge and follow-up, helps to promote better patient care. One way to achieve this is through the utilization of continuous quality improvement (CQI).[6, 7] CQI is used to evaluate patient outcomes and prevent potential problems from developing or reoccurring.[8] This concept involves every level of the health care organization including pulmonary rehabilitation. It utilizes every employee in committing to the same goal—improving the quality of patient care.

CQI emphasizes improving the system or work process, not the employee. As cited in Scholtes (1992), Deming and others analyzed various system problems and they suggest that 85% of an organization's inefficiency is the result of systematic problems (e.g., a lack of communication among departments).[9] Deming suggests that health care professionals develop a new attitude toward continuous quality improvement by using some of the strategies listed next.[9]

- Create a constancy of purpose toward improvement.
- Adapt a new philosophy. Be ready to take the challenge and learn new responsibilities.
- Communicate with other departments.
- Build quality into patient care.
- Minimize cost while still promoting improved quality of care.
- Motivate staff through job training and education.
- Utilize leadership to improve quality of care.
- Eliminate fear to improve efficiency.
- Involve all employees in improving quality of care.[10]

In addition to the strategies just listed, the interdisciplinary pulmonary rehabilitation team may consider several other steps to improve patient care and encounter fewer barriers within the organization:[9]

- *Maintain communication.* Communication among pulmonary rehabilitation staff and other departments is critical. All involved need to know exactly why, what, how, and when the CQI data will be collected. Communication encourages cooperation from coworkers and often leads to suggestions for improving quality of care.

- *Fix obvious problems.* Explore any problems in depth. Develop appropriate solutions once problems are identified.

- *Look upstream.* If your team is faced with a problem, mentally walk through the entire process. See if you can identify any problems.

- *Monitor changes.* Careful planning reduces chances of unanticipated data and minimizes error.

- *Document progress and problems.* Keep good records of every process tried. They can provide valuable data for future efforts.

Outcomes

In developing opportunities to measure outcomes, selecting effective tools to monitor program performance is essential. Various processes may be used to help individuals and departments improve their system. One process the AACVPR Outcomes Committee identified was Green's PRECEDE Framework, which is based on three outcome domains. These domains are health, clinical, and behavioral outcomes.[11] In pulmonary rehabilitation the health outcomes represent general or primary indicators that include morbidity, mortality, and quality of life.[12] These outcomes are influenced by clinical outcomes that include physiological,[13, 14] psychosocial, and medical utilization indices.[7] Clinical outcomes are often influenced by patient behaviors as a result of lifestyle changes. Behavioral outcomes may include adherence to medical regimen, diet and exercise routines, smoking cessation, breathing retraining, and relaxation skills.

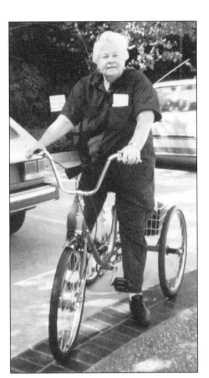

Another process that may improve program outcomes is suggested by the Joint Commission on Accreditation of Health Care Organizations (JCAHO).[4] This process of improving performance involves planning, designing, measuring, and assessing program components. This method evaluates not only what is done but also how well it was done to help improve the quality of care. The performance dimensions as suggested by JCAHO are listed here:

- Appropriateness: Are steps being taken to accomplish goals?
- Availability: Does the program meet patient needs?
- Timeliness: Are needs met in a timely manner?
- Continuity: Is there a continuum of care? Are other departments involved?
- Safety: Has safety been considered?
- Efficiency: Are all departments working together to meet their desired outcomes?

Indicators

No matter which process is chosen to improve program outcomes, the overall goal of CQI is to improve the patient's outcome.[15, 16, 29] In helping to meet these goals, indicators are also very effective.[5] Indicators are tools used to measure the performance of various functions in a pulmonary rehabilitation program over a period of time. It is important that indicators reflect the standard of care or practice based on current norms, if available. These indicators should identify opportunities to improve the quality of care and must be valid and measurable. The staff should understand the indicator being monitored, including its structure, process, and how it will be measured. Indicators may be either clinical or statistical. Clinical indicators are often more subjective. Statistical indicators are more objective and often easier to measure. Tables 6.1 and 6.2 contain various examples of clinical and statistical indicators, respectively.

The overall goal of CQI is to improve the patient's outcome.

For each indicator data are collected and organized to allow the staff to assign acceptable thresholds. An example of an acceptable threshold would be that 10 out of 12 charts show proper documentation of oxygen saturation when the patients begin the exercise component. The results of the data will show if the threshold was met and determine if further follow-up is needed. The source of the data varies depending on the indicator to be measured. Table 6.3 lists resources where data can be collected. The data should reflect the interaction of patient care staff with other departments and involve the total organization whenever possible.

Outcomes are the end result of CQI and should be reliable and valid. Table 6.4 gives examples of specific patient outcomes to monitor. Outcomes must be measured objectively to assess the progress of the patient and to evaluate the effectiveness of the rehabilitation program and staff.[11] Patient outcomes can include improvements in activities of daily living (ADLs), healthy behavior, and involvement in health care decisions. Various forms may be utilized to track outcomes. Tables 6.5 and 6.6 and

Outcomes must be measured objectively to assess the progress of the patient and to evaluate the effectiveness of the rehabilitation program and staff.

Table 6.1 Clinical Indicators for Pulmonary Rehabilitation Program

Staff Clinical Indicators	Expectations/Methods
Medication update	Staff update any changes in participants' medications every month and document.
Oxygen saturation checks	Staff check and document participants' O_2 saturations during exercise.
Patient problems	Staff document and send notification to participants' referring physician.
Preadmission work complete	Preadmission work is completed before participant starts program.

Participant Clinical Indicators	Expectations/Methods
Exercise safety (e.g., treadmill safety)	Participant can increase, decrease, and stop the treadmill safely by self. Document accordingly.
Patient education	Participants' retention of instructional material is demonstrated on a pre/post questionnaire.
Diaphragmatic breathing	Participants will be able to utilize and demonstrate diaphragmatic breathing and pursed-lip breathing by specified time.
Proper hand washing	Participants wash hands prior to starting each exercise period. Document accordingly.

Table 6.2 Statistical Indicators for Pulmonary Rehabilitation Program

Staff Statistical Indicators	Expectation/Methods
Preventative maintenance	All machines are checked every six months for cleanliness and proper working.
Crash cart	Documentation of checking crash cart is completed per hospital protocol.
Tracking of incident/notification forms	Record keeping of incidents with responses sent, if appropriate
Safety check	Quarterly checks by safety committee are done regarding all safety issues in the department. Document safety check and corrected deficiencies when applicable.
Medication errors	Documentation of any errors.
Medical record deficiencies	All pertinent information present in chart.

Participant Statistical Indicators	Expectation/Methods
Rehospitalization	Audit of participants' hospitalizations[17] 2 yr prior to/2 yr after the program.
Participant's complaints	Record keeping of participant's complaints and documentation of department's response.
Measuring weight maintenance /loss	Documentation of participant's weight.

Table 6.3   Data Collection

- Patient records
- Laboratory reports
- Exercise logs
- Medication logs
- Direct observation and measurement

- Departmental logs
- Infection control reports
- Incident/notification reports
- Utilization review findings
- Autopsy reports

Table 6.4   Evaluating Participants' Outcomes

Changes in Exercise Tolerance

- Pre- and post 6- or 12-minute walk
- Pre- and postpulmonary exercise stress test
- Home exercise training logs
- Strength measurement
- Flexibility and posture
- Performance on specific training modalities (e.g., ventilatory muscle, upper extremity)

Changes in Symptoms

- Dyspnea measurements comparison
- Frequency of cough, sputum production, or wheezing
- Weight gain or loss

Other Changes

- Activities of daily living
- Postprogram follow-up questionnaires
- Pre- and postprogram knowledge test
- Pulmonary rehabilitation medication regimen compliance
- Frequency and duration of respiratory exacerbations
- Frequency and duration of hospitalizations
- Frequency of emergency room visits
- Return to productive employment

Adapted, by permission, from L. Beytas and G.L. Connors, 1993, Organization and management of a pulmonary rehabilitation program. In *Pulmonary rehabilitation: Guidelines to success,* 2nd ed., edited by J.E. Hodgkin, G.L. Connors, and C.W. Bell. Copyright 1993 by J.B. Lippincott.

appendix C contain examples of indicator, measurement, and outcome tools that will help with the development of a CQI program.

JCAHO Guidelines

The pulmonary rehabilitation personnel should communicate with the education and CQI departments, if available, to remain current on the everchanging guidelines suggested by JCAHO.[4] Key suggestions from JCAHO are described here:

Develop a competency plan for your pulmonary rehabilitation program. The purpose is to ensure that quality care is delivered. All members of the rehabilitation

Table 6.5   Examples of the Process of CQI—Pulmonary Rehabilitation Clinical Indicators

Clinical Indicator	Expectation/Method	Data Analysis	Outcome
1. Treadmill safety	Participant can increase, decrease, and stop treadmill by self. Method: chart review, flow sheet, documentation.	10 out of 15 participants were able to increase, decrease, and stop by self safely.	Documentation was lacking on three participants. Two participants were unable to handle treadmill safely. Improvement is needed in documentation. Will continue to monitor.
2. Patient education	Participant will fill out pre/post questionnaires to evaluate comprehension of the instruction given. Method: pre/post questionnaires.	6 out of 10 participants completed the pre/post questionnaires.	Findings revealed more instruction was needed in bronchial hygiene. All participants need to complete questionnaires. Will continue to monitor.
3. Medication updated	Participants are to have their medication updated monthly and documented on their exercise charts. Method: Medication flow sheet documentation.	5 out of 20 charts randomly audited were compliant.	Improvement is needed in documentation of participants' change of medication to help improve participant safety and staff communication. Will continue to monitor.

Table 6.6   Examples of the Process of CQI—Pulmonary Rehabilitation Statistical Indicators

Statistical Indicator	Expectation/Method	Data Analysis	Outcome
1. Rehospitalization[*]	Staff will audit hospitalization 2 yr pre and 2 yr post rehab. Method: Medical records	Out of 59 charts audited, 372 hospital days 2 yr prior, 227 hospital days 2 yr post. 65 admissions 2 yr prior. 30 admissions 2 yr post.	Marked decrease in hospital admissions and length of stay for patients with pulmonary diagnosis after attending a six-week program.
2. Preventive maintenance on all exercise equipment	All machines are to be checked every 6 mo for cleanliness and proper working order. Method: Visual inspection and record keeping	All machines were clean and documentation of preventive maintenance was done on 8/16.	Preventive maintenance had been done on all machines. Documentation was present. Opportunity for improvement at this time: none.
3. Crash cart	Crash cart is to be checked and documented every exercise day. Method: Crash cart log	Staff documentation of crash cart was done every day of exercise.	Crash cart had been properly checked and documented. Opportunity for improvement: none.

[*] Taken from retrospective study done by St. Rose Hospital, Hayward, CA. Abstract presented at AACVPR annual meeting 10/95 and published in 1995 *J Cardiopulm Rehabil* 15 (5):349.

staff must be competent to fulfill their assigned responsibilities. The evaluation and documentation of competency should include staff knowledge and skill, effective and safe use of equipment, prevention of contamination and transfer of infection, CPR, and other lifesaving interventions. The competency plan may also include hospitalwide measures such as nursing/staff orientation, general hospital orientation, reorientation, quality care meetings, and educational tracking for all staff.

▌ Determine pulmonary rehabilitation program and staff competency (see appendix D) through[17, 18]

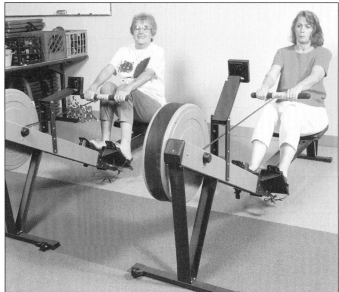

- maintaining staff credentials,
- orientation and skills checklist,
- ongoing educational tracking,
- inservices,
- continuing education,
- incident/variance reports,
- performance appraisals,
- peer reviews,
- staff meetings,
- committee meetings,
- communicating with staff and other departments,
- student and cross-training competency,
- reviewing scope of care, and
- reviewing age-specific learning principles.

▌ Evaluate pulmonary rehabilitation manager competency by evaluating the managers'[18]

- participation in leadership, management, and clinical education programs;
- clinical skills;
- knowledge of personnel policies;
- managing of personnel; and
- delegation and supervision skills.

▌ JCAHO also recommends that participants' rehabilitation training can be further enhanced if the interdisciplinary team has the ability to

- assess participants' needs,
- know what and how to teach,
- evaluate and document knowledge gained by participants, and
- assist participants in setting realistic goals.

The pulmonary rehabilitation personnel should review the current guidelines recommended by JCAHO annually. This helps staff to continue to improve the quality of care.

FOLLOW-UP

Pulmonary rehabilitation is an ongoing process of lifestyle changes that begins with the participant's entrance into the program and continues throughout the follow-up component.[19, 20] Follow-up is needed for pulmonary rehabilitation graduates to continue to improve their quality of life and physical and functional activities. Pulmonary rehabilitation programs have implemented various types of follow-up options for their graduates. These activities, described in table 6.7, help to promote compliance with rehabilitation goals, maintain long-term benefits, and provide psychosocial support. One of the key options is maintenance exercise, which has been demonstrated to improve outcomes.[21, 22]

Table 6.7   Follow-Up Options
• Maintenance exercise program
• Physician's office visits
• Keeping the primary care physician informed and updated on progress
• Support/educational groups
• Transplant support groups
• Family support groups
• Participants' phone tree
• Social events including parties, outings, and trips
• Newsletters
• Volunteering with rehabilitation program
• Referral to community groups (ALA and Better Breathers' Club)
• Phone follow-up by rehabilitation program staff
• Postprogram questionnaires
• Home visits by rehabilitation staff
• Reevaluation by rehabilitation staff
• National Pulmonary Rehabilitation Week (observed during the first week of spring)
• Home health referral to home care company and/or home health agency
• Referral to vocational rehabilitation

Adapted, by permission, from L. Beytas and G.L. Connors, 1993, Organization and management of a pulmonary rehabilitation program. In *Pulmonary rehabilitation: Guidelines to success*, 2ed., edited by J.E. Hodgkin, G.L. Connors, and C.W. Bell. Copyright 1993 by J.B. Lippincott.

Lasting long-term success requires long-term follow-up that could last several months or years. Staff should encourage participants to continue the rehabilitation process by giving them interesting and creative options for exercise and life-style changes.[23] It is important to provide participants with a written individualized home exercise plan prior to completion of the program. This written plan should include

▌ self-monitoring guidelines for target heart rate and appropriate dyspnea levels during exercise;

▌ current level of exercise and exercise goals;

▌ specific instructions in completing their exercise log; and

▌ reminders to follow their medication, nutrition, breathing techniques, and other home recommendations.[24, 25, 26]

Continued physical and functional gains are the goals of follow-up care. These goals cannot be achieved if exercise is discontinued.[27] The saying "variety is the spice of life" is not just a cliché, but it is a useful guideline for keeping participants interested and motivated to exercise on a consistent basis. An enthusiastic, creative, and supportive rehabilitation staff is critical in getting pulmonary rehabilitation participants to continue in a maintenance exercise program. Appealing and innovative options for maintenance exercise include

▌ stationary bicycling,

▌ upper body ergometry and circuit weight training,

▌ elastic bands,

▌ modified low-impact aerobic exercise routines and/or dance steps,

▌ group game activities, and

▌ pool exercise.

Another innovative option for maintenance exercise is the local, national, and international Transplant Olympic Games program. This program encourages lung transplant recipients of all ages to undergo extensive physical training before participating in competitive athletic events such as basketball, tennis, golf, swimming, and track and field. The Transplant Olympic Games are sponsored biannually by the National Kidney Foundation. Any solid organ recipient is eligible to participate in the games. Other options for the graduates may be enrollment in a fitness club, YMCAs, and senior centers.[28] In all of the above options, an individualized, goal-oriented physical activity program is extremely valuable in improving compliance and continuing physical and functional gains.

Psychosocial follow-up should not be overlooked. Some examples of psychosocial follow-up include[29, 30]

▌ support groups for participants and significant others,

▌ well spouses' support groups,

▌ Better Breathers' Club of the American Lung Association,

▌ social outings (e.g., bus trips, parties, picnics, movies, cruises),

▌ newsletters,

▌ cards (e.g., birthday, get well), and

▌ volunteer work in the pulmonary rehabilitation program.

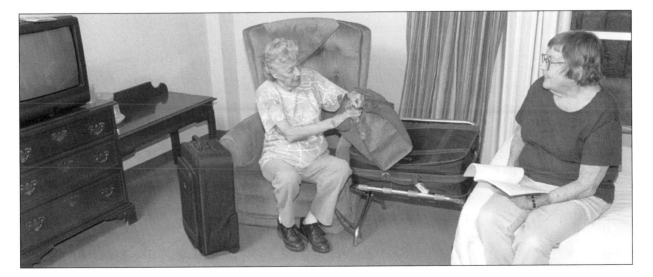

These follow-up examples help facilitate communication and fellowship, increase self-esteem, and improve compliance.

Home care is another follow-up option for pulmonary participants when needed. It allows the continuation of medical services to be rendered in the comfort and convenience of the patient's home.[26, 31, 32, 33] These services may consist of

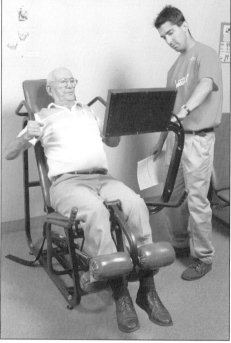

- evaluation of the participant's need for adaptive equipment and medical supplies;

- home ventilator management;

- IV therapy;

- wound care;

- respiratory equipment evaluation, use instruction, and cleaning;

- nutritional intervention;

- psychosocial support; and

- monitoring of the pulmonary rehabilitation home recommendations.

The need for home care has been well established and continues to grow. With the increasing emphasis being placed on providing care in a less costly setting, the rehabilitation team can be an essential part of the overall reduction in health care expenditures and must keep abreast of the services available to their participants in the community.

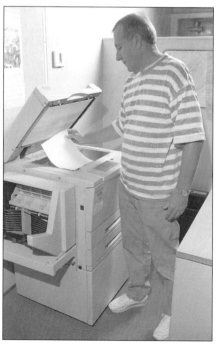

A postprogram follow-up questionnaire may be used to gather information relative to how the participant is complying with the home program. The information gathered may be tabulated and used for continuous quality improvement.[34] An example of a follow-up questionnaire is shown in figure 6.1.

An additional advantage of follow-up is the opportunity it provides for ongoing interaction between the participant's primary care physician and your program. This can be accomplished by sending the physician updated reports regarding the patient's progress, compliance with the home exercise program, and additional information gathered from follow-up activities and questionnaires. In addition to improving participant compliance because of the individual's continued interaction with his or her physician, this process helps to ensure a continued excellent relationship with the physician and your program.

CONCLUSION

A CQI program can be used to help the rehabilitation program provide excellence in pulmonary patient care by correcting any identified problems. If your facility is accredited by JCAHO, your CQI program must conform to their requirements as well as the Medicare Conditions of Participation.

PULMONARY REHABILITATION PROGRAM FOLLOW-UP QUESTIONNAIRE

Name: _____

Evaluation Date: _____ Response date: _____

Your thoughts about your health and quality of life are important to us in helping to determine the effectiveness of the training and exercise components in our pulmonary rehabilitation program. This questionnaire will help us to understand how our program affected you. We appreciate your time and cooperation in answering the questions. Please read each question carefully. Thank you!

Health

1. How would you rate each of the following *now* as compared to *before* you participated in the pulmonary rehabilitation program? (Circle one per line)

   A. Shortness of breath   Better   No change   Worse
   B. Cough   Less   No change   More
   C. Sputum amount   Less   No change   More
   D. Sputum consistency   Thinner   No change   Thicker
   E. Wheezing   Less   No change   More
   F. Swelling of feet/ankles   Less   No change   More
   G. Appetite   Better   No change   Worse
   H. Sleep   Better   No change   Worse
   I. Getting out of the house   More   No change   Less
   J. Sexual activity   Better   No change   Worse

2. Have you had any respiratory infections in the past 3 months?   No   Yes   If yes, please answer the following:

   a) How many have you had? _____

   b) Did you use an antibiotic for your respiratory infection?   No   Yes

   If yes, name the antibiotic used _____

3. Do you smoke?   No   Yes   If yes, how much per day? _____

4. Do you drink alcohol?   No   Yes   If yes, how much per day? _____

5. How many days have you been hospitalized in the past 3 months? _____

6. List the medications you are currently using:

   _____

   _____

   _____

7. Are you using supplemental oxygen?   No   Yes   If yes, how many hours per day? _____

Work

1. Has there been any change in your work situation since you graduated from the pulmonary rehabilitation program? (Circle one)

   A.   No   Yes   A change in job (explain) _____

   B.   No   Yes   Have you quit your job?

   C.   No   Yes   Have you reduced the number of hours worked?

   D.   No   Yes   Have you increased the number of hours worked?

   E.   No   Yes   Have you retired?

2. Has your spouse's working situation changed since you graduated from the pulmonary rehabilitation program? (Circle one)

   A.   No   Yes   Started working?

   B.   No   Yes   Stopped working?

(continued)

Figure 6.1   Pulmonary rehabilitation program follow-up questionnaire.

"Pulmonary Rehabilitation Program Follow-Up Questionnaire" is reprinted courtesy of the Pulmonary Rehabilitation Program at St. Helena Hospital, Deer Park, CA.

Home and Family

1. Has there been any change in your living situation since you graduated from the pulmonary rehabilitation program? (Circle one)

   A.   No   Yes   Change in address? If yes, please write below:

                         _____

   B.   No   Yes   Change in marital status? If yes, circle one:

                1)   Married

                2)   Divorced

                3)   Death of a spouse

Diet

1. How would you compare your diet (eating habits) *now* as compared to *before* the pulmonary rehabilitation program?

A. Food portions	More	No change	Less
B. Eating whole grains	More	No change	Less
C. Eating vegetables	More	No change	Less
D. Eating fruits	More	No change	Less
E. Eating foods high in fat	More	No change	Less
F. Drinking fluids	More	No change	Less
G. Use of salt	More	No change	Less

2. What is your current weight? _____

Exercise

1. How would you rate your exercise (activity) level *now* as compared to *before* the pulmonary rehabilitation program? (Circle one)

                                   More   No change   Less

2. List the type of exercise you do (walk, golf, bicycle, etc.):

   _____

3. How many days per week do you exercise? _____

4. How many minutes do you exercise on these days? _____

Figure 6.1 *(continued)*

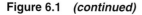

CQI is a never-ending process; no matter how good you are, you can always improve.

CQI is a never-ending process; no matter how good you are, you can always improve.[6] CQI works best when all are involved and committed to the same goals. Following the CQI process helps to justify the resources the team uses in the program.

Follow-up care provides the opportunity for the participants to improve their quality of life and continue working on their goals. The long-term support from the interdisciplinary team helps inspire "the pulmonary athlete" to strive for the gold and obtain his or her individual goals. For comprehensive pulmonary rehabilitation to occur, follow-up is necessary. It is one of the essential components of pulmonary rehabilitation.

REFERENCES

1. Sneider, R., J.A. O'Malley, and M. Kahn. 1988. Trends in pulmonary rehabilitation at Eisenhower Medical Center: Our 11 years experience. *J Cardiopulm Rehabil* 11:453-61.

2. Hodgkin, J. 1990. Prognosis in chronic obstructive pulmonary disease. *Clin Chest Med* 11 (3): 555-69.

3. Ries, A.L. 1990. Position paper of the American Association of Cardiovascular and Pulmonary Rehabilitation. *J Cardiopulm Rehabil* 10:418-41.

4. Joint Commission for Accreditation of Hospital Organizations (JCAHO). 1996. *Accreditation manual for hospitals*. Chicago: Author.

5. Patton, S., and J. Stanley. 1993. Bridging quality assurance and continuous quality improvement. *J Nurs Care Qual* 7 (2): 15-23.

6. Kirk, R. 1992. The big picture: Total quality management and continuous quality improvement. *Jona* 22 (4): 24-28.

7. Masters, F., and J.A. Schmele. 1991. Total quality management: An idea whose time has come. *J Nur Qual Assur* 5 (4): 7-16.

8. Roos, L. et al. 1990. Post surgical mortality in Manitoba and New England. *Jama* 263 (18): 2453-58.

9. Scholtes, P. 1992. *Team hand book*. Madison, WI: Joiner Associates.

10. Goldman, R.L. 1992. The reliability of peer assessment of quality of care. *Jama* 267 (7): 958-59.

11. Pashkow, P. et al. 1995. Outcome measurement in cardiac and pulmonary rehabilitation. *J Cardiopulm Rehabil* 15 (6): 394-405.

12. Emery, C., N. Leatherman, N. MacIntyre, and E. Burker. 1991. Psychological outcomes of a pulmonary rehabilitation program. *Chest* 100 (3): 613-17.

13. Anthonisen, N.R., E.C. Wright, and J.E. Hodgkin. 1986. Prognosis in chronic obstructive pulmonary disease. *Am Rev Respir Dis* 133:14-20.

14. Ferguson, G.T., and R.M. Cherlack. April 8, 1993. Management of chronic obstructive pulmonary disease. *N Engl J Med* 328:1017-22.

15. Creps, L.B. et al. August 1992. Integrating total quality management and quality assurance at the University of Michigan Medical Center. *QRB* 250-58.

16. Goldstein, R.S. et al. November 1994. Randomized controlled trial of respiratory rehabilitation. *Lancet* (344): 1394-97.

17. Schlintz, V. 1993. *Staff development train the trainer for managers hospital manual*. Hayward, CA: St. Rose Hospital.

18. American Association of Cardiovascular and Pulmonary Rehabilitation (AACVPR). 1993. *Guidelines for pulmonary rehabilitation programs*. Champaign, IL: Human Kinetics.

19. Hodgkin, J.E., G.L. Connors, and C.W. Bell, eds. 1993. *Pulmonary rehabilitation: Guidelines to success*. 2d ed. Philadelphia: Lippincott.

20. Ries, A.L. 1988. Pulmonary rehabilitation. In *Pulmonary diseases and disorders*. 2nd ed. Edited by A.P. Fishman, 1325-31. New York: McGraw-Hill.

21. Lopes, D., S. Hung, L. Marino, P. Lopes, and R. Zinati. 1995. Pulmonary rehabilitation program. (Abstract). *J Cardiopulm Rehabil* 15 (5): 349.

22. Ries, A.L. 1995. Effects of pulmonary rehabilitation on physiologic and psychosocial outcomes in patients with chronic obstructive pulmonary disease. *Ann Intern Med* 122:823-32.

23. Rodrigues, J.C., and J.S. Ilowite. 1993. Pulmonary rehabilitation in the elderly patient. *Clin Chest Med* 14:429-36.

24. Zadai, C.C. 1985. Rehabilitation of the patient with chronic obstructive pulmonary disease. In *Cardiopulmonary physical therapy*, edited by S. Irwin and J.S. Tecklin, 367-81. St. Louis: Mosby.

25. Frownfelter, D. 1996. The patient in the community. In *Principles and practice of cardiopulmonary physical therapy*. 3d ed. Edited by D. Frownfelter and E. Dean, 721-33. St. Louis: Mosby.

26. O'Ryan, J.A. 1984. Home care. In *Pulmonary rehabilitation: From hospital to home*, edited by J.A. O'Ryan and D.G. Burns, 199-210. Chicago: Year Book.

27. Make, B.J., and J. Buckolz. 1991. Exercise training in COPD patients improves cardiac function. *Am Rev Respir Dis* 143:80A.

28. Staats, B.A., and P.M. Simon. 1996. Comprehensive pulmonary rehabilitation in chronic obstructive pulmonary disease. In *Pulmonary rehabilitation, Lung biology in health and disease,* edited by A.P. Fishman. Vol. 91, 651-81. New York: Marcel Dekker, Inc.

29. Burns, M. 1993. Social and recreational support of the pulmonary patient. In *Pulmonary rehabilitation*: *Guidelines to success.* 2d ed. Edited by J.E. Hodgkin, G.L. Connors, and C.W. Bell, 392-402. Philadelphia: Lippincott.

30. Petty, T.L., and L.M. Nett. 1984. *Enjoying life with emphysema.* Philadelphia: Lea & Febiger.

31. Dunne, P.J., S.L. McIntruff, and C. Darr. 1993. The role of home care. In *Pulmonary rehabilitation: Guidelines to success.* 2d ed. Edited by J.E. Hodgkin, G.L. Connors, and C.W. Bell, 332-358. Philadelphia: Lippincott.

32. Wijkstra, P.J. et al. 1994. Quality of life in patients with chronic obstructive pulmonary disease improves after rehabilitation at home. *Eur Respir J* 7:269-73.

33. AARC Clinical Practice Guideline. 1995. Discharge planning for the respiratory care patient. *Respir Care* 40 (12): 1308-12.

34. O'Leary, D. 1990. "CQI—A step beyond QA," *Joint Commission Perspective.* March/April, 2-3.

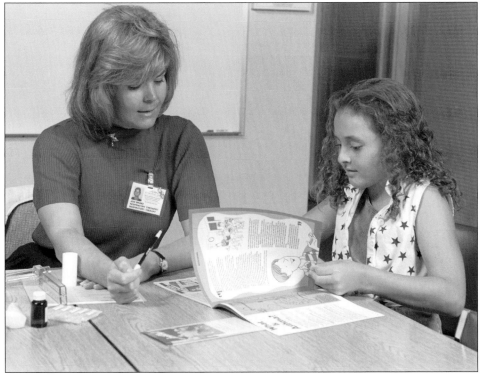

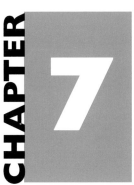

CHAPTER 7

Pulmonary Rehabilitation for Patients With Special Conditions

Traditionally, pulmonary rehabilitation has focused on patients with COPD (usually due to cigarette smoking) because it is the most common type of chronic lung disease. During the past decade, advances in the diagnoses and treatment of chronic respiratory failure have led to the emergence of additional subgroups of patients who may benefit from pulmonary rehabilitation (see table 7.1). [1-6]

While patients with special conditions have the potential to benefit from participation in a pulmonary rehabilitation program, they also pose new challenges for the rehabilitation professional. Although the components of a comprehensive pulmonary rehabilitation program (i.e., assessment, patient training, exercise, psychosocial intervention, and follow-up) are the same for these patients as for the COPD population, modification of the program components is essential to meet their specific needs. One factor to consider is the tremendous emotional issues patients with special conditions experience that may impede rehabilitation or even their willingness to participate in a program. These emotional issues must be assessed and treated for pulmonary rehabilitation to succeed. The purpose of this chapter is to inform the pulmonary rehabilitation specialist of the need to design pulmonary rehabilitation programs for patients with special conditions.

Although the components of a comprehensive pulmonary rehabilitation program are the same for patients with special conditions as for the COPD population, modification of the program components is essential to meet their specific needs.

Table 7.1   Pulmonary Rehabilitation for Patients with Special Conditions
Obstructive Lung Disease
• Asthma
• Alpha 1 antitrypsin deficiency (a1AT)
• Cystic fibrosis
Nonobstructive Lung Disease
• Interstitial lung disease
• Neuromuscular and neurologic conditions
• Primary pulmonary hypertension
Other Conditions
• Before and after volume reduction surgery (VRS)
• Before and after lung transplant
• Lung cancer
• Ventilator dependency
• Pediatric patients with pulmonary disease

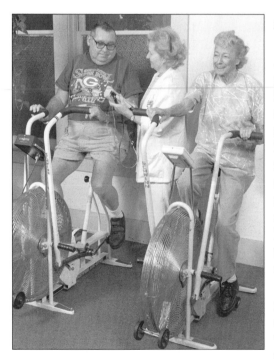

ASTHMA

Although many patients with asthma have long asymptomatic periods, some have extreme airway hyperreactivity that results in frequent exacerbations and others have chronic airflow obstruction. Often these patients utilize a disproportionate percentage of the medical resources devoted to asthma care and are limited by their lung disease. Such patients are likely to benefit from pulmonary rehabilitation[7, 8] with an emphasis on the recognition of known triggers (e.g., exposure to allergens and irritants, viral upper respiratory syndromes, bacterial otitis and sinusitis, allergic and nonallergic rhinitis, and esophageal reflux). It is equally important to discuss with patients peak flow monitoring, the role of various forms of medical therapy,[9-11] and the use of a self-management plan during acute exacerbations.[12]

Evidence shows that exercise training is also beneficial for patients with asthma.[13] Many asthmatics become deconditioned due to chronic inactivity as a result of dyspnea or efforts to prevent exercise-induced bronchospasm (EIB). Proper instruction regarding warm-up and cool-down routines and the use of medications such as beta agonist, cromolyn sodium, or nedocromil prior to exercise can help to prevent EIB. This allows the asthmatic to participate in the prescribed exercise training program.

Obesity resulting from chronic or frequent systemic corticosteroid administration can also contribute to the symptom of exertional dyspnea. Dietary intake should be evaluated and nutritional counseling should be provided, especially for those on chronic systemic steroid therapy. Endurance training of the upper and lower extremities can promote weight loss and possibly reverse some of the muscle weakness caused by chronic steroid use.

Endurance training may also benefit patients who are not overweight by delaying the occurrence of the anaerobic threshold. In patients with well-controlled asthma, the training intensity may be set near the anaerobic threshold or at a high percentage (i.e., 60% to 80%) of the maximal heart rate or $\dot{V}O_2$max, as determined by pulmonary exercise stress testing. Table 7.2 summarizes the components and program content that need to be emphasized or modified for patients with asthma.

Table 7.2   Program Modifications for Patients With Asthma
• Age-specific patient/family training
• Recognition of triggers
• Peak flow monitoring
• Role of medical therapy
• Exercise training
• Self-management plan
• Importance of exercise warm-up and cool-down
• Premedication prior to exercise to prevent exercise-induced bronchospasm
• Dietary intake and evaluation for patients on chronic systemic steroids

ALPHA I ANTITRYPSIN DEFICIENCY

Approximately 2% to 3% of cases of emphysema develop in patients with alpha 1 antitrypsin deficiency (a1AT).[14, 15] Patients with a1AT tend to develop COPD at a younger age than those patients with emphysema not related to this congenital deficiency.[16, 17] Differences in the radiograph and lung morphology are seen when comparing patients with and without a1AT. There are no significant differences between these two groups in the symptoms or mechanisms that result in dyspnea, and, in general, no significant modifications are necessary when designing an exercise regimen

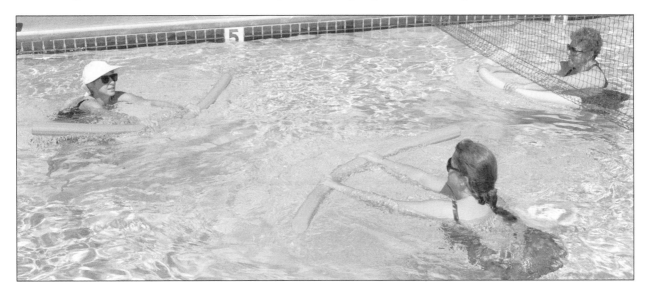

for patients with a1AT. Smoking cessation is imperative for these patients, as continued cigarette smoking in the face of low a1AT levels accelerates the deterioration in pulmonary function.

Some data have suggested that replacement therapy with intravenous infusions of plasma-purified a1AT may reduce mortality and slow the decline in lung function, although reports from controlled randomized studies are still pending.[15] Intravenous replacement therapy is currently only recommended for patients with lung impairment (FEV_1 < 80% predicted) and a1AT levels that are lower than 11 μmol/L. Lung transplantation has been a successful treatment option in patients with end-stage disease. As with other lung transplant candidates, pulmonary rehabilitation can be helpful in maintaining overall function pretransplant and facilitating recovery in the posttransplant period. See table 7.3 for a summary of the program components and content that need to be emphasized or modified for patients with alpha 1 antitrypsin deficiency and available options.

Table 7.3   Program Modifications and Options for Patients With Alpha 1 Antitrypsin Deficiency
• Exercise program same as for COPD patients
• Smoking cessation imperative
• Intravenous replacement therapy
• Lung transplantation

CYSTIC FIBROSIS

Cystic fibrosis (CF) is the most common genetic disease among Caucasian populations.[18, 19] Over the last several decades, median survival rates in CF have improved; therefore, pulmonologists who specialize in adult care can expect to see patients with CF.[18, 20] Respiratory complications due to mucus retention and recurrent respiratory tract infections are the main cause for deterioration of lung function in patients with CF. Compared to older patients with COPD and similar degrees of airflow obstruction, exercise tolerance is usually greater in patients with CF due to their younger age. Exercise tolerance is extremely variable among CF patients, however, and is most limited at times of exacerbation due to recurrent infections. Dyspnea and cough are common symptoms that frequently cause patients to reduce their physical activity, which may lead to greater difficulty clearing secretions. Peripheral muscle weakness is also frequently seen due to problems with postural habits (e.g., prolonged forward leaning), corticosteroid use, self-limitation in activity, and poor nutritional status leading to deconditioning. As a result, nutritional evaluation and counseling are of great importance.[21-23] Strength and endurance training using techniques described in chapter 4 have generally resulted in improved symptoms of dyspnea and functional status.[24]

The role of exercise in aiding mucous clearance is controversial. Exercise does lead to more sputum expectoration, although it should not be considered a replacement for conventional postural drainage therapy. Patients with CF and the personnel working with them should understand that vigorous coughing often accompanies exercise. These patients need to be especially conscious of replacing sodium and chloride when exercising in the heat due to abnormalities in sweat production.

Table 7.6   Program Modifications for Patients With Neuromuscular and Neurologic Conditions

- Age-specific patient/family training
- Treatment of underlying disorders
- Assessment of severity of disease
- Psychological support for patient and family
- Strength training
- Ambulation and cycle exercise for early disease states
- Interval training
- Orthotics
- Postural drainage therapy
- Proper body positioning
- Suctioning
- Mechanical ventilation

PRIMARY PULMONARY HYPERTENSION

Primary pulmonary hypertension (PPH) is associated with a significant reduction in five-year survival after diagnosis, with mortality being closely related to the severity of the pulmonary hypertension and the performance of the right ventricle.[44] The only therapeutic options available to these patients are lung transplantation and prostacyclin infusion.[45] Exercise training is generally thought to be contraindicated in this population due to concerns of low cardiac output, arrhythmias, pulmonary venous congestion, and hypoxemia, which may occur when the heart rate goes up during exercise. Participation in a modified pulmonary rehabilitation program, however, that includes assessment, patient training, psychosocial intervention, follow-up, and no exercise training may be beneficial for patients during the pretransplant waiting period. In general, these patients can participate in regular exercise after lung transplantation. See table 7.7 for a summary of the program components and content that need to be emphasized or modified for patients with primary pulmonary hypertension.

Table 7.7   Program Modifications and Options for Patients With Primary Pulmonary Hypertension

• No exercise prior to transplant	• Lung transplantation
• Prostacyclin infusion	• Exercise after lung transplantation

VOLUME REDUCTION SURGERY/PNEUMOPLASTY FOR EMPHYSEMA

A greater understanding of the pathogenesis of dyspnea in COPD, along with observations of COPD patients who have undergone single-lung transplant, has led to a renewed interest in the surgical excision of lung tissue from patients with diffuse emphysema and hyperinflation. This surgery, which is referred to as volume reduction surgery (VRS) pneumoplasty, has been performed via median sternotomy and video-assisted thoracoscopy (VATS). Early results suggest that some patients experience significant improvements in dyspnea, breathing mechanics, lung function, inspiratory muscle strength, maximal walk distance, and self-selected walking velocity after this procedure.[46, 47] Additional research is needed to determine the efficacy of VRS and which patients are most likely to benefit from the procedure. The Health Care Financing Administration (HCFA) has stopped payment through Medicare for VRS pending the outcome of a National Heart, Lung and Blood Institute prospective collaborative study. In this study HCFA recognizes pulmonary rehabilitation as the standard of care for the study groups involved.

Although the precise role of pulmonary rehabilitation in VRS has not been clearly defined, most experts agree that patients should only be considered for surgical therapy if they remain symptomatic despite maximal medical therapy and pulmonary rehabilitation. In fact, the assessments done in pulmonary rehabilitation may be of great value in determining the selection of the surgical candidate. Some patients who participate in a rehabilitation program may experience enough improvement to postpone or cancel surgical therapy. As with pretransplant rehabilitation, exercise training may potentially reduce some of the postoperative complications, and postoperative training may hasten recovery.

Good communication between the referring pulmonary rehabilitation program and the surgical team is crucial for optimal results. The rehabilitation team should be familiar with the patient's goals, the planned duration of therapy, and preferences of exercise intensity and modality set by the pulmonary/surgical team. Special factors that may require modification of the immediate postoperative rehabilitation training regimen may include prolonged air leaks requiring extended tube thoracostomy and concurrent medical conditions that precluded transplantation. Pulmonary rehabilitation following VRS is helpful in monitoring the patient to determine changes in the patient's exercise tolerance, medication program, and need for oxygenation. One must always keep in mind that the patients who are interested in VRS are indeed candidates for pulmonary rehabilitation regardless of surgery. The program content and components that need to be emphasized and modified for patients undergoing volume reduction surgery/pneumoplasty for emphysema are summarized in table 7.8.

Table 7.8   Program Modifications for Patients Undergoing Volume Reduction Surgery (VRS)/Pneumoplasty for Emphysema

- Pulmonary rehabilitation assessments to help determine selection of surgical candidate
- Communication between referring pulmonary rehabilitation team and surgical team
- Preoperative exercise training to reduce postoperative complications
- Postoperative exercise training
- Modification of immediate postoperative rehabilitation due to
    - prolonged air leaks,
    - extended tube thoracostomy, and
    - concurrent medical conditions that precluded transplantation.
- Post-VRS changes needed in exercise, medication, and oxygenation

LUNG TRANSPLANTATION

Due to improvements in surgical techniques and immunosuppressive regimens thousands of single- and double-lung transplants have been successfully performed since this surgery was re-introduced in the early 1980s. Lung transplantation is an option for patients with severe chronic respiratory diseases such as COPD, pulmonary fibrosis, cystic fibrosis, bronchiectasis, pulmonary hypertension, and a1AT.[48] Following is an explanation of the role of pulmonary rehabilitation before and after transplantation.[49, 50]

Before Transplantation

The primary goal of pretransplant rehabilitation is to maintain the patient's functional status.[51] Even patients with severe respiratory impairment may experience a reduction in dyspnea and an improvement in functional status.[52, 53] It is unusual, however, for sufficient improvement to occur as to eliminate the need for transplant. It is possible that pretransplant pulmonary rehabilitation may decrease the risk of perioperative pulmonary complications and even decrease the duration of hospitalization after transplant.[51, 53] The structure of the rehabilitation program is ordinarily quite similar to programs that are designed to treat the underlying pulmonary diseases as has been described throughout this book. Some modifications, however, may need to be considered.

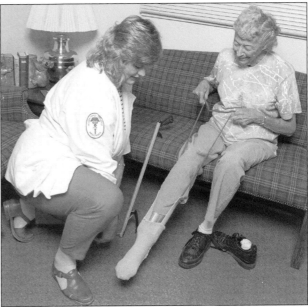

Patients who are awaiting lung transplant are typically those with the most severe underlying pulmonary diseases. As a result, the intensity of exercise training may need to be reduced. Usually patients exercise close to the highest workload that can be tolerated from the standpoint of dyspnea.[54, 55] Prior to transplant the patients should exercise in a supervised environment to ensure that the prescribed workload can be safely tolerated but is intense enough to have a beneficial effect. Consequently, pulmonary rehabilitation is essential for these patients. Some stable patients may be able to continue their exercise at home with equipment that is practical for the home setting (e.g., stationary bicycle, free weights, inspiratory muscle trainer).

The waiting time to transplant is unknown when the patient is placed on the transplant list but is generally between six months and two years. During the time the patient is waiting for a transplant, the disease can progress requiring reassessment and modifications in the patient's exercise program, medications, and oxygen prescription. Periodic review of the home exercise prescription and the patient's ongoing attendance in the pulmonary rehabilitation maintenance exercise program allow reassessment by the pulmonary rehabilitation team and may also improve compliance. See table 7.9 for a summary of the program content and components that need to be modified for patients both before and after lung transplantation.

After Transplantation

Postoperative rehabilitation can begin as early as 24 to 48 hours after surgery. The goals of rehabilitation in this phase include optimizing airway clearance and lung

Table 7.9 Program Modifications for Patients Before and After Lung Transplantation

Pretransplant

- Age-specific patient/family training
- Intensity of exercise training reduced
- Exercise as tolerated by dyspnea
- Stable patient may exercise at home
- Waiting time to transplant unknown, so disease can progress, requiring reassessment and modification of exercise and medical program
- Periodic review of home exercise program and maintenance exercise attendance

Immediate Posttransplant

- Optimizing airway clearance and lung expansion
- Decreasing requirement for supplemental oxygen
- Improving stability in erect posture
- Range of motion, basic transfer activities
- Breathing pattern efficiency
- Upper and lower extremity strengthening
- Functional mobility
- Postural drainage therapy
- Directed cough
- Special walker to facilitate walking with chest tubes
- Analgesia titrated to exercise
- Stable gait

Postdischarge

- Oxygen saturation monitored
- Postural awareness
- Back protection
- Increased tolerance for activities of daily living
- Reassurance
- Signs of infection or rejection (e.g., decrease in exercise tolerance)

expansion postextubation, decreasing the requirements for supplemental oxygen, and improving stability in the erect posture.[56] Rehabilitation in this early period should include range of motion, basic transfer activities (e.g., sitting to standing), breathing pattern efficiency, upper and lower extremity strengthening, functional mobility (e.g., ambulation), and postural drainage therapy. Directed coughing is especially important because of the impairment in the cough reflex that results from denervation of the donor lung. Resistive exercise of the upper and lower extremities can be performed in addition to simple ambulation. Special walkers can be used to facilitate walking while chest tubes are still in place. Analgesia needs to be titrated so exercise can be performed without worsening incisional pain. When surgery has been performed via a median sternotomy or antero-lateral thoracotomy, adequate time (i.e., four to six weeks) should be allowed before the patient can engage in strenuous upper extremity exercises such as arm cycling and wall pulley weights. Prior to discharge, it is important to check that the patient's gait is stable (i.e., at low risk for falls) and that lower extremity strength is adequate (i.e., for such tasks as transferring into and out of bed/chairs, stair climbing, etc.). Oxygen saturation should be monitored during different levels of exertion so that patients and their families are aware of oxygen requirements during activities of daily living and exercise at home.

After discharge from the hospital, patients may return to the rehabilitation program site for additional training and evaluation of exercise tolerance. Postural awareness and back protection measures need to be addressed to prevent spinal compression fractures secondary to osteoporosis due to prolonged use of immunosuppression medications. The major goal of rehabilitation during this phase is to achieve increased tolerance for activities of daily living. Patients may need reassurance that they can safely perform activities that are more strenuous than those performed prior to transplant. It may be helpful to follow parameters that reflect functional status such as the 6-minute walk test and maximum $\dot{V}O_2$ measured during a pulmonary exercise stress test. [57-59] The 6-minute walk test is simpler to perform and can usually be completed by the patient prior to resuming outpatient rehabilitation. It is frequently difficult for patients to perform a symptom-limited maximal exercise study shortly after discharge. Serial repetition of these studies at regular intervals (e.g., 3, 6, or 12 months after transplant) can be helpful in following the patient's progress; a decrease in exercise tolerance may be an early indicator of infection or rejection.

LUNG CANCER

Lung cancer and its treatments are associated with multiple physical and psychological symptoms including dyspnea, reduced exercise, activities of daily living intolerance, depression, and anxiety. Symptoms of cough and dyspnea may be caused by a number of factors including persistent obstruction of a central airway by tumor, lung injury due to radiation or chemotherapy, or underlying cardiopulmonary disease. For patients who have been treated for lung cancer, participation in a pulmonary rehabilitation program may improve both functional status and quality of life.

Patient training should stress self-management strategies and teach patients when to seek health care services. Physical training should be included to increase muscle strength and endurance. As these goals are identical to those of patients with COPD, patients with cancer can easily be integrated into any comprehensive pulmonary rehabilitation program. However, pulmonary rehabilitation performed concurrently with radiation and chemotherapy is usually not tolerated by the patient due to the side effects of the cancer treatment. During this time the pulmonary rehabilitation professional should work with the patient one on one covering the areas of breathing retraining, pacing, energy conservation, and addressing nutritional issues. The patient may be able to participate in a comprehensive pulmonary rehabilitation program when feeling better. For the lung cancer patient undergoing surgical treatment (i.e., pneumonectomy), pulmonary rehabilitation both before and after surgery may be comparable to undergoing lung transplant and VRS. Communication with the patient's oncologist is necessary because patients need to be medically stable before they can be admitted into the rehabilitation program. A summary of the program content and components that need to be emphasized or modified for patients with lung cancer is listed in table 7.10.

Table 7.10 Program Modifications for Patients With Lung Cancer
• Self-management strategies
• Exercise training to increase muscle strength and endurance
• Patient training covering the following areas:
- One-on-one training while patient is receiving cancer treatment
- Breathing retraining
- Pacing
- Energy conservation
- Nutritional issues
- When to seek health care services
• Attending the pulmonary rehabilitation program when patient is feeling better
• Pulmonary rehabilitation pre/post surgery may be comparable to lung transplant/VRS patients

VENTILATOR DEPENDENCY

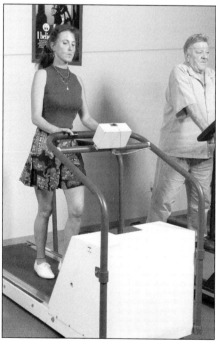

An increasing number of patients with chronic respiratory failure are returning to their home environment while still receiving intermittent, continuous, or nocturnal ventilatory support.[60-63] These patients, who are often discharged after long stays in acute or extended care facilities, typically suffer from significant atrophy of the peripheral skeletal muscles. Critical illness, suboptimal nutritional support, and corticosteroid and other medication usage may contribute to muscle weakness. Measures to improve peripheral muscle strength may increase patient independence and thus quality of life. The nutritional assessment is important for these patients to determine if supplementation, that is, a feeding tube and so forth, is needed, which will also increase muscle strength and exercise tolerance.

Strength training can be accomplished by using free weights, gravity, manual resistance, elastic bands as well as other methods described in chapter 4. In patients who receive intermittent ventilatory support, it may be advantageous to begin training during periods of mechanical ventilation. Adjustments in ventilator settings, including the F_IO_2, may be required. As strength and endurance improve, exercise training with the usual modalities during periods of spontaneous breathing may be added.

Patients who require chronic tracheotomy placement have limitations in their speech and are at risk for swallowing dysfunction. Evaluation by a speech therapist can identify problems in these areas. The use of cuffless or fenestrated tracheotomy tubes or Passey Muir valves can allow for speech, while compensatory swallowing maneuvers can often prevent aspiration. See table 7.11 for a summary of the program content and components that need to be emphasized or modified for patients who are ventilator dependent.

Table 7.11	Program Modifications for Patients Who Are Ventilator Dependent

- Age-specific patient/family training
- Nutrition assessment
- Strength training
- Intermittent ventilatory support
- Exercise training during periods of mechanical ventilation
- Adjustment in ventilator setting during exercise (F_IO_2)
- Speech therapist evaluation

PEDIATRIC PATIENTS WITH PULMONARY DISEASE

Asthma and CF have been discussed earlier in this chapter; however, a few considerations should be noted in the pediatric population. Children with these disorders are often kept from participating in athletic activities. Optimal medical therapy and preexercise warm-up routines can result in normal tolerance for athletic activities in children with asthma. Family members, school teachers, coaches, and physical education teachers all require instruction regarding the importance of exercise and safety issues for children with lung disease. Achieving normal or near normal pulmonary function is unlikely in the child with CF, except at a very young age. Bronchodilator therapy, postural drainage therapy when indicated, and the early treatment of respiratory tract infections can help children with CF remain active. The benefits of regular exercise training have been discussed previously and apply to children as well. Table 7.12 has a summary of the program content and components that need to be modified for pediatric patients with pulmonary disease.

Table 7.12	Program Modifications for Pediatric Patients With Pulmonary Disease

- Age-specific patient/family training
- Optimal medical therapy
- Preexercise warm-up routines
- Family member, school teachers, coaches, and physical education teacher instructed in the following:
  - Exercise and safety issues
  - Benefits of regular exercise training
  - Bronchodilator therapy
  - Postural drainage
  - Early treatment of respiratory tract infections

CONCLUSION

Most of the experience in the field of pulmonary rehabilitation has been in working with patients with COPD; however, patients with special conditions also need to be considered. These patients benefit from improved respiratory symptoms, functional status, and tolerance of activities of daily living. Close evaluation of the patient's pathophysiology and good communication with the patient's primary care physician or pulmonologist will allow for an individually designed program for these special patients. We must expand our knowledge and understanding to help optimize life for patients with all types of lung disease.

REFERENCES

1. Foster, S., and H.M. Thomas, III. 1990. Pulmonary rehabilitation in lung disease other than chronic obstructive pulmonary disease. *Am Rev Respir Dis* 141:601-04.

2. Bach, J.R. 1993. Pulmonary rehabilitation. In *Rehabilitation medicine principles and pulmonary practice,* edited by J.D. Delisa, 952-72. Philadelphia: Lippincott.

3. Bach, J.R. 1993. Mechanical exsufflation, noninvasive ventilation, and new strategies for pulmonary rehabilitation and sleep disordered breathing. *NY Acad Med* 68:321-40.

4. Bach, J.R. 1993. Pulmonary rehabilitation in neuromuscular disorders. *Neurology* 14:515-29.

5. Novitch, R.S., and H.M. Thomas, III. 1995. Pulmonary rehabilitation in patients with interstitial lung disease. *Am Rev Respir Dis* A684.

6. Cowley, R.S. et al. 1994. The role of rehabilitation in the intensive care unit. *J Head Trauma Rehabil* 9 (1): 32-42.

7. Make, B. 1994. Collaborative self-management strategies for patients with respiratory disease. *Respir Care* 39: 566-579.

8. Strunk, R.C. et al. 1991. Rehabilitation of a patient with asthma in the outpatient setting. *J Allergy Clin Immunol* 87:601-11.

9. Mayo, P.H., J. Richman, and W. Harris. 1990. Results of a program to reduce admissions for adult asthma. *Ann Intern Med* 112:864-71.

10. Guidelines for the diagnosis and management of asthma. 1991. *J Allergy Clin Immunol* 88(3):424-534.

11. National Asthma Education Program et al. 1991. Guidelines for the diagnosis and management of asthma. *J Allergy Clin Immunol* 88(3). St Louis: Mosby.

12. Beasley, R., M. Cushley, and S.T. Holgate. 1989. A self-management plan in the treatment of adult asthma. *Thorax* 44:200-204.

13. Cochrane, L.M., and C.J. Clark. 1990. Benefits and problems of a physical training program for asthmatic patients. *Thorax* 45:345-51.

14. Crystal, R.G. 1990. A_1 antitrypsin deficiency, emphysema and liver disease: Genetic basis and strategies for therapy. *J Clin Invest* 85:1343-52.

15. Stoller, J.K. 1989. Alpha 1 antitrypsin deficiency and augmentation therapy in emphysema. *Clev Clin J Med* 56:683-89.

16. Perlmutter, D.H., and J.A. Pierce. 1989. The a_1 antitrypsin gene and emphysema. *Am J Physiol* 257:147-62

17. Snider, G.L. 1989. Pulmonary disease in alpha 1 antitrypsin deficiency. *Ann Intern Med* 111:957-59.

18. FitzSimmons, S. 1993. The changing epidemiology of cystic fibrosis. *J Paediatr* 122:1-9.

19. Scanlin, T. 1988. Cystic fibrosis. In *Pulmonary diseases and disorders*. 2d ed. Edited by A. Fishman, 1273-94. New York: McGraw-Hill.

20. Murphy, S. 1987. Cystic fibrosis in adults: Diagnosis and management. *Clin Chest Med* 8:695-710.

21. Shepherd, R.W., and G.J. Cleghorn. 1989. Nutritional management. In *Cystic fibrosis: Nutritional and intestinal disorders,* edited by R.W. Sheperd, 53-65. Boca Raton, FL: CRC Press.

22. Luder, E. 1991. Nutritional care of patients with cystic fibrosis. *Top Clin Nutr* 6:39-50.

23. Daniels, L.A., and G.P. Davidson. 1989. Current issues in the nutritional management of children with cystic fibrosis. *Aust Paediatr J* 25:261-66.

24. De Jong, W. et al. 1994. Effect of a home exercise training program in patients with cystic fibrosis. *Chest* 1105:463-68.

25. Dear, C.L. et al. 1994. Impact of preoperative pulmonary rehabilitation on the cystic fibrosis lung transplant recipients. *Am J Respir Crit Care Med* 149 (4): A740.

26. Fiel, S.B. 1991. Heart-lung transplantation for patients with cystic fibrosis: A test of clinical wisdom. *Arch Intern Med* 151:870-72.

27. Heart-Lung Transplant Advisory Group to the Cystic Fibrosis Foundation. 1988. *Indications and contraindications for heart-lung transplantation in cystic fibrosis patients.* Rockville, MD: Cystic Fibrosis Foundation.

28. Scott, J. et al. 1988. Heart-lung transplantation for cystic fibrosis. *Lancet* 2:192-94.

29. Fulmer, J.D. 1990. Interstitial lung diseases. In *Internal medicine*. 2nd ed. Edited by J.H. Stein, 675-83. Norwalk, CT: Appleton & Lange.

30. King, Jr., T.E., R.M. Cherniac, and M.I. Schwarz. 1994. Idiopathic pulmonary fibrosis and other interstitial lung disease of unknown etiology. In *Textbook of respiratory medicine,* edited by J.F. Murray and J.A. Nadel, 2:287-303. Philadelphia: W.B. Saunders.

31. Novitch, R.S., and H.M. Thomas III. 1996. Pulmonary rehabilitation in chronic pulmonary interstitial disease. In *Pulmonary rehabilitation, Lung biology in health and disease,* edited by A.P. Fishman. Vol. 91, 683-700. New York: Marcel Dekker, Inc.

32. Siegler, E.L., M.G. Stineman, and G. Maislin. 1994. Development of complications during rehabilitation. *Arch Intern Med* 145:2185-90.

33. Marciniuk, D.D., and C.G. Gallagher. June 1994. Clinical exercise testing in interstitial lung disease. In *Clin Chest Med Clin Exer Testing*, 15 (2): 287-303.

34. Bach, J.R., and A.S. Alba. 1991. Pulmonary dysfunction and sleep disordered breathing as post-polio sequelae: Evaluation and management. *Orthopedics* 14: 1329-37.

35. Brooke, M.H. et al. 1989. Duchenne muscular dystrophy: Patterns of clinical progression and effects of supportive therapy. *Neurology* 39:475-81.

36. Bach, J.R., D.I. Campagnolo, and S. Hoeman. 1991. Life satisfaction of individuals with Duchenne muscular dystrophy using long-term mechanical ventilatory support. *Am J Phys Med Rehabil* 70:129-35.

37. Bach, J.R. 1992. Pulmonary rehabilitation considerations for Duchenne muscular dystrophy: The prolongation of life by respiratory muscle aids. *Crit Rev Phys Rehabil Med* 3:239-69.

38. Staas, W.E. et al. 1993. Rehabilitation of the spinal cord injured patient. In *Rehabilitation medicine: Principles and practice.* 2d ed., edited by J.A. DeLisa, 886-915. Philadelphia: Lippincott.

39. Bach, J.R. 1996. Conventional approaches to managing neuromuscular ventilatory failure. In *Pulmonary rehabilitation: The obstructive and paralytic conditions,* edited by J.R. Bach, 285-303. Philadelphia: Hanley and Belfus.

40. Kaplan, L.M., and D. Hollander. 1994. Respiratory dysfunction in myasthenia gravis. *Clin Chest Med* 15:683-91.

41. American Association for Respiratory Care. l991. Postural drainage therapy. *Respir Care* 36 (12): 1418.

42. Kigin, C.M. l990. Breathing exercises for the medical patient: The art and the science. *Phys Ther* 70:700-706.

43. Anderson, F., J. Bardach, and J. Goodgold. 1979. Sexuality and neuromuscular disease. *Rehabilitation Monograph No. 56.* New York: Institute of Rehabilitation Medicine.

44. D'alonzo, G.E. et al. 1991. Survival in patients with primary pulmonary hypertension: Results from a national prospective registry. *Ann Intern Med* 115:343-49.

45. Rubin, L.J. et al. 1990. Treatment of primary pulmonary hypertension and continuous intravenous cyclin (epoprostenol). *Ann Intern Med* 112:485-491.

46. Cooper, J.D. et al. 1995. Bilateral pneumectomy (volume reduction) for chronic obstructive pulmonary disease. *J Thorac Cardiovasc Surg* 109:106-19.

47. Sciurba, F.C. et al. 1996. Improvement in pulmonary function and elastic recoil after lung reduction surgery. *N Engl J Med* 334:1095-99.

48. American Thoracic Society. 1993. American thoracic society statement: Lung transplantation. *Am Rev Respir Dis* 147:772-76.

49. Goldstein, R.S., and M.J. Hall. 1996. Pulmonary rehabilitation before and after lung transplantation. In *Pulmonary rehabilitation, Lung biology in health and disease,* edited by A.P. Fishman. Vol. 91, 683-700. New York: Marcel Dekker, Inc.

50. Manzetti, J.D. et al. 1994. Exercise, education and quality of life in lung transplant candidates. *J Heart Lung Transplant* 13:297-305.

51. Sheldon, J.B. et al. 1993. Pulmonary rehabilitation prior to lung transplantation. *Am Rev Respir Dis* 147:A597.

52. Niederman, M.S. et al. 1991. Benefits of a pulmonary rehabilitation program: Improvements are independent of lung function. *Chest* 99: 798-804.

53. Biggar, D. et al. 1993. Medium term results of pulmonary rehabilitation prior to lung transplantation. *Am Rev Respir Dis* 47 (4): A33.

54. Foster, S.D., D. Lopez, and H.M. Thomas, III. 1988. Pulmonary rehabilitation in COPD patients with elevated PCO_2. *Am Rev Respir Dis* 138:1519-23.

55. Punzal, P.A. et al. 1991. Maximum intensity exercise training in patients with COPD. *Chest* 100:618-23.

56. Biggar, D.G., J. Mallen, and E.P. Trulock. 1993. Pulmonary rehabilitation before and after transplantation. In *Principles and practice of pulmonary rehabilitation*, edited by R. Casaburi and T. Petty, 459-469. Philadelphia: W.B. Saunders.

57. Orens, J.B. et al. 1995. Cardiopulmonary exercise testing following allogeneic lung transplantation for different underlying disease states. *Chest* 107:144-49.

58. Otulana, B.A., T.W. Higenbottam, and J. Wallwork. 1992. Causes of exercise limitation after heart-lung transplantation. *J Heart Lung Transplant* 11:S244-51.

59. Menard-Rothe, D. et al. March/April 1997. Self-selected walking velocity for functional ambulation in patients with end-stage emphysema. *J Cardiopulm Rehabil* 17 (2): 85-91.

60. Make, B. et al. 1984. Rehabilitation of ventilator-dependent subjects with lung diseases: The concept and initial experience. *Chest* 86 (3): 358-65.

61. Jackson, N.C. 1991. Pulmonary rehabilitation for mechanically ventilated patient. *Crit Care Nurs Clin North Am* 3 (4): 365-591.

62. O'Donohue, W.J. et al. 1986. Long-term mechanical ventilation: Guidelines for management in the home and alternate sites. *Chest* 90:15-375.

63. Make, B.J., and M.E. Gilmartin. 1991. Care of ventilator-assisted individuals in the home and alternate sites. In *Respiratory care: A guide to clinical practice*, edited by G.G. Burton, J.E. Hodgkin, and J.J. Ward, 669-690. Philadelphia: Lippincott.

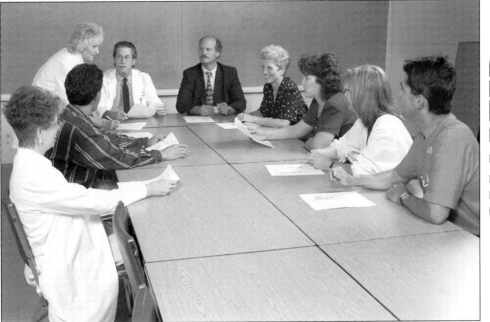

Program Management

This chapter covers the basic principles of pulmonary rehabilitation management, which include the structure of the interdisciplinary team, the team members' qualifications and responsibilities, as well as the administrative aspects of program management. The structure of the team is determined by your facility's needs and available resources. Specific management areas to consider include program location, facility, group size and structure, equipment needs, time constraints, patient populations served, adherence to the Joint Commission on Accreditation of Health Care Organizations (JCAHO) standards, and policies and procedures. It is essential that the program coordinator/director be familiar with all areas of reimbursement and the importance of thorough documentation. Developing a marketing strategy and plan with your interdisciplinary team members is also a key ingredient to promoting awareness of your program. By applying these basic principles of management, success with your pulmonary rehabilitation program can be achieved.

The structure of the interdisciplinary pulmonary rehabilitation team is determined by your facility's needs and available resources.

INTERDISCIPLINARY PULMONARY REHABILITATION TEAM

Providing excellence in the care of the patient with pulmonary disease requires health care professionals who are compassionate, caring, enthusiastic, and motivated. They should also be patient advocates with a strong belief and understanding in the goals of pulmonary rehabilitation. The number of team members and their professional backgrounds will vary considerably from one facility to another. It is not necessary for

It is not necessary for
every member of an
interdisciplinary team
to assess each patient;
however, the collective
knowledge, skills, and
clinical experiences of
the team should reflect
the interdisciplinary
expertise necessary to
achieve the desired
patient and program
goals and outcomes.

every member of an interdisciplinary team to assess each patient; however, the collective knowledge, skills, and clinical experiences of the team should reflect the interdisciplinary expertise necessary to achieve the desired patient and program goals and outcomes.[1-4] Team communication and interaction are vital to successful rehabilitation of the pulmonary patient. In pulmonary rehabilitation we do not just treat the disease, we treat the patients as human beings with empathy and compassion.

Structure

The structure of an interdisciplinary team begins with the patient as the nucleus. Team structure depends upon a number of factors such as patient population and characteristics, program budget and reimbursement, and the availability of team members and resources. A pulmonary rehabilitation team must have a medical director and a designated coordinator/director. Team members may work full- or part-time, on call, or as consultants or volunteers and may include both licensed and nonlicensed health care professionals. It is very helpful to have at least one full-time team member (usually the coordinator/director). The pulmonary rehabilitation team always includes the patient, primary-care physician, program coordinator/director, and the medical director. Additional members of the team may include the following:

Patient
Primary-care physician
Program coordinator/director
Medical director

▌ Respiratory therapist or technician	▌ Chaplain or pastoral-care associate
▌ Registered or licensed vocational nurse	▌ Biofeedback technician
	▌ Speech therapist
▌ Physical therapist	▌ Physiatrist
▌ Occupational therapist	▌ Recreational therapist
▌ Exercise physiologist	▌ Pulmonary laboratory technologist
▌ Dietitian	▌ Rehabilitation program graduate volunteers
▌ Pharmacist	
▌ Social worker	▌ Home-care personnel
▌ Clinical psychologist	▌ Business office representative
▌ Psychiatrist	▌ Vocational rehabilitation counselor

Pulmonary rehabilitation is a personal experience for both the patient and the team members. As stated by Dr. Brian Tiep,

An outstanding and
successful pulmonary
rehabilitation program
results from a dedicated
interdisciplinary team.

> *The human drama of struggle and achievement unfolds with each new patient who enters a program. Those team members who participate in this drama are rewarded with the joys of accomplishment and of knowing that they have contributed to making the lives of their patients more livable.*[5]

An outstanding and successful pulmonary rehabilitation program results from a dedicated interdisciplinary team.[6]

Responsibilities

To achieve the patient and program goals, the interdisciplinary team must have the knowledge, communication skills, and technical skills necessary to carry out the following responsibilities:

- Assess the patient
- Determine realistic patient goals
- Develop an individualized treatment plan
- Conduct patient training sessions
- Initiate department emergency procedures as necessary
- Evaluate patient progress
- Document the need for the skilled level of care and services provided
- Reassess the treatment plan
- Develop a home program plan for collaborative self-management
- Monitor patient outcomes
- Understand the continuous quality improvement (CQI) principles (see chapter 6)
- Provide in-services to other departments
- Attend pulmonary rehabilitation team meetings
- Recommend pulmonary rehabilitation to potential patients
- Serve as role models through attitude, communication style, and professionalism

Conferences

The effectiveness of the interdisciplinary team depends on an adequate system of communication. The team conference provides the opportunity for this interaction to occur. Team conferences are often held biweekly. The purpose of the conference is for the team to present and discuss the following information:

- History and physical examination data
- Medical test results
- Team members' assessment
- Patient goals
- Specific target/problem areas identified
- Individualized treatment plan
- Evaluation of patient progress
- Revision of treatment plan if necessary
- Postprogram needs and outcomes

The effectiveness of the interdisciplinary team depends on an adequate system of communication.

The interdisciplinary team concept provides the patient with the highest quality care possible through the expertise of the many disciplines involved and also enhances CQI. Documentation of the team conference information is necessary to show the patient's progress toward his or her established goals and outcomes. This documentation, which is included in the medical records, must be signed by either the medical director, program coordinator/director, or both, as determined by the program's policies and procedures.

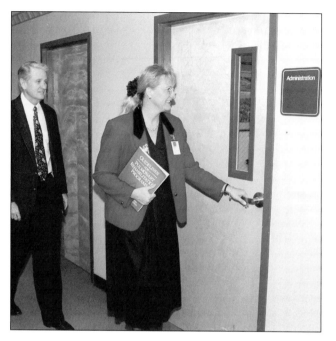

Qualifications

All personnel should be trained in basic life-support techniques. The following sections describe the minimum guidelines for core personnel and can be found in the *AACVPR Clinical Competency Guidelines for Pulmonary Rehabilitation Professionals* in appendix D. It is important that the staff and team members demonstrate a sense of responsibility to their employer and profession. They can accomplish this through knowledge and implementation of the mission, vision, and values of their department and facility and joining and becoming active in their local, state, regional, or national organizations. In this era of health care reform, it is important to be proactive for change not reactive.

Medical Director

The medical director should be a licensed physician with an interest in pulmonary rehabilitation and knowledge of pulmonary function and exercise testing. The role of the medical director may vary from program to program. He or she often functions as an administrator, diagnostician, clinician, educator, liaison, consultant, or research coordinator. The JCAHO requires that the medical director be involved in the budget process with periodic review of the program's policy and procedures.[7] The medical director acts as a liaison among the pulmonary rehabilitation team, the medical community,[8] and the facilities administration. The medical director's support and enthusiasm for the program is essential. As a proponent of rehabilitation, he or she should educate health care professionals and colleagues about the benefits of pulmonary rehabilitation.

Program Coordinator/Director

The program coordinator/director should be trained in a health-related profession and have clinical experience and expertise in the care of patients with pulmonary diseases. She or he should understand the philosophy and goals of pulmonary rehabilitation[1] and be knowledgeable in the program's administration,[9-12] marketing, patient training,[13] and reimbursement.[14, 15]

Other Team Members

Each team member is responsible for his or her specific specialty but should also be able to work as part of the interdisciplinary team.

At least one team member should have a national certification or a state license in a health-related specialty (e.g., respiratory care, nursing, physical therapy, occupational therapy). This person may or may not be the program coordinator. All team members should have training or experience in working with patients with pulmonary disease.[6] Each team member is responsible for his or her specific specialty but should also be able to work as part of the interdisciplinary team. All individuals should contribute to developing and implementing program goals and strategies. The ability to communicate effectively with patients, colleagues, and the general public is an important attribute.

POLICIES AND PROCEDURES

The pulmonary rehabilitation staff must be familiar with the department's policies and procedures. These may include

- the mission statement of the facility and program;
- scope of care including program location, hours of operation, content, description and program schedule, patient selection criteria and admission to the program, and emergency procedures;
- staff requirements including job descriptions, responsibilities, in-service attendance, evaluations, dress code, and so forth;
- documentation;
- continuous quality improvement; and
- patient rights.

The pulmonary rehabilitation staff must also be familiar with the facility's policies and procedures, which may include

- administrative policies including patients' rights, organizational ethics, and management of information (e.g., confidentiality, security, integrity, retention, availability of medical records, etc.);
- infection surveillance/control;
- safety; and
- facility orientation including confidentiality, payroll, security, employee benefits, risk management, and so on.

FACILITIES

The facilities and equipment used for the pulmonary rehabilitation program should meet state, federal, and JCAHO safety code standards. Sufficient space should be available for the multiple services provided. The equipment budget should address equipment expenses in relation to purchase, maintenance, and depreciation. The physical area can vary greatly depending upon program structure, patient population, needs, and resources. The program may often be the first contact for patients and the general public with the health care facility; therefore, the program plays an important role in public relations for the entire organization. An organized, clean, and well-maintained facility provides patients with a sense of ownership and enhances patient satisfaction and safety. The following considerations for the pulmonary rehabilitation environment should be addressed:

The physical area can vary greatly depending upon program structure, patient population, needs, and resources.

- Adequate and convenient parking, including handicapped parking spaces
- Access for individuals with disabilities
- Easily accessible water/drinking source
- Restrooms with handicap access
- Sufficient space for classroom, exercise, clinical, and administrative activities

❚ Oxygen source (e.g., piped in, liquid, concentrators, E-cylinder, etc.)

❚ Optimal light, temperature, and ventilation

❚ Storage space for equipment (oxygen, wheelchairs, walkers, respiratory therapy equipment)

❚ Hand washing facilities

❚ Activities of daily living (ADLs) facilities such as a teaching kitchen, bed, washer/dryer, tool bench, and so on, to help train patients in their specific ADLs needs

❚ Avoidance of chemical odors from cleaning agents, new paint, and white board markers (odorless white board markers are available)

❚ Fans in the classroom/exercise area (provide a sense of openness and lessen patients' feeling of claustrophobia)

❚ A copy of the Patient's Bill of Rights displayed in the department (see figure 8.1)

❚ Confidentiality of patient records and patient privacy

❚ Emergency equipment including an oxygen source and delivery apparatus, resuscitation mask, first-aid supplies, and bronchodilator medications

❚ Strict avoidance of scented perfumes, deodorants, hair sprays, and so forth, by staff and patients

Regardless of the equipment and space used in pulmonary rehabilitation, the environment must be safe and comfortable. But also consider that the dedication and enthusiasm of the interdisciplinary team are the most important elements of the program, not solely the facility and equipment available.

LOCATION

Pulmonary rehabilitation programs may be conducted in a variety of locations. Typically the programs are located within a hospital setting. However, clinics, comprehensive outpatient rehabilitation facilities (CORFs), YMCAs and YWCAs, community

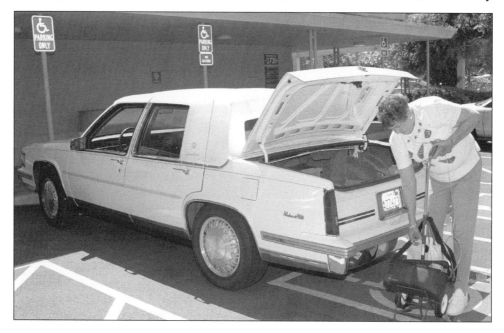

STATEMENT OF PATIENT RIGHTS

Thank you for choosing our pulmonary rehabilitation program for your outpatient rehabilitation needs. In order to receive the most out of your program, we want you to know the following information.

YOUR RIGHTS

You have the right to

- Exercise these rights without regard to sex, culture, economic, educational, or religious background or the source of payments for your care.
- Considerate and respectful care at all times and under all circumstances, with the recognition of personal dignity.
- Knowledge of the name of the pulmonary rehabilitation coordinator/director who has primary responsibility for coordinating your pulmonary rehabilitation program and the names and professional relationships of the interdisciplinary team members who will see you.
- Receive information about your illness and the course and outcome of treatment in terms that you can understand.
- Receive as much information as you need about the pulmonary rehabilitation program and the components that it entails in order for you to give informed consent or to refuse this course of treatment.
- Participate actively in decisions regarding your care. This includes the right to refuse treatment.
- Full consideration of privacy when attending the pulmonary rehabilitation program. Some of the areas are not as private as we would like them to be. Let us know if you are not comfortable discussing issues with the team members in this setting. You have the right to be advised as to the reason for the presence of an individual.
- Confidential treatment of all communications and records pertaining to your care. You will need to provide written permission before medical records can be released.
- Reasonable responses to any reasonable requests you may make for service.
- Reasonable continuity of care and to know in advance the time and location of appointments as well as the identity of persons providing the care.
- Be advised of any research affecting your care. You have the right to refuse to participate in such research projects. Any experimental or research activities will require your informed consent.
- Be informed of any continuing health care requirements following your discharge from the pulmonary rehabilitation program.
- Examine and receive an explanation of your bill regardless of source of payment.
- Know that all patient rights apply also to the person who may have legal responsibility to make decisions regarding medical care on your behalf.
- Wear appropriate personal clothing and religious or other symbolic items, if desired, as long as they do not interfere with diagnostic procedures or treatment.
- Expect reasonable safety insofar as the pulmonary rehabilitation program practices and environment are concerned.
- To discuss/resolve ethical issues surrounding your care.

YOUR RESPONSIBILITIES

We ask you to assist us by

- Providing complete and accurate information regarding your medical history.
- Reporting changes in your condition to the pulmonary rehabilitation team members.
- Providing written consent for treatment as requested.
- Complying with your instructions and letting the pulmonary rehabilitation staff know if you have concerns about the treatment program.
- Asking questions of the pulmonary rehabilitation staff and actively participating in your care.
- Being considerate of others and respecting their confidentiality and privacy. Our space is not always as private as we would prefer. Please leave the information you may overhear or see here at our facility.
- Being on time or calling if you are unable to attend the pulmonary rehabilitation program as scheduled.
- Meeting financial responsibilities, including provision of appropriate insurance and billing information.

COMPLIMENTS/CONCERNS:

- If you have a compliment regarding the pulmonary rehabilitation program or a specific team member please share it with the staff and/or the Pulmonary Rehabilitation Program Coordinator/Director. You may also want to write a letter to the facility administrator.
- Direct any concern or complaint regarding your treatment while in the pulmonary rehabilitation program to the Pulmonary Rehabilitation Program Coordinator/Director. If you do not feel it was adequately addressed, please ask for the manager. If you still do not feel your concern has been adequately addressed, contact the Quality Review Department at the facility. You have the right to expect a response within a reasonable time frame.

Figure 8.1   Sample statement of patient rights for a pulmonary rehabilitation program

The essential require-
ments in selecting a site
are accessibility for the
patient, a conducive
environment to good
health, and appropriate
medical and emergency
supervision as well as
the ability to provide
all of the components
of a comprehensive
rehabilitation program.

centers, and a myriad of other settings also provide potential sites for rehabilitation programs.[16, 17] The essential requirements in selecting a site are accessibility for the patient, a conducive environment to good health, and appropriate medical and emergency supervision. Additionally, the site must be able to provide all of the components of a comprehensive rehabilitation program including assessment, patient training, exercise, psychosocial intervention, and follow-up care. The program setting depends upon the patient populations you serve, your geographic location, and your program finances. See table 8.1 for program location options.

Table 8.1   Location Options for Pulmonary Rehabilitation Programs

Hospital Setting (Inpatient)
- Acute care during hospitalization
- Transitional care unit
- Rehabilitation hospital

Hospital Setting (Outpatient)
- Outpatient hospital setting
- Clinic setting
- Residential outpatient facility
- Comprehensive outpatient rehabilitation facility (CORF)
- Shared facility with other programs (e.g., cardiac rehabilitation, wellness program)

Alternate Sites
- Physician's office
- Storefront
- Home residence
- Wellness center
- Fitness center or spa
- Senior citizen center
- Local high school or community college
- Adult education center
- Places of worship
- Club meeting halls

Adapted, by permission, from L. Beytas and G.L. Connors, 1993, Organization and management of a pulmonary rehabilitation program. In *Pulmonary rehabilitation: Guidelines to success*, 2ed., edited by J.E. Hodgkin, G.L. Connors, and C.W. Bell. Copyright 1993 by J.B. Lippincott.

GROUP SIZE AND SCHEDULE

Pulmonary rehabilitation programs are typically conducted in small groups of approximately four to six patients, although some programs work with the patient on a one-on-one basis. In a national survey of pulmonary rehabilitation programs published in 1995, the average group size was nine patients. The mean program length was 45 hours, 2 hours per day, 2.5 days per week, for 9 weeks.[18]

Regardless of program size or design, it should be individualized to meet each patient's specific needs. Program schedules will vary according to staff, facilities, resources, budget, and patient needs (e.g., degrees of impairments, limitations, ages, job schedules). It is difficult to set specific guidelines; however, a typical program may include 30 to 50 hours over a 4- to 12-week period, 2 to 4 hours per day, meeting 2 to 3 days per week, with patient training, psychosocial intervention, and exercise incorporated into the sessions. Dr. Philip Corsello stated, "There is a failure to appreciate that pulmonary rehabilitation is not accomplished in three weeks. It is a lifetime process."[6] See figure 8.2 for a sample outpatient program schedule.

Regardless of program size or design, it should be individualized to meet each patient's specific needs.

DOCUMENTATION

Accurate and thorough charting facilitates effective communication among the team, primary care physician, and third-party payers. Documentation is used to monitor

---

OUTPATIENT PULMONARY REHABILITATION SCHEDULE

Weeks 1-4 meet twice per week.

Tuesday			Thursday	
Date:			Date:	
Week 1	12-1	Introduction & Pre-Testing	12-1	The Respiratory System: Structure and Function
	1-2	Exercise	1-2:30	Exercise
	2-3	Support Group	2:30-4	Activities of Daily Living
	3-4	Breathing Exercises		
Date:			Date:	
Week 2	12-1	Exercise Principles	12-1	Disease Process/Oxygen as a Drug
	1-2	Exercise	1-2:30	Exercise
	2-3	Support Group	2:30-3	Smoking Cessation
	3-4	Metered Dose Inhaler	3-4	Support Group/Sexuality
Date:			Date:	
Week 3	11:30-12	Dietary Evaluations	12-1	Your Food Life (Nutritional Training)
	12-1	Medications (Part I)	1-2:30	Exercise
	1-2	Exercise	2:30-3:30	Home Equipment/Travel
	2-3	Support Group/Stress Management	3:30-4	Secondhand Smoke
	3-4	Self-Assessment Techniques		
Date:			Date:	
Week 4	12-1	Medications (Part II)	12-1	Post Testing/Home Exercise Prescription
	1-2	Exercise	1-2:30	Exercise
	2-3	Support Group/ Relaxation Management	2:30-3:30	Choices: The Key is You (support group)
	3-4	COPD Training Review	3:30-4	Review Exercise Schedule

Weeks 5 and 6 consist of exercise three days per week.

Monday	Wednesday	Friday
Date:	Date:	Date:
Week 5 12:30-1:45	12:30-1:45	12:30-1:45
Date:	Date:	Date:
Week 6 12:30-1:45	12:30-1:45	12:30-1:45

Physical Therapy Follow-Up

Support/Educational Group: Last Wednesday of every month 2:00-3:30 P.M.

Family and Significant Other Support Group: 3rd Monday of every month 3:00-4:00 P.M.

Figure 8.2   Sample outpatient pulmonary rehabilitation program schedule.

Reprinted courtesy of the Pulmonary Rehabilitation Program at Mt. Diablo Medical Center, Concord, CA.

Documentation must
reflect the need for
professional supervi-
sion of the treatment
and the high level of
skilled care required to
perform it.

patient progress, demonstrate outcomes, and provide CQI. Documentation is also a
necessary precursor for reimbursement. It must reflect the need for professional supervision of the treatment and the high level of skilled care required to perform it. The
medical necessity of the patient's treatment must be reflected in the team's documentation.[5]

Documentation for pulmonary rehabilitation should include

▌ physician's orders for the prescribed treatment program;

▌ patient assessment and delineation of patient goals, target areas, and outcomes;

▌ progress notes of patient's response toward attainable goals;

▌ team conferences at regular intervals;

▌ recommendations for a home program plan for collaborative self-management;

▌ discharge summary; and

▌ postprogram evaluation.

A patient's chart is a convenient way to organize documentation. Specific forms
should adhere to the requirements of the medical records department in your institution. The staff's documentation should convey the patient's response to the treatment
given. The format for charting may vary, but it should always refer to the specific
problem or target area being treated. One form of documentation may be accomplished
by using a narrative commentary, or SOAP charting (subjective, objective, assessment data, and plan).[19] See figure 8.3 for an explanation and example of SOAP charting. Other documentation forms and format may include

The format for charting
may vary, but it should
always refer to the
specific problem or
target area being
treated.

▌ flow sheets,

▌ individualized progress notes,

▌ periodic progress updates,

▌ team conference documentation, and

▌ discharge summaries.

The discharge summary may include

▌ recommendations in self-care maintenance and symptom management techniques,

▌ a home exercise program that addresses progression and guidelines for change,
and

▌ a medication record and treatment program to reinforce the physician's orders
and copies of diagnostic studies performed.

REIMBURSEMENT

Billing and documentation requirements of third-party payers must be followed carefully to ensure appropriate reimbursement for services rendered.[20] Program directors
and staff should be familiar with current Health Care Financing Administration (HCFA)
guidelines and the Medicare intermediaries' policies pertaining to pulmonary rehabilitation,[21] as these guidelines and policies are often used as a basis for reimbursement
by other third-party payers. It is important to know that Medicare does not cover some
services such as health promotion; maintenance care; documentation time; duplica-

---

(S) Subjective data documents the patient's verbalized feelings or complaints.

"I am using my yellow inhaler whenever I need it, at least eight times a day. I put it in my mouth and then do two squirts, and most of the time I cough."

(O) Objective data documents measurable responses and observations of the rehabilitation staff.

Patient was observed using the yellow inhaler (bronchodilator) with the following errors: 1. Placed inhaler in his mouth, which initiates an immediate cough response. 2. Squirted two puffs at a time. 3. Unable to coordinate inhalation with the actuation of the inhaler. 4. Did not hold breath after medication was inhaled.

(A) Assessment data documents results of the intervention as determined by the provider.

Improper inhaler use; patient was never instructed prior to program.

(P) Plan documents the next steps in the rehabilitation intervention based on patient performance as documented in the assessment data.

1. Patient to be trained in correct inhaler use with a holding chamber.

2. Reassess patient technique to verify correct use of inhaler with holding chamber.

Figure 8.3 SOAP charting.

tion of services with an occupational therapist, physical therapist, registered nurse, or respiratory therapist; films or videos; treatment not medically necessary; and so on. Differences exist throughout the United States in how reimbursement guidelines are applied by various intermediaries and third-party payers. The reimbursement arena is constantly changing in the current environment of managed care. The pulmonary rehabilitation coordinator/director must be familiar with the process of obtaining prior authorization for the pulmonary rehabilitation program by the insurance companies as coverage varies depending on the patient's policy. They must also become involved with the managed-care contracting department to ensure that pulmonary rehabilitation is included during negotiations. Networking with other program directors is critical in providing the awareness, knowledge, and support needed to obtain appropriate reimbursement.

> The reimbursement arena is constantly changing in the current environment of managed care.

It is also recommended that the program have a close liaison with its facility's business office to ensure that billing information is complete and accurate and that if problems with reimbursement occur, they are addressed promptly and effectively. A representative from the business office should be a member of the interdisciplinary team. A close working relationship with the medical records department is also helpful to ensure that complete records are kept and made available for third-party payer audit or other review, if requested.

MARKETING

Program success depends upon consumer awareness, which is accomplished through developing a marketing strategy. Marketing is not just advertising, it is an organized and structured process that determines who the customer is (patients, patients' significant others, physicians) and what the customer needs (a comprehensive pulmonary rehabilitation program). From this information a marketing plan is created and put into action to ensure the success of the program. Numerous texts have included chapters on marketing strategies and plans.[22, 23] The marketing plan involves assessing and auditing the external environment; looking at the internal system for providing the product; defining the product; pricing the product; and finally, planning for promotion

> Program success depends upon consumer awareness.

of the product. Implementation is the final phase of the plan. Marketing plans often fail because homework is not done in researching the following:

▮ Is there a need for the program in this market area?

▮ What are the consumer needs relative to this program?

▮ Will the physicians support the program with referrals?

▮ Can the program provide what the consumer needs?

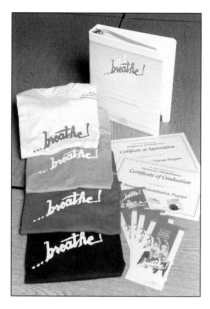

The most critical marketing expert in pulmonary rehabilitation is the interdisciplinary team member who interfaces with the patient and program graduates. This individual's participation in community activities provides marketing opportunities for pulmonary rehabilitation that include newspaper; television and radio interviews; wellness fairs; and speaking engagements to groups such as senior citizens, Elks, Kiwanis, and Chambers of Commerce. These activities contribute to successful marketing and enhance the public's awareness of pulmonary rehabilitation.

An example of a national marketing idea that may be used by local programs is the utilization of National Pulmonary Rehabilitation Week, which occurs the first week of spring. Figure 8.4 is an example of a proclamation that may be used to promote community awareness of lung disease and rehabilitation. This proclamation is often signed by the mayor or the governor. The AACVPR has marketing packets available at the national office to assist programs in recognizing this week. The pulmonary rehabilitation program must be viewed and marketed from a global perspective, remembering that prevention is integrated into every component of the program.

CONCLUSION

A successful pulmonary rehabilitation program results from effective management techniques and program structure; a supportive and actively participating medical director; and a dedicated, knowledgeable, and enthusiastic interdisciplinary team. A motivated and inspiring program coordinator/director and good leadership and team-building techniques enhance the success of the program.

Location, program schedule, and equipment may vary as dictated by the needs of the patients, the significant others, the community, and the facility. Thorough documentation assists communication among team members as the patient proceeds through

---

Whereas, lung disease constitutes a critical, social, and economic health problem in the United States; and

Whereas, pulmonary rehabilitation is a vital component of comprehensive quality care of the lung patient, but both the public and medical communities are generally unaware of its physical, emotional, and economic benefits; and

Whereas, the incidence of lung disease can be reduced through earlier detection, treatment, prevention, and rehabilitation; and

Whereas, the establishment of a special week each year to promote lung disease awareness, prevention, and rehabilitation will greatly assist in decreasing its incidence;

Now, therefore, I, _____ , do hereby proclaim the first week of spring as Pulmonary Rehabilitation Week in our community and urge all citizens to generously support this most worthy effort.

Figure 8.4   Proclamation for National Pulmonary Rehabilitation Week.

Reprinted, by permission, from G.L. Connors, S. Schnell-Hobbs, and W. Syvertsen, 1993, Marketing the pulmonary rehabilitation program. In *Pulmonary rehabilitation: Guidelines to success,* 2ed., edited by J.E. Hodgkin, G.L. Connors, and C.W. Bell. Copyright 1993 by J.B. Lippincott.

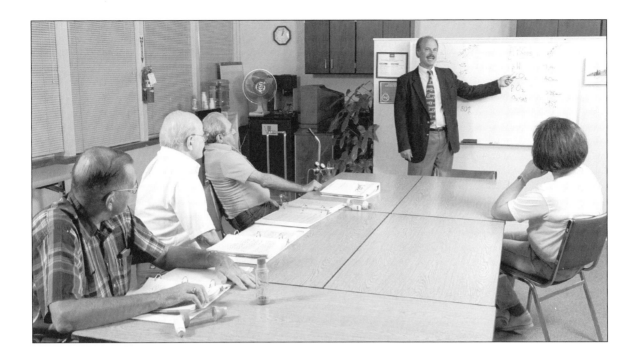

the rehabilitation program. Documentation is also necessary to demonstrate outcomes and it is essential for ensuring appropriate reimbursement.

Marketing the program is essential from the beginning. Market planning assists in designing a program by providing analysis of the customers and their needs and the community within which the program will exist. A strategic marketing plan also enhances operations and assists in making plans for future expansions.

The program location, structure, documentation, reimbursement, marketing, and all of the essential components of pulmonary rehabilitation are only as successful as the people who put them into operation. Successful pulmonary rehabilitation programs result from the development of a team of specialized individuals who come together with the common goals of enhancing the lives of this unique and challenging group of patients with pulmonary diseases.

Successful pulmonary rehabilitation programs result from the development of a team of specialized individuals who come together with the common goals of enhancing the lives of this unique and challenging group of patients with pulmonary diseases.

REFERENCES

1. American Thoracic Society. 1995. Standards for the diagnosis and care of patients with chronic obstructive pulmonary disease. *Am J Respir Crit Care Med* 152:S77-120.

2. Beytas, L.J., and G.L. Connors. 1993. Organization and management of a pulmonary rehabilitation program. In *Pulmonary rehabilitation: Guidelines to success.* 2d ed. Edited by J.E. Hodgkin, G.L. Connors, and C.W. Bell, 32-49. Philadelphia: Lippincott.

3. Ries, A.L. 1990. Position paper of the American Association of Cardiovascular and Pulmonary Rehabilitation: Scientific basis of pulmonary rehabilitation. *J Cardiopulm Rehabil* 10:418-41.

4. Hodgkin, J.E. 1986. Organization of a pulmonary rehabilitation program. *Clin Chest Med* 7 (4): 541-49.

5. Tiep, B.L. 1993. Pulmonary rehabilitation program organization. In *Principles and practice of pulmonary rehabilitation,* edited by R. Casaburi and T.L. Petty, 302-16. Philadelphia: W.B. Saunders.

6. Corsello, P.R. 1991. Rehabilitation of the chronic obstructive pulmonary disease patient: General principles. *Pulmonary therapy and rehabilitation: Principles and practice.* 2d ed. Edited by F. Haas and K. Axen, 196-212. Baltimore: Williams & Wilkins.

7. Joint Commission for Accreditation of Hospital Organizations. 1996. *Accreditation manual for hospitals.* Chicago: Author.

8. Haas, F., and A. Haas. 1991. History of pulmonary rehabilitation, or, the more things change, the more they remain the same. *Pulmonary therapy and rehabilitation: Principles and practice.* 2d ed. Edited by F. Haas and K. Axen, 179-94. Baltimore: Williams & Wilkins.

9. Hall, L. 1996. On the road toward managed health and wellness. *J Respir Care Prac* (February/March): 16-18.

10. Williams, W. 1996. Equipment review data management choices. *Adv/Respir* (March): 53-64.

11. Horowitz, A.C. 1996. Legal issues in respiratory care. *Adv/Respir* (March): 43-44.

12. Bezold, C. 1992. Five futures. *Healthcare Forum J* (May/June): 101-16.

13. Make, B. 1994. Collaborative self-management strategies for patients with respiratory disease. *Respir Care* 39 (5):5 66-83.

14. Brown, C. July 1995. HCFA releases cost data report on Medicare payments. *AARC Times*, 6.

15. Connors, G.L. 1994. Keys to the payors' vault. *Respir Ther* 7 (2): 41-46.

16. Kravetz, H.M. 1993. How the office-based pulmonary rehabilitation program works. *Principles and practice of pulmonary rehabilitation*, Edited by R. Casaburi and T.L. Petty, 483-86. Philadelphia: W.B. Saunders.

17. Sutton, F.D. 1993. The proprietary pulmonary rehabilitation program. *Principles and practice of pulmonary rehabilitation,* edited by R. Casaburi and T.L. Petty, 478-82. Philadelphia: W.B. Saunders.

18. Bickford, L.S., J.E. Hodgkin, and S.L. MacIntruff. 1995. National pulmonary rehabilitation survey, update. *J Cardiopulm Rehabil* 15:406-11.

19. Fink, J.B., and A.K. Fink. 1986. *The respiratory therapist as manager.* Chicago: Year Book Medical.

20. Elkousy, N.M. et al. 1988. Outpatient pulmonary rehabilitation: A Medicare fiscal intermediary's viewpoint. *J Cardiopulm Rehab* 8 (11): 492-97.

21. Connors, G.L., L. Hilling, S. Grindal, and W.K. Wilkinson. 1993. A determinant of program survival. In *Pulmonary rehabilitation: Guidelines to success.* 2d ed. Edited by J.E. Hodgkin, G.L. Connors, and C.W. Bell, 562-86. Philadelphia: Lippincott.

22. Kotler, P., and R.N. Clark. 1987. *Marketing for health care organizations.* Englewood Cliffs, N.J.: Prentice Hall.

23. Kotler, P., and A.R. Andreasen. 1987. *Strategic marketing for non-profit organizations.* 3d ed. Englewood Cliffs, N.J.: Prentice Hall.

Pulmonary Rehabilitation: Joint ACCP/AACVPR Evidence-Based Guidelines*

ACCP/AACVPR Pulmonary Rehabilitation Guidelines Panel*

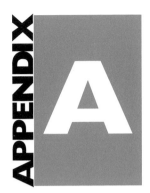

Key words: chronic obstructive pulmonary disease, dyspnea, exercise training, guidelines, health-care utilization, psychosocial, pulmonary rehabilitation, quality of life, survival, ventilatory muscle training.

Abbreviations: AACVPR = American Association of Cardiovascular and Pulmonary Rehabilitation; ACCP = American College of Chest Physicians; ADLs = activities of daily living; BDI = baseline dyspnea index; CRQ = chronic respiratory disease questionnaire; HR = heart rate; IPPB = intermittent positive pressure breathing; MRC = Medical Research Council; NIH = National Institutes of Health; OCD = oxygen cost diagram; PFSDQ = pulmonary functional status and dyspnea questionnaire; PImax = maximal Inspiratory pressure; QOL = quality of life; QWB = quality of well-being scale; SGRQ = St. George's Respiratory Questionnaire; SOBQ = University of California, San Diego Shortness of Breath Questionnaire; TDI = transitional dyspnea index; VAS = visual analog scale; VE = minute ventilation; VMT = ventilatory muscle training; VO_2 = oxygen consumption.

Chronic pulmonary diseases have become increasingly important causes of morbidity and mortality in the modern world. The COPDs are the most common chronic lung diseases and the major impetus for the development of pulmonary rehabilitation programs over the past half century. The purpose of this document is to review the current "state of the evidence" for the scientific basis of pulmonary rehabilitation as a foundation on which to make recommendations for practice.

EPIDEMIOLOGY OF COPD

In the United States, the overall prevalence of COPD in adult white populations is 4 to 6% in men and 1 to 3% in women. In persons older than 55 years, COPD is recognized in approximately 10 to 15%.[1,2] As of 1985, the prevalence rates of COPD in adults 65 years and older was 167/1,000 in men and 126/1,000 in women.[3] Recent trends suggest that disease prevalence is stable to decreasing in men, but increasing among women. The 1993 National Health Interview Survey estimated that 14 million adults had chronic bronchitis and 2 million had emphysema.[4]

As of 1990, COPD became the fourth leading cause of death in the United States.[5,6] In 1991, there were 85,544 deaths due to COPD.[5] In 1993, the age-adjusted death rate was 21.4/100,000, representing a 46.6% increase from 1979.[6] In the age group 55 to 74 years, COPD ranked third in men and fourth in women as a cause of death.

*Andrew L. Ries, MD, MPH, FCCP (Chair); Brian W. Carlin, MD, FCCP (AACVPR Representative); Virginia Carrieri-Kohlman, RN, DNSc (AACVPR Representative); Richard Casaburi, PhD, MD, FCCP (ACCP Representative); Bartolome R. Celli, MD, FCCP (ACCP Representative); Charles F. Emery, PhD (AACVPR Representative); John E. Hodgkin, MD, FCCP (AACVPR Representative); Donald A. Mahler, MD, FCCP (ACCP Representative); Barry Make, MD, FCCP (ACCP Representative); and Judah Skolnick, MD, FCCP (Liaison from ACCP Health and Science Policy Committee).

Reprint requests: Andrew L. Ries, MD, MPH, UCSD Rehabilitation Program, 269 Washington Street (West), San Diego, CA 92103-8377.

Reprinted, by permission, from A.L. Ries, et. al., 1997, "Pulmonary rehabilitation: Joint ACCP/AACVPR evidence-based guidelines," *CHEST* 112.

The impact of COPD on morbidity is even greater than on mortality. In the 1985 National Health Interview Survey, COPD accounted for 5% of office visits to physicians and >13% of hospitalizations.[2] COPD is an enormous cause of disability among affected individuals. Morbidity and mortality from COPD continue to increase despite reduced cigarette smoking rates due to the long latency period before clinical disease. Lower smoking rates, ultimately, will reduce the burden of COPD, but not for many years. With increased life expectancy and lower mortality from other diseases, the impact of COPD will be magnified in our aging population.

PULMONARY REHABILITATION

Background

Rehabilitation for patients with chronic lung diseases is well established and widely accepted as a means of enhancing standard therapy in order to alleviate symptoms and optimize function.[7-13] The primary goal of rehabilitation is to restore the patient to the highest possible level of independent function. This goal is accomplished by helping patients to increase their activity through exercise training and to reduce and gain control of their symptoms. Patients and significant others learn more about their disease, treatment options, and coping strategies. Patients are encouraged to become actively involved in providing their own health care, more independent in daily activities, and less dependent on health professionals and expensive medical resources. Rather than focusing solely on reversing the disease process, rehabilitation attempts to improve disability from disease.

Historically, pulmonary rehabilitation has been used primarily for patients with COPD. However, it has also been applied successfully to patients with other chronic lung conditions such as interstitial diseases, cystic fibrosis, bronchiectasis, thoracic cage abnormalities, and neuromuscular disorders as well as part of the evaluation, preparation for, and recovery from surgical interventions such as lung transplantation and lung volume reduction surgery.[12] Pulmonary rehabilitation is appropriate for any patient with stable disease of the respiratory system and disabling symptoms. Even patients with severe disease can benefit if they are selected appropriately and if realistic goals are set.

DEFINITIONS

In 1974, the American College of Chest Physicians (ACCP) Committee on Pulmonary Rehabilitation adopted the following definition quoted in an ATS statement:

"Pulmonary rehabilitation may be defined as an art of medical practice wherein an individually tailored, multidisciplinary program is formulated which through accurate diagnosis, therapy, emotional support, and education, stabilizes or reverses both the physio- and psychopathology of pulmonary diseases and attempts to return the patient to the highest possible functional capacity allowed by his pulmonary handicap and overall life situation."[13]

This definition focuses on three important features of successful rehabilitation:

Individual

Patients with disabling lung disease require individual assessment of needs, individual attention, and a program designed to meet realistic individual goals (mutually developed by both the patient and the health-care professionals).

Multidisciplinary

Pulmonary rehabilitation integrates expertise from various health-care disciplines integrated into a comprehensive, cohesive program tailored to the needs of each patient.

Attention to Physiopathology and Psychopathology

To be successful, pulmonary rehabilitation addresses psychological as well as pathophysiologic problems.

A newer definition was developed by a National Institutes of Health (NIH) Workshop on Pulmonary Rehabilitation Research that reviewed the scientific evidence and future research opportunities. It emphasizes key aspects as the multidimensional activities, continuum of services that may be applied in different sites, interdisciplinary team, involvement of patients and families, and individual goals for independence and function in the community.

"Pulmonary rehabilitation is a multidimensional continuum of services directed to persons with pulmonary disease and their families, usually by an interdisciplinary team of specialists, with the goal of achieving and maintaining the individual's maximum level of independence and functioning in the community."[14]

The interdisciplinary team of health-care professionals in pulmonary rehabilitation may include physicians, nurses, respiratory, physical, and occupational therapists, psychologists, exercise specialists, dieticians, and others with appropriate expertise.

Method for the Guidelines Panel

The Guidelines Panel was organized under the joint sponsorship of the ACCP and the American Association of Cardiovascular and Pulmonary Rehabilitation (AACVPR). In addition to the Chair (Dr. Ries), each organization appointed four representatives: Drs. Casaburi, Celli, Mahler, and Make represented the ACCP; Drs. Carlin, Carrieri-Kohlman, Emery, and Hodgkin represented the AACVPR. Dr. Judah Skolnick served as the Liaison from the ACCP Health and Science Policy Committee.

The primary purpose of this document is to review the scientific basis for pulmonary rehabilitation. The review focuses on adults with COPD in whom most of the research in this area has been conducted. The panel recognized that pulmonary rehabilitation may also be applied to patients with other lung diseases and significant outcomes have been demonstrated in such diseases.

The document is organized by topics including both therapeutic components and important health outcomes of pulmonary rehabilitation. Component topics include lower extremity training, upper extremity training, ventilatory muscle training (VMT), and psychosocial/behavioral interventions. Health outcome topics include psychosocial/behavioral

measures, dyspnea, quality of life (QOL), health-care utilization, and survival. For the component topics, the panel reviewed studies addressing the rationale for including these modalities in comprehensive rehabilitation programs. For the outcome topics, the panel focused on studies in which pulmonary rehabilitation was used as the intervention. For these purposes, pulmonary rehabilitation was considered to include individual patient assessment and multimodality treatment.

Although education is an important component included in comprehensive pulmonary rehabilitation programs, this topic was not reviewed separately. Education is generally considered to be a necessary, but not sufficient, part of pulmonary rehabilitation. The Panel agreed with this assessment, but could not identify a sufficient number of studies focused solely on education independent of other interventions. Discussion of relevant articles on education in chronic lung disease is included in the section on psychosocial interventions.

In selecting articles to be reviewed in this document, the Panel relied on several sources: (1) computer searches of National Library of Medicine databases; (2) bibliographies from recently published studies and review articles; and (3) input solicited from experts in pulmonary rehabilitation. All relevant studies were reviewed; however, only selected ones were included in the evidence tables. The criteria used in selecting articles are highlighted in each section.

In presenting results of the review, the Panel used a standard format incorporating evidence tables. For each section, two members of the Panel assumed primary responsibility for reviewing the scientific literature and identifying appropriate studies and articles to be included. Articles selected represented original scientific work. Abstracts, review articles, expert opinions, and position papers were used as source documents but were not included in the formal review.

In preparing and evaluating recommendations, the Panel assigned a letter grade designating the overall strength of the scientific evidence for each recommendation.[15] Ratings reflect both the quality of the studies, including study design and methods used, and the consistency of the results of the scientific evidence. The following rating scale was used: A—scientific evidence provided by well-designed, well-conducted, controlled trials (randomized and nonrandomized) with statistically significant results that consistently support the guideline recommendation; B—scientific evidence provided by observational studies or by controlled trials with less consistent results to support the guideline recommendation; and C—expert opinion that supports the guideline recommendation because the available scientific evidence did not present consistent results or because controlled trials were lacking.

Table 1 summarizes the recommendations and evidence grades in this document.

LOWER EXTREMITY TRAINING

Introduction

Exercise programs for the muscles of ambulation are a part of virtually every program of pulmonary rehabilitation. A large body of literature supports the effectiveness of these programs[8,16-22] and supports the following conclusions:

1. Measures of lung function do not improve as a result of exercise programs for the lower extremities.

2. Patients indicate that their functional capabilities for ambulation improve as a result of these exercise programs.

3. The tolerance of a given submaximal task involving the muscles of ambulation generally improves.

Recommendation

Patients with COPD who undergo a program of lower extremity exercise training consistently improve measures of exercise tolerance without evi-

Table 1.	Summary of Recommendations and Evidence Grades for Pulmonary Rehabilitation Guidelines for Patients With COPD	
Component/Outcome	**Recommendations**	**Grade**
Lower extremity training	Lower extremity training improves exercise tolerance and is recommended as part of pulmonary rehabilitation	A
Upper extremity training	Strength and endurance training improves arm function; arm exercises should be included in pulmonary rehabilitation	B
Ventilatory muscle training	Scientific evidence does not support the routine use of VMT in pulmonary rehabilitation; it may be considered in selected patients with decreased respiratory muscle strength and breathlessness	B
Psychosocial, behavioral, and educational components and outcomes	Evidence does not support the benefits of short-term psychosocial interventions as single therapeutic modalities; longer-term interventions may be beneficial; expert opinion supports inclusion of educational and psychosocial intervention components in pulmonary rehabilitation	C
Dyspnea	Pulmonary rehabilitation improves the symptom of dyspnea	A
Quality of life	Pulmonary rehabilitation improves health-related QOL	B
Health-care utilization	Pulmonary rehabilitation has reduced the number of hospitalizations and days of hospitalization	B
Survival	Pulmonary rehabilitation may improve survival	C

dence of adverse outcome. A program of exercise training of the muscles of ambulation is recommended as a part of pulmonary rehabilitation for patients with COPD.

Strength of Evidence = A

Scientific Evidence.   Many patients with COPD entering a rehabilitation program are deconditioned.[23] Physiologic improvements in muscle function are desirable and achievable goals in most patients with COPD. However, improvements in motivation and exercise technique are also likely results of most exercise programs; these nonphysiologic benefits are worthwhile and highly desirable.

A recent comprehensive review examined the literature published in this area through 1991;[16] other recent reviews have appeared.[17-22] The current review focuses on the results of 14 randomized controlled trials that have appeared in the peer-reviewed literature; eight of these studies have been published since 1991. However, it must be acknowledged that such trials cannot be blinded. Effort-dependent out-

come measures in such studies may be influenced by the motivation of the participants. Therefore, as a second focus, uncontrolled trials of exercise training in patients with COPD whose outcome measures are unequivocally effort independent are also examined.

Controlled Trials: Table 2 presents the features of published controlled trials of lower extremity exercise training.[24-37] This has been an international effort, with six countries being represented among the 14 trials. Sample size averages 40 (range, 13 to 119). Most participants have been men, though recent studies have tended to include more women. The average age of the patients in almost all studies is 60 to 70 years. The average FEV_1 of the participants is reported in all studies and can be used as an index of disease severity. In all but three studies, average FEV_1 is in the range of 0.8 to 1.2 L or 33 to 39% predicted, indicating severe airflow limitation. In the other three studies,[24,26,35] disease severity was more moderate.

Most studies administered exercise programs predominantly in an outpatient, supervised setting.

Table 2.   Controlled Trials of Lower Extremity Exercise Training Programs

Source/Country	Patients	Intervention/Follow-up	Outcome
Randomized controlled trials			
Chester et al[24] (1977) United States	Sample size: 29 (21 intervention, 8 control) Gender: 100% male Age: mean, 51 yr (intervention group) FEV_1: mean, 1.27 L	Intervention: 4-wk inpatient daily treadmill and other exercise modalities; 15 min on treadmill; intensity: mean HR, 125 ± 8 beats/min. Follow-up: 4 wk	Intervention group: In treadmill testing, decreased $\dot{V}E$ and $\dot{V}O_2$ at a given exercise level, but not in cycle ergometer testing; no changes in hemodynamics; increase in total work performed in incremental treadmill protocol. Control group: no significant changes
McCavin et al[25] (1977) Great Britain	Sample size: 24 (12 intervention, 12 control) Gender: 100 % male Age: mean, 59 yr (range, 40-69 yr) FEV_1: mean, 1.06 L	Intervention: 3-mo unmonitored home stair climbing exercise program; up to10 min at least once daily for at least 5 d/wk; intensity: increased as tolerated. Follow-up: 3 mo	Intervention group: 6% increase in 12-min walk distance; in incremental cycle ergometer test, 23% increase in peak work rate, but no significant change in peak $\dot{V}O_2$: no significant change in $\dot{V}E$ or HR at submaximal work rate Control group: no significant improvements

(continued)

Table 2. *(continued)*

Source/Country	Patients	Intervention/Follow-up	Outcome
Cockcroft et al[26] (1981) Great Britain	Sample size: 34 (18 intervention, 16 control) Gender: 100% male Age: mean, 61 yr FEV_1: mean, 1.43 L	Intervention, 6 wk in rehabilitation center, followed by unsupervised home exercise for 6 mo; cycle ergometer, walking, and other modalities exercise; daily exercise, duration and intensity unspecified Follow-up: 8 mo	Intervention group: at 6 wk, 12-min walk distance increased 33%; in progressive treadmill test, no significant increase in peak $\dot{V}O_2$; no change in submaximal $\dot{V}E$ or HR Control group: no significant improvements
Busch and McClements[27] (1988) Canada	Sample size: 14 (7 intervention, 7 control) Gender: 79% male Age: mean, 65 yr FEV_1: mean, 0.81 L (26% pred)	Intervention: 18-wk home, unsupervised exercise with walking or stair-stepping program; mean duration 5 min at least 5 d/wk; Intensity: symptom-limited Follow-up: 18 wk	Intervention group: no significant change in peak work rate in incremental cycle ergometer protocol; no significant change in multistage stepping test Control group: significant decrease in cycle ergometer endurance
Lake et al[28] (1990) Australia	Sample size: 13 (6 lower extremity intervention, 7 control) Gender: 92% male Age: mean, 59 yr FEV_1: mean, 0.86 L (32% pred)	Intervention: 8-wk supervised outpatient walking exercise program, 3 sessions per week, 20 min per session; Intensity: unspecified Follow-up: 8 wk	Intervention group: average 122-m increase in 6-min walk distance; no significant change in peak work rate or $\dot{V}O_2$ in incremental cycle ergometer test Control group: no significant changes
Weiner et al[29] (1992) Israel	Sample size: 24 (12 intervention, 12 control) Gender: 50% male Age: mean, 63 yr (range, 45-80 yr) FEV_1: mean, 36% pred	Intervention: 6-mo supervised outpatient cycle ergometer exercise program, 3 times per week, 20 min per session, intensity advanced to 50% of peak work rate Follow-up: 6-mo	Intervention group: no change in 12-min walk distance; 102% increase in endurance time in constant work rate cycle ergometer test Control group: no significant changes
Reardon et al[30] (1994) United States	Sample size: 20 (10 rehabilitation intervention, 10 control) Gender: 50% male Age: mean, 66 yr (range, 52-75 yr) FEV_1: mean, 0.87 L	Intervention: 6-wk outpatient comprehensive rehabilitation program (12 3-h sessions with education and lower/upper extremity plus inspiratory resistive exercise) vs control; stair climbing, treadmill, cycle exercise three times per week; intensity: moderate	Intervention group: in incremental treadmill protocol, 40% increase in duration but no change in peak $\dot{V}O_2$ or other physiologic variables: dyspnea ratings decreased Control group: no significant changes

(continued)

Source/Country	Patients	Intervention/Follow-up	Outcome
Reardon et al[30] *(continued)*		dyspnea or HR 70-85% maximum Follow-up: 6 wk	
Goldstein et al[31] (1994) Canada	Sample size: 89 (45 intervention, 44 control) Gender: 49% male Age: mean, 66 yr FEV$_1$: mean 35% pred	Intervention: 8-wk inpatient multidisciplinary rehabilitation program (upper and lower extremity exercise, education) + 16 wk supervised outpatient program vs conventional community care control; treadmill exercise, 20 min per session three times per week; intensity increased as tolerated Follow-up: 24 wk	Significant difference in improvement between intervention and control group in 6-min walking distance (approximately 10%) and tolerance of a submaximal cycle ergometer work rate Control group: 9% decrease in peak work rate, decrease in peak $\dot{V}O_2$
Wijkstra et al[32] (1994) The Netherlands	Sample size: 43 (28 rehabilitation intervention, 15 control) Gender: 86% male Age: mean, 63 yr FEV$_1$: mean, 1.33 L (44% pred)	Intervention: 12-wk outpatient rehabilitation program (24 sessions with cycle, upper extremity and inspiratory muscle exercise) with monthly nurse and physician visits vs control; exercise intensity: up to 76% of initial peak work rate Follow-up: 12 wk	Intervention group: in incremental cycle ergometer test, 10% increase in peak work rate, significant increase in peak $\dot{V}O_2$ Control group: 9% decrease in peak work rate, decrease in peak $\dot{V}O_2$
Ries et al[33] (1995) United States	Sample size: 119 (57 rehabilitation intervention, 62 education control) Gender: 73% male Age: mean, 63 yr FEV$_1$: mean, 1.23 L	Intervention: 8-wk outpatient comprehensive rehabilitation program (12 4-h sessions with treadmill/walking exercise, education and psychosocial support) + monthly visits for 1 yr vs education control program (four 2-h sessions); Intensity: highest tolerated symptom-limited level Follow-up: 6 yr	Intervention group: at 8 wk, in incremental treadmill test, 9% increase in peak $\dot{V}O_2$, 33% increase in maximum treadmill workload, endurance treadmill test 85% increase in duration; breathlessness ratings decreased Control group: no significant changes
Strijbos et al[34] (1996) The Netherlands	Sample size, 45 (15 outpatient rehabilitation, 15 home rehabilitation, 15 control) Gender: 84% male Age: mean, 61 yr FEV$_1$ mean,	Intervention: 12-wk outpatient rehabilitation (24 1-h exercise sessions + three nurse education and three physician visits) vs home rehabilitation (24 1-h exercise sessions + three nurse and three physician visits) vs control, walking, stair climbing and cycle	Intervention group: in both rehabilitation groups, improvements in 4-min walk distance and peak work rate in incremental cycle ergometer test and decreases in dyspnea score; however, at 18-mo follow-up, gains better maintained in home exercise group *(continued)*

Table 2. *(continued)*

Source/Country	Patients	Intervention/Follow-up	Outcome
Strijbos et al[34] *(continued)*	1.23 L (43% pred)	exercise; intensity: unspecified Follow-up: 18 mo	Control group: no significant changes
Berry et al[35] (1996) United States	Sample size: 17 (9 intervention, 8 control) Gender: 71% male Age: mean, 71 yr FEV_1: mean, 1.47 L (46% pred)	Intervention: 12-wk supervised outpatient walking exercise program, three times per week, 20 min per session; Intensity 50-75% of HR reserve Follow-up: 12 wk	Intervention group: significant increase in 12-min walk distance; in incremental treadmill testing, no significant increase in treadmill time, and no significant changes in Borg dyspnea ratings Control group: no significant changes
Nonrandomized controlled trials			
Sinclair and Ingram[36] (1980) Great Britain	Sample size: 33 (17 intervention [in city], 16 control [outside city]) Gender: NA* Age: mean, 65 yr (range, 46-83 yr) FEV_1: mean, 1.06 L	Intervention outpatient daily home exercise program supervised weekly, 12-min plus stair climbing; average duration 14 min; intensity according to individual ability Follow-up mean, 11 mo	Intervention group: 22% increase in 12-min walk distance, increased stride length Control group: no significant changes
O'Donnell et al[37] (1995) United States	Sample size 60 (30 intervention, 30 control self-selected) Gender: 72% male Age: mean, 68 yr FEV_1: mean, 0.96 L (38% pred)	Intervention: 6-wk outpatient exercise program (18 2.5-h sessions with multimodality upper and lower extremity training with some education) vs control group that chose to defer exercise training; intensity "high-intensity" perceived exertion (Borg scale) Follow-up: mean, 6 wk	Intervention group: 18% increase in 6-min walk distance; in incremental cycle ergometer test, 33% in peak work rate but no significant increase in peak $\dot{V}O_2$; at standardized work rate, 10% decrease in $\dot{V}E$; decrease in breathlessness ratings Control group: no significant changes

*NA = not available. This abbreviation applies for all tables.

Three studies examined the effectiveness of unsupervised home exercise programs; two of these programs were conducted in an inpatient rehabilitation center.[24,31] Another study compared the effectiveness of a supervised outpatient and home exercise program.[34] A variety of lower extremity exercise modalities were employed in these studies: the predominant exercise was walking in three studies, treadmill in two studies, stationary bicycle in two studies, stair climbing in one study, and a combination of modalities in five studies.

The studies varied considerably in the standard parameters of the training prescription: duration, frequency, and intensity. The duration of the exercise programs ranged from 4 weeks to 46 weeks, with the majority of 6 to 8 weeks (five studies) or 12 to 24 weeks (six studies). Session frequency was most commonly three per week (five studies); "daily" sessions, conducted in four studies, were usually in the context of unsupervised programs conducted at home. Duration of exercise sessions was poorly described in some programs. It is of concern that in five studies, daily duration of the predominant exercise mode was <15 min and in three others the duration was 20 min since studies in healthy subjects have shown that these durations are likely too short to elicit a substantial training effect in the exercising muscles.[38,39] Also, most studies failed to describe the intensity of training objectively. In six studies, intensity targets were either unspecified or denoted non-specifically (eg, "advanced as tolerated"). In three studies, intensity was set primarily on perceived breathlessness ratings. In three additional studies, work rate targets were set as fixed fractions (50%, 70%, and 75%) of the peak work rate tolerated in a preprogram incremental exercise test. In healthy subjects, there is posited to be a "critical training intensity" below which a training program will not elicit physiologic effects;[38,40] this is likely to be true in patients with COPD though quantitative differences are probable. The work rate targets in the published pulmonary rehabilitation studies may be suboptimal. Ries and Archibald[41] have posited that exercise intensities near maximal levels are well tolerated in this patient group.

Outcome measures in these studies included timed walking tests, incremental treadmill and stationary bicycle protocols, and constant work rate treadmill and cycle studies. Of the nine studies that employed timed walking tests, all but one reported significant increases. However, as mentioned above, the results of these tests are substantially effort and practice dependent. Although it has been recommended that timed walking tests be repeated up to three times at baseline to achieve reproducible results,[42] none of these eight studies followed this procedure. In the five studies utilizing incremental treadmill protocols, only one[33] reported an increased peak oxygen consumption ($\dot{V}O_2$). In the six studies utilizing incremental cycle ergometer protocols, only one[32] reported an increased peak $\dot{V}O_2$. Seven studies reported the responses to submaximal treadmill or cycle ergometer exercise. In three of these studies, the observation was that the tolerated duration of exercise was increased; these results are difficult to interpret unequivocally as increased motivation may play a role. In four studies, changes in physiologic responses to submaximal exercise levels were observed. In two cases, no changes were detected. In one study, a proportional decrease in both $\dot{V}O_2$ and minute ventilation ($\dot{V}E$) was observed

during treadmill exercise; this was interpreted as likely a result of improved pacing strategy.[24] In the remaining study, a decrease in $\dot{V}E$ at a given cycle ergometer work rate was observed without a significant decrease in $\dot{V}O_2$.[37]

All three studies demonstrating relatively convincing evidence of a physiologic training effect[32,33,37] incorporated supervised exercise programs with high-intensity targets. However, review of these randomized trials fails to yield firm recommendations on optimal specific training regimens for patients with COPD.

Uncontrolled Trials: Although not included in the evidence table, noncontrolled studies in which outcome measures feature an effort-independent measure of a physiologic training effect were also reviewed. Several studies reported physiologic responses to identical exercise stimuli before and after training and utilized the cycle ergometer (a relatively strategy-independent mode of exercise). In eight studies (previously reviewed[16]), no significant changes in physiologic responses were detected. However, in six studies,[43-48] a fall in pulmonary ventilation and/or blood lactate level was noted, which may be a manifestation of improved aerobic function of the exercising muscles as a result of training.[49] The study of Casaburi and coworkers[47] is of special interest because patients were randomized to exercise at moderate or heavy exercise intensities (with session duration adjusted so that the total work per exercise session did not vary with group assignment). Significant decrease in lactate, $\dot{V}E$, and heart rate (HR) in response to identical exercise stimuli were seen only in the group that trained at the high exercise intensity.

Other evidence that a physiologic training effect can be achieved is available in a recent report by Maltais and coworkers[50] that the aerobic enzymes increase in concentration in muscle biopsy specimens obtained from patients with COPD as a result of a rigorous program of exercise training. This is in contrast to the earlier report by Belman and Kendregan[51] who detected no changes in muscle enzyme concentrations after a less rigorous exercise program.

Unresolved Issues in Recommending a Training Prescription in Pulmonary Rehabilitation: Although a large body of evidence supports the benefit of lower extremity training in patients with COPD, there are several unresolved issues in reviewing the literature that make it difficult to provide specific recommendations regarding exercise prescription in the context of pulmonary rehabilitation. These issues include the following.

1. The majority of literature regarding rehabilitative exercise deals with one variety of lung disease—COPD. The reader is referred to summaries of the responses to exercise programs in patients with asthma,[52] cystic fibrosis,[53] and restrictive lung diseases.[54-56] The relatively sparse literature regarding the effectiveness of non-COPD exercise programs leaves open the possibility that direct extrapolation of approaches used in COPD to these other lung disorders may not be appropriate.

2. The benefits of rehabilitative exercise programs are multifactorial and "success" will be defined by the set of benefits that are desired. In particular, exercise programs have both psychological and physiologic benefits.[16] Psychological benefits include improved motivation, the antidepressant effects of exercise, loss of fear of dyspnea, and desensitization to dyspnea.[57] Another related benefit is improved "efficiency" of movement (eg, longer stride length) that may decrease the metabolic cost of performing a given task. Physiologic benefits include structural and biochemical changes in the exercising muscles that improve the capacity of the muscle to tolerate a given rate of work. A substantial body of literature has determined the characteristics of an exercise program required to yield these "training" effects in healthy subjects.[58] Exercise mode, frequency of exercise sessions, duration of sessions, length of the exercise program, and exercise intensity are important determinants. It seems likely that the characteristics of effective training programs for patients with COPD are qualitatively similar, although quantitative differences may be present.

3. Much of the literature dealing with the effect of exercise programs on patients with COPD utilizes measures of exercise tolerance that are effort, motivation, and strategy dependent. Timed walking distances and treadmill walking protocols are such tests. Improvement in these measures can be due to the psychological effects of a training program and cannot be taken as clear evidence of a physiologic training effect.

4. Particularly in literature prior to 1990, the characteristics of rehabilitative programs were often insufficiently described to allow definition of an effective training program. In particular, studies in which exercise intensity or session durations were "increased as tolerated" are difficult to interpret.

Conclusions

There is substantial evidence that lower extremity exercise training should be included in rehabilitation programs for patients with COPD. Benefits may be both physiologic and psychological. However, the optimal specific exercise prescription guidelines for the muscles of ambulation cannot be defined with certainty at this time.

UPPER EXTREMITY TRAINING

Introduction

Patients with COPD may use some muscles of the shoulder girdle to partake in pulmonary ventilation, especially when the arms are anchored. These muscles can then provide support to pull on the ribcage.[59] In addition, arm elevation increases oxygen uptake and carbon dioxide production in these patients, and will also decrease the participation in ventilation of some of the muscles of the shoulder girdle.[60] Arm training has the potential to improve arm exercise performance by decreasing ventilatory demand during arm work, and by improving arm endurance. When the arms are braced, arm training improves the ventilatory contribution of those muscles by increasing shoulder girdle muscle strength.[61]

There is no standard way to train the arms, but two basic forms of training have received the most attention. Arm training with an arm ergometer is achieved by having patients cycle with the arms at approximately 50 rpm, initially without resistive load. The load is then typically increased at 5-W intervals until 20 to 30 min of exercise are tolerated. The response is monitored in terms of arm fatigue and dyspnea. The arms can also be trained by repetitively lifting weights up to shoulder level. The weights are increased as tolerated until 20 to 30 min of exercise are tolerated. The response is also monitored in terms of fatigue and dyspnea.

Recommendation

Strength and endurance training of the upper extremities improves arm function in patients with

COPD. Arm exercises are safe, and should be included in rehabilitation programs for patients with COPD.

Strength of Evidence = B

Scientific Evidence. The evidence supporting the benefit of upper extremity exercise is based on the results of one controlled study of patients with airflow obstruction due to cystic fibrosis[62] and five controlled trials in patients, with COPD.[28,51,63-65] One of these studies compared upper extremity training with leg exercise.[51] Two uncontrolled trials, one in patients with low cervical cord injury quadriplegia[66] and the other one in patients with COPD[67] also support the use of upper extremity exercise in the rehabilitation of patients with lung disease.

The results of all five randomized studies (Table 3) [28,51,63-65] and one observational study (Table 4) [67] in patients with COPD show that arm training is specific for the arms. Arm training also increases the capacity to perform arm work and decreases oxygen uptake for a similar amount of work. The exact reason for these changes is not clear. Possible mechanisms include desensitization to dyspnea, better coordination of the muscles partaking in arm elevation, and true metabolic adaptations.

In the study that compared arm with leg training, training of the lower extremities improved leg function, but did not improve upper extremity exercise capacity. The converse was also true: arm training did not result in improved leg performance.[51] Two controlled studies had several training groups, including arm and leg combined.[28,64] The conclusion of both studies is that arm training alone is less effective than leg training in improving overall function. In one of the studies,[28] the addition of arm training to leg training resulted in significant improvement in functional status when compared to either exercise alone.

One study compared unsupported arm exercise (arm elevation against gravity with progressive increase in weights) vs arm cranking in 45 patients with COPD. The improvement in work capacity and decreased oxygen uptake at similar work levels suggests greater benefit from unsupported exercise vs arm cranking.[65] In one other study, patients were randomized to backpacking while walking or the same regimen plus arm training using weight lifting.[63] There was a significant improvement in work

capacity and lower ventilatory requirement at the same work level in the upper extremity training group compared to simple walking. One study compared baseline O_2 uptake, CO_2 production, and $\dot{V}E$ values during arm elevation with posttraining results.[67] After unsupported arm training, metabolic and ventilatory requirements for arm elevation decreased significantly (18%).

Arm strength and endurance training may also improve respiratory muscle function. This concept is supported by two reports that did not involve patients with COPD. The first one is a study of quadriplegic patients with decreased vital capacity. Training of the pectoralis muscle against progressive loads increased vital capacity and decreased residual volume by 20%.[66] One older study of patients with airflow obstruction due to cystic fibrosis compared intense upper extremity exercise (rowing, swimming, canoeing), VMT (using isocapneic hyperventilation), and no training in control subjects. Arm training increased maximal sustained ventilatory capacity to the same degree as specific VMT.[62] The results of both studies suggest that training of the muscles of the shoulder girdle has a beneficial effect on respiratory muscle function.

Conclusions

There are beneficial effects of upper extremity exercise. They include increased exercise capacity of the arms, and decreased metabolic and ventilatory demand for similar arm work after training. Only two studies[28,64] have evaluated the effect of arm training on other outcomes, such as functional status and performance. Neither study found a significant effect of arm training when used alone. One of the studies[28] found improved functional score when combined arm and leg exercise was performed compared to either form of exercise alone. Arm cranking is the most common form of training. It is better standardized and easier to test, compared to other forms of exercise. In the only comparative study, unsupported arm training resulted in better improvement in physiologic outcomes when compared to arm cranking.[65] The exact form of training that results in the best outcomes remains unknown.

Future Research Directions: Available studies of upper extremity training in pulmonary rehabilitation are promising. This is an area that warrants further investigation. Future directions for research

Table 3. Randomized Controlled Trials of Arm Exercise Training*

Source/Country	Patients	Intervention/Follow-up	Outcome
Belman and Kendregan[51] (1981) United States	Sample size: 15 (8 arm training, 7 leg training) Gender: 73% male Age: mean, 61 yr FEV_1: mean, 1.06 L	Intervention: 6-wk each outpatient cycle ergometry exercise program, four times per week; starting at 1/3 of maximum on incremental test and increased as tolerated up to 20 min per session Follow-up: 6 wk	Improvement in exercise endurance in 9 of 15 patients; the endurance increase was specific for the limb trained; no increase in the aerobic enzymes measured in muscle by biopsy
O'Hara et al[63] (1984) United States	Sample size: 14 (7 intervention, 7 control) Gender: 79% male Age: mean, 57 yr FEV_1: mean, 1.15 L	Intervention: 6-wk home weightlifting program (wrist curls, arm curls, leg squats, calf raises, supine dumbbell press), daily exercise, weekly supervision; 10 repetitions, three sets of each exercise; initial load 4.3 ± 0.9 kg increased weekly to 10.4 ± 2.6 kg; both groups walked with a small backpack weight a few minutes each day Follow-up: 6 wk	12-min walk distance improved significantly only in the arm trainers (16%); it improved but not significantly in control subjects; ventilation at same workload during cycle ergometry decreased only in the arm trainers (18%); no improvement in arm exercise in control subjects
Ries et al[64] (1988) United States	Sample size: 28 (8 GR training, 9 PNF training, 11 control) Completed: 28 Gender: NA Age: NA FEV_1: mean, 0.86 L (35% pred)	Intervention: all subjects participated in 8-wk pulmonary rehabilitation program with walking exercise; both arm training groups (GR and PNF) performed isokinetic arm cycle training 12 times for 15 min each session; GR included five low-resistance, high-repetition exercises with 1-2 sets of 10 repetitions each with hand weights; PNF included 4 exercises with hand weights in 3 sets of 4-10 repetitions each; daily training in both groups. Follow-up: 8 wk	Compared to control subjects, both upper extremity training groups demonstrated improvement on performance of specific training tests; no differences in isotonic arm cycle or ventilatory muscle endurance exercise; breathlessness decreased for all tests in all groups after pulmonary rehabilitation
Lake et al[28] (1990) Australia	Sample size: 26 (6 upper limb, 6 lower limb, 7 combined, 7 control) Gender: 85% male	Intervention: 8-wk outpatient exercise program, 3 times per week, 1 h per session; 20 min of upper-limb circuit training or walking exercise (combined group had 15	Significant improvement in 6-min walking distance in lower limb training and combined training groups; significant improvement in arm ergometry endurance in arm training and combined training

(continued)

Source/Country	Patients	Intervention/Follow-up	Outcome
Lake et al[28] (continued)	Age: mean, 66 yr FEV$_1$: mean, 0.88 L	min each) Follow-up: 8 wk	groups; significant improvement in scale of well-being only in the combined arm and leg training group
Martinez et al[65] (1993) United States	Sample size: 35 (18 arm exercise with weighted dowels, 17 arm ergometry) Gender: 40% male Age: mean, 66 yr FEV$_1$: mean, 32% pred	Intervention: 10-wk outpatient rehabilitation program; all patients underwent leg ergometry and ventilatory muscle training with threshold device; training 3 times per week Follow-up: 10 wk	Endurance time and work capacity (in watts) increased significantly for both groups (40%); there was greater increase for unsupported arm exercise in the dowel training group; there was decreased $\dot{V}O_2$ (15%) during arm exercise only in the dowel-trained group

*GR = gravity resistance; PNF = proprioceptive neuromuscular facilitation.

Table 4. Nonrandomized Trial of Arm Exercise

Source/Country	Patients	Intervention/Follow-up	Outcome
Couser et al[67] (1993) United States	Sample size: 14 Gender: 86% male Age: 65 yr FEV$_1$: 1.12% L	Intervention: 8-wk outpatient rehabilitation program 3 times per week (9 patients) or 3-wk inpatient program 5 d/wk (5 patients); leg cycle ergometry, arm cycle ergometry, and unsupported arm exercise training Follow-up: 8 wk (outpatients) or 3 wk (inpatients)	After training $\dot{V}O_2$ CO_2 production, and $\dot{V}E$ were significantly lower during arm elevation than before training

might include the following: (1) establish better criteria to select patients who would benefit most from arm training; (2) determine the effect of arm training on functional outcomes; (3) evaluate different forms of arm exercise training programs; this includes exploring the effect of the type, duration, frequency, and intensity of the program on the outcome variables; and (4) determine the effect of intense arm exercise training on respiratory muscle function.

VENTILATORY MUSCLE TRAINING

Introduction

Respiratory muscle weakness may contribute to dyspnea and exercise limitation.[68,69] The rationale for VMT is that enhancing respiratory muscle function will potentially reduce the severity of breathlessness and improve exercise tolerance. The two major types of VMT are sustained hyperpnea and inspiratory resistance breathing. Training systems for sustained hyperpnea are not generally portable and require monitoring so that patients need to train at a medical facility. Inspiratory resistance training uses small, hand-held devices and has been studied more extensively. For these reasons, this review considers only inspiratory resistance training as a method of VMT.

Published articles of VMT in patients with COPD were identified from a MEDLINE literature search and from a meta-analysis of VMT by Smith and coworkers[70] published in 1992. For this review, articles were selected to assess the effects of VMT based on the following criteria: randomized trial involving treatment and control groups; use of a resistance or pressure device for VMT; and consideration of appropriate outcomes such as inspiratory muscle strength, measured as maximal inspiratory pressure (PImax), exercise, or functional capacity (eg, 6- or 12-min walking distance), dyspnea ratings, and/or health status.[71] The 11 individual studies selected are described in Tables 5 [72-77] and 6.[29,35,78-80]

One important question in examining the scientific evidence of VMT studies is, "Was the training stimulus adequate to induce an appropriate physiologic response?" This question relates to the overload principle of training (ie, the training load must exceed the daily load encountered by the muscle).[81] Thus, a VMT program designed to enhance strength should lead to an increase in PImax.

Recommendation

The scientific evidence at the present time does not support the routine use of VMT as an essential component of pulmonary rehabilitation. However, VMT may be considered in selected patients with COPD who have decreased respiratory muscle strength and breathlessness.

Strength of Evidence = B

Scientific Evidence.   In a meta-analysis of 17 "relevant randomized trials" of VMT, Smith and coworkers[70] reported nonsignificant changes in PImax in 11 studies in which it was evaluated and in respiratory muscle endurance in nine studies in which it was evaluated. These findings demonstrate that the training stimulus (mode, frequency, intensity, and/or duration) was inadequate in these studies to induce the expected physiologic training responses. However, in five studies in which respiratory strength or endurance did improve, a moderate treatment effect was observed for improved functional exercise capacity (p = 0.007). These findings emphasize the importance of the training stimulus.

Additional analyses by Smith and coworkers[70] suggested that VMT may lead to appreciable improvements in respiratory muscle strength and/or endurance if the breathing pattern is controlled. This would ensure that substantial pressures are generated during inspiration. As an example, there was a significant difference (p = 0.02) for improvement

in PImax when the inspiratory flow rate was controlled (five studies) compared with an uncontrolled flow rate (six studies).

An AACVPR committee has recommended that dyspnea ratings, functional status, and health-related QOL are three important outcome measures that should be included in the evaluation of pulmonary rehabilitation.[71] Many of the 17 trials of VMT examined by Smith and coworkers[70] considered only physiologic responses and did not include various clinical outcomes. Of the eight randomized controlled trials of VMT (Table 5),[72-77] three studies measured dyspnea ratings, five studies included functional or exercise capacity (eg, 6- or 12-min walking distance), and two studies considered components of health-related QOL.

There was a significant reduction in the severity of dyspnea as measured by the Baseline and Transition Dyspnea Indexes after VMT reported by Harver and coworkers[74] and Lisboa and coworkers.[76] Most importantly, both studies showed significant correlations between the changes in PImax and changes in dyspnea ratings with VMT. These results support the described rationale for VMT. In the study by Larson and coworkers,[73] there was no change in "shortness of breath" as measured on a five-point scale. However, the authors did not provide evidence that this instrument was appropriate (validity, reliability, and sensitivity) for measuring dyspnea.

There were variable changes in exercise capacity with VMT. Two studies found an increase in a timed walking distance test,[72,73] whereas two studies showed no change in the VMT group.[75,77] Further analysis revealed a significant increase in PImax with VMT in those groups who improved exercise capacity; in contrast, there was no change in PImax after VMT in the two studies that reported no change in the 6- or 12-min walking distance. Collectively, these four studies are consistent: when the stimulus or load placed on the respiratory muscles with resistance training is sufficient to augment PImax, there is an associated increase in exercise capacity.

Health-related QOL was considered in only two investigations.[73,75] Neither study showed significant improvements in health status. However, in the study by Guyatt and coworkers,[75] there was no significant improvement in PImax with VMT; therefore, an impact on physical or emotional function would

Table 5. Randomized Controlled Trials of VMT

Source/Country	Patients	Intervention/Follow-up	Outcome
Pardy et al[72] (1981) Canada	Sample size: 17 (8 physiotherapy, 9 inspiratory muscle training) Gender: 88% male Age: mean, 62 yr FEV_1: mean 28% pred	Intervention: 2-mo outpatient training program; VMT: inspiring against resistance for two 15-min periods; physiotherapy: cycle ergometer, treadmill, stairs, and lifting weights three times per week Follow-up: 2 mo	VMT group increased 12-min walk distance and exercise endurance time; physiotherapy group showed no changes
Larson et al[73] (1988) United States	Sample size: 22 (12 light and 10 heavier inspiratory load trainers) Gender: 91% male Age: mean, 64 yr FEV_1: mean, 31% pred	Intervention: 8-wk outpatient training program; pressure threshold device at 15% (light) or 30% (heavier) of PImax for 15 min/d for first week and 30 min/d for 7 wk Follow-up: 8 wk	30% PImax group increased PImax, endurance time for breathing against inspiratory resistance, and 12-min walk distance, 15% PImax group showed no changes; no change in functional impairment, mood, health status, or symptoms in either group
Harver et al[74] (1989) United States	Sample size: 19 (10 intervention, 9 control) Gender: 84% male Age: 63 yr (range, 48-76 yr) FEV_1: 1.06 L (38% pred)	Intervention: 8-wk outpatient program with daily home training; VMT: inspiratory resistance exercise for 15 min twice daily with resistance gradually increased; control group: sham training with minimal resistance Follow-up: 8 wk	Training group increased PImax and decreased severity of dyspnea compared with control group
Guyatt et al[75] (1992) Canada	Sample size: 82 (43 intervention, 39 control—each group divided into use or nonuse of nose clips) Gender: 71% male Age: mean, 66 yr FEV_1: 1.02 L	Intervention: 12-wk outpatient program with daily home training, VMT: inspiratory resistance exercise for 10 min 5 times per day, resistance increased as tolerated; control group: sham training with minimal resistance Follow-up: 6 mo	No differences between groups for PImax, progressive exercise, 6-min walk distance, physical or emotional factors
Lisboa et al[76] (1994) Chile	Sample size: 20 (10 intervention, 10 control) Gender: 50% male Age: mean, 70 yr FEV_1: 37% pred	Intervention: 5-wk outpatient program with home training 6 d/wk; VMT: pressure threshold device at 30% PImax for 15 min twice per day, load increased as tolerated, control group: sham training with minimal load (12% PImax) Follow-up: 5 wk	Training group increased PImax, inspiratory muscle power output, and maximal inspiratory flow rate and decreased severity of dyspnea compared with control group

(continued)

Table 5. *(continued)*

Source/Country	Patients	Intervention/Follow-up	Outcome
Preusser et al[77] (1994) United States	Sample size: 20 (12 high resistance, 8 low resistance training) Gender: 35% male Age: mean, 65 yr (range 45-82 yr) FEV$_1$: 34% pred	Intervention: 12-wk supervised outpatient training program three times per week; threshold loading device a high (52% PImax) or low (22% PImax) load; training for 5 min per session at week 1 to 18 min per session at week 12 Follow-up: 12 wk	PImax increased in high-intensity training group only; both groups improved inspiratory muscle endurance and 12-min walk distance; no differences between groups for PImax, inspiratory muscle endurance, or 12-min walk distance

Table 6. Randomized Controlled Trials of VMT and Exercise Training*

Source/Country	Patients	Intervention/Follow-up	Outcome
Goldstein et al[78] (1989) Canada	Sample size: 11 (6 inspiratory muscle training, 5 control subjects in addition to pulmonary rehabilitation) Gender: 83% male Age: mean, 66 yr (range, 56-73 yr) FEV$_1$: mean, 33% pred	Intervention: 4-wk inpatient pulmonary rehabilitation program; VMT with pressure threshold device with initial load sustained for 10 min up to 20 min, then load increased; control group performed sham training with nominal load; training 2 times per day 15 d/wk Follow-up: 1 mo	Training group increased inspiratory muscle endurance but no change in PImax; control group showed no changes
Dekhuijzen et al[79] (1991) The Netherlands	Sample size: 40 (20 inspiratory muscle training, 20 control subjects in addition to pulmonary rehabilitation) Gender: 75% male Age: mean, 59 yr FEV$_1$: mean, 50% pred	Intervention: 10-wk outpatient pulmonary rehabilitation program 5 d/wk; VMT: target flow with added resistance at 70% PImax held for 3 s for 15 min twice daily, load adjusted twice per week based on PImax; control group: no VMT Follow-up: 10 wk	Training group had increased PImax and greater increase in 12-min walk distance compared with control group; both groups improved maximum cycle ergometer exercise and symptoms
Weiner et al[29] (1992) Israel	Sample size: 36 (12 inspiratory muscle training + general exercise, 12 general exercise alone, 12 control) Gender: 50% male	Intervention: 6-mo outpatient training program 3 times per week; VMT exercise group used a threshold device for 15 min at 15% of PImax for 1 wk, increased to 60% of PImax by the end of first month, and then continued; general	VMT + exercise group had significant increase in PImax and respiratory muscle endurance, and significantly greater increase in the 12-min walk distance and endurance on the cycle ergometer than general exercise only or control groups *(continued)*

Source/Country	Patients	Intervention/Follow-up	Outcome
Weiner et al[29] *(continued)*	Age: mean, 65 yr (range, 45-80 yr) FEV_1: mean, 35% pred	exercise consisted of increasing load of cycle ergometer to 50% of maximal work for 20 min, with rowing ergometry for 10 min, and resistance training of upper and lower extremities for 15 min; exercise only group—as described with sham VMT; control group—no training Follow-up: 6 mo	
Wanke et al[80] (1994) Austria	Sample size: 42 (21 inspiratory muscle + cycle ergometry training, 21 cycle ergometry training only) Gender: 52% male Age: mean, 56 yr FEV_1: 1.33 L (46% pred)	Intervention: 8-wk outpatient training program, VMT group exercised daily with 12 maximal static inspiratory efforts (strength) and 10 min at 70% of maximal Pdi (endurance); both groups performed cycle ergometry exercise consisting of 20-30 min of cycle ergometry at 60% of maximal HR reserve for 4 d/wk for 8 wk Follow-up: 8 wk	VMT + cycle exercise group had significant increase in PImax, Pdimax, and inspiratory muscle endurance time, and greater increase in $\dot{V}O_2$max, maximal power output, and $\dot{V}$Emax compared with cycle exercise only group
Berry et al[35] (1996) United States	Sample size: 25 (8 inspiratory muscle training with general exercise, 9 general exercise only, 8 sham breathing exercise) Gender: 64% male Age: mean, 69 yr FEV_1: mean, 1.44 L (47% pred)	Intervention: 12-wk supervised outpatient program three times per week; VMT + exercise group used a pressure threshold device at 15% (2 wk), 30% (2 wk), 60% (2 wk), and 80% (6 wk) of PImax for 7 d/wk for 12 wk; exercise consisted of walking up to 20 min at 50-75% of maximal HR reserve and upper extremity resistance training of five different exercises using hand-held weights, 3 d/wk; exercise group: as described with sham VMT (15% of PImax); control group: 10-15 min of flexibility training, 15-20 min of breathing exercises, and sham VMT (15% of PImax) Follow-up: 12 wk	VMT + exercise and exercise groups had significantly greater 12-min walk distance than control group, but no differences in PImax, $\dot{V}O_2$max, treadmill time, or other variables for the three groups

*Pdimax = maximum transdiaphragmatic pressure.

not be expected. Although Larson and coworkers[73] achieved an increase in PImax with VMT, there were no changes in the Sickness Impact Profile or Health Perceptions Questionnaire in the training group. Two possibilities are that VMT does not affect health-related QOL or that these instruments are not sensitive to measure small changes in components of health status.

Four other studies have examined VMT concurrent with general exercise training (lower and upper extremities) in patients with COPD (Table 6).[29,35,78-80] In three studies, the groups who performed VMT and exercise exhibited significant increases in PImax and had significantly greater increases in exercise performance compared with the groups who did exercise only.[29,79,80] In the other study, patients who performed VMT did not improve PImax; therefore, the training stimulus appeared to be inadequate.[35]

Conclusions

Most randomized controlled trials of inspiratory resistance training in patients with COPD do not provide conclusive scientific evidence of benefit. However, many of these studies did not include a sufficient training stimulus to achieve the expected increase in respiratory muscle function. Selected randomized, controlled trials that included adequate training loads (ie, an intensity of at least 30% of PImax)[74,76,81] and measured clinical outcomes have showed improvements in dyspnea and/or exercise tolerance with VMT.[29,73,74,76-79,81] Accordingly, VMT may be considered in individual patients with COPD who remain symptomatic despite optimal therapy.

PSYCHOSOCIAL, BEHAVIORAL, AND EDUCATIONAL COMPONENTS AND OUTCOMES

Introduction

Most studies of psychological factors in patients with COPD indicate that depression, anxiety, and selected psychiatric symptoms are common,[82-85] although methods of psychological/psychiatric evalu-

ation have varied considerably across studies. The data generally confirm that depression and anxiety may affect a substantial number of patients with COPD,[83,84] but that depression and anxiety are not necessarily concomitants of chronic lung disease. In some patients with COPD, there appear to be few, if any, significant psychological symptoms.[48] Overall, the data suggest a positive association of psychological distress with pulmonary impairment and that COPD associated with poor body image, increased loneliness, reduced social support, dissatisfaction with social support, and negative self-concept.[87-89] In addition, several studies of patients with COPD have found that psychological distress predicts restricted activities of daily living (ADLs), with emotional/psychosocial factors (eg, depression, anxiety, somatization, low self-esteem, attitudes toward treatment, social support) being more predictive of functional capacity than traditional physiologic indicators.[85,90-92] Further, Kaplan and colleagues[93] found that self-efficacy for walking (ie, the patient's belief that he/she will be able to complete a walking task) predicted survival over a 5-year period. However, at least one study found no relationship of depression and anxiety with 12-min walk distance,[84] and other studies have found that psychosocial factors are not necessarily adequate predictors of longer-term physical functioning. Thus, COPD appears to be associated with psychological distress and poor self-image, which predict restricted ADLs on a short-term basis, but disease indicators and self-efficacy for walking, rather than psychosocial distress, appear to be more strongly associated with long-term functioning and survival. In addition, several studies have documented impairment on tests of cognitive or neuro-psychological functioning among hypoxemic patients with COPD,[94-96] indicating deficits in higher-level cognitive tasks such as attention, complex visual-motor processes, abstraction ability, and verbal tasks.

Many pulmonary rehabilitation programs include a psychosocial or behavioral component in addition to exercise training. The psychosocial component is sometimes included in the context of patient education[97] or is conducted separately as a support group or stress management group.[33,98] Typically, the goals of the psychosocial components are to address specific psychological factors such as depression and anxiety, teach relaxation skills, address pertinent issues such as sexual relations as well as family and work relationships, and facilitate information sharing and emotional support among group members.[33,98] In addition, behavioral strategies may be incorporated into the psychosocial component to reinforce positive health behaviors such as smoking cessation, dietary change, and exercise maintenance.

Recommendation

Evidence to date does not support the benefits of short-term psychosocial interventions as single therapeutic modalities, but longer-term interventions may be beneficial. Although scientific evidence is lacking, expert opinion supports the inclusion of educational and psychosocial interventions as components of comprehensive pulmonary rehabilitation programs for patients with COPD.

Strength of Evidence = C

Scientific Evidence. Psychosocial Intervention Components:

1. Psychosocial Interventions: Several studies evaluating psychosocial interventions among patients with COPD are summarized in Table 7. [99-103] Results of two studies were generally negative, indicating that stress management alone had minimal impact on psychosocial functioning as measured by the Sickness Impact Profile,[101] and progressive muscle relaxation had no persistent impact on dyspnea or anxiety.[100] Although acute improvements in dyspnea and anxiety have been observed immediately following relaxation interventions, studies have not demonstrated longer-term benefits of brief interventions.[100,104] Only the study of Tandon[99] of a 9-month yoga intervention was associated with positive outcomes (increased exercise tolerance, decreased symptoms). However, the studies with negative findings are limited by the brief length of time allotted to the intervention, and the inherent limitations in both depth and breadth of training. Overall, the data do not support the efficacy of short-term focused psychosocial interventions for patients with COPD, but provide limited support for the benefits of a more intensive single-component intervention. In addition, more work is needed to better define the appropriate outcome measures to assess the results of such interventions.

2. Health Behavior Interventions: Behavioral factors are important in the preventive care and rehabilitation of patients with COPD. Specifically, smoking is well known to be the primary risk factor for the onset of COPD. Although data suggest benefits of smoking cessation early in the course of COPD,[105] most patients have quit smoking by the time they initiate a pulmonary rehabilitation program. Thus, the data regarding smoking cessation interventions in pulmonary rehabilitation are sparse. Two studies (including one randomized controlled study) report modest success with smoking cessation among both inpatient[106] and outpatient[107] smokers with COPD. Intervention techniques include brand fading and stimulus control[107] as well as use of a behavioral treatment manual with follow-up problem-solving sessions.[106] The generally poor results suggest that the presence of COPD does not facilitate the process of smoking cessation. Indeed, to the extent that smoking is perceived by the patient as a way of coping with depression, anxiety, and loneliness, smoking cessation may be extremely difficult to achieve without addressing specific areas of related psychological distress. With regard to diet and nutrition, to our knowledge, no studies have evaluated the effects of behavioral weight management (gain or loss) among patients with COPD enrolled in a pulmonary rehabilitation program.

3. Adherence Intervention: Probably the most important behavioral aspect of pulmonary rehabilitation is the extent to which patients comply with the exercise program or with other medical therapies. Atkins and colleagues[108] investigated the effects of three types of cognitive and behavioral interventions on exercise compliance (walking) among 76 patients with COPD (37% men) who were randomly assigned to one of five groups: (1) behavior modification (eg, scheduling, contracting, reinforcement principles, relaxation, breathing exercises); (2) cognitive modification (eg, increased awareness of negative self-statements, substitution of positive statements); (3) cognitive-behavior modification (eg, combination of the first two components); (4) attention control (subjects met with researchers for same length of time discussing general principles about COPD); or (5) no-treatment control (subjects advised to start a walking program). Results indicated that the combined cognitive-behavioral group achieved a greater time spent

Table 7. Effects of Select Psychosocial/Behavioral/Educational Interventions in Pulmonary Rehabilitation*

Source/Country	Patients	Intervention/Follow-up	Outcome
Randomized controlled trials			
Tandon[99] (1978) Australia	Sample size: 22 (11 yoga, 11 standard physiotherapy) Gender: 100% male Age: mean, 60 yr (range, 52-65 yr) FEV_1: mean, 0.90 L	Intervention: 9-mo outpatient program, 3 times per week × 4 wk, 2 times per week × 4 wk, then 1 time per week × 7 mo; yoga: breathing exercises and 10 yogic postures; physiotherapy; relaxation exercises, breathing exercises, leg and trunk exercises. Follow-up: 9 mo	Significant increase in maximum exercise tolerance on a cycle ergometer in yoga group; slight (not significant) decrease in physiotherapy group; significantly higher number of yoga subjects reported decrease in symptoms of lung disease
Renfroe[100] (1988) United States	Sample size: 20 (12 intervention, 8 control) (14 COPD, 6 asthma) Gender: 50% male Age: mean, 61 yr (range, 20-84 yr) FEV_1: NA	Intervention: 4-wk program of PMR with weekly 1-h supervised sessions and daily home practice; control group had four 1-h sessions of relaxing on their own Follow-up: 4 wk	Anxiety measured with State Trait Anxiety Inventory reduced within sessions, but not between sessions in PMR group; dyspnea measured with VAS; reduced within sessions but not between sessions in PMR group; changes in PMR group significantly better than control subjects
Blake et al[101] (1990) United States	Sample size: 94 (45 intervention, 49 control) Gender: 80% male Age: mean, 63 yr FEV_1: mean $FEV_1/FVC = 0.44$	Intervention: one to three 60- to 90-min nurse-administered stress management sessions; individualized plan including education, relaxation techniques, identifying social support, and coping strategies Follow-up: 12 mo	No significant difference between treatment and control groups on Sickness Impact Profile measures of physical function, psychosocial function, or overall functional status; no significant group differences in morbidity (hospital days, days of restricted activity, physician visits)
Sassi-Dambron et al[102] (1995) United States	Sample size: 89 (46 dyspnea management treatment, 43 health education control) Gender: 55% male Age: mean, 67 yr FEV_1: mean, 1.15 L (50% pred)	Intervention: 6-wk, 6-session outpatient dyspnea management treatment (lung disease and dyspnea education, PMR, breathing retraining, pacing, self-talk, panic control) vs general health education control group who received lectures not directly related to lung disease Follow-up: 6 mo	Only significant difference between groups was decreased dyspnea in BDI/TDI for experimental group compared to control group at 6 mo; both groups showed decreased dyspnea on SOBQ up to 6 mo; no changes in six other measures of dyspnea, 6-min walk distance, QWB, State-Trait Anxiety Inventory, or Center for Epidemiologic Studies' Depression (CES-D) scale

(continued)

Source/Country	Patients	Intervention/Follow-up	Outcome
Observational study			
Janelli et al[103] (1991) United States	Sample size: 30 Gender: 27% male Age: mean, 68 yr FEV$_1$: NA	Intervention: 6-wk COPD educational program at a private hospital for 1 h/wk Follow-up: 6 wk	No change on scale assessing coping behavior
*PMR = progressive muscle relaxation.			

walking than the other groups. Furthermore, the three experimental groups achieved a larger percent average increase in exercise tolerance and a greater increase in self-efficacy for walking than did the combined control groups, although at 6 months of follow-up, group differences in exercise tolerance were no longer statistically significant. These data suggest the short-term effects of cognitive and behavioral interventions for enhancing exercise adherence among patients with COPD.

4. Education Interventions: Patient education is a central component of pulmonary rehabilitation. Education classes are generally conducted in a class format and may cover a wide variety of topics, including anatomy and physiology, COPD pathophysiology, breathing retraining, diet and nutrition, medication regimens (including drug action, side effects, administration with inhaler technique, and self-care algorithms), energy conservation with ADLs, importance of exercise, strategies for managing dyspnea, symptom assessment and knowledge about when to seek medical treatment, travel, and safe use of oxygen. Amount of time allotted to each topic varies considerably across programs.[109] In addition to lectures, the education component often includes printed handouts, demonstrations, and active coaching.

Because educational content is intrinsic to most pulmonary rehabilitation programs, few studies have evaluated the effects of education alone on patient outcomes. Only five studies have empirically evaluated the effects of focused education interventions among patients with COPD. Three of the studies demonstrated at least mild improvements in dyspnea,[102,110,111] although one of these studies indicated improvement on only one of six dyspnea indicators.[102] Two additional studies indicated negative results. One study found no benefit of education on

coping skills,[103] and another study indicated that psychological distress levels were increased rather than decreased following an education intervention.[112] Thus, education outside the context of a multicomponent pulmonary rehabilitation program that includes exercise training may not be sufficient to improve the well-being of patients with COPD.

Psychosocial Outcomes of Comprehensive Pulmonary Rehabilitation: Thirty-eight studies of psychosocial outcomes among patients with COPD were reviewed. Twenty-one of the studies were correlational, helping to describe the typology of psychosocial phenomena among patients with COPD. A total of seven studies of psychosocial outcomes of pulmonary rehabilitation satisfied the following criteria: (1) conducted with a sample of patients with COPD; (2) involved a multicomponent pulmonary rehabilitation program with at least a brief description of the intervention; and (3) either included a detailed description of the psychosocial outcome measures utilized or used reliable and valid outcome measures. Three of the studies were randomized controlled studies and are summarized in Table 8;[33,113,114] and the other four were observational studies, summarized in Table 9.[82,97,98,115] All of the interventions included exercise rehabilitation as the primary component, with additional components of education and psychosocial support.

Results from the randomized interventions suggest no significant decreases in depression associated with pulmonary rehabilitation.[33,113] Similarly, changes in anxiety observed in the study of Gayle and colleagues[113] were observed in both the exercise and the control groups; hence, there appeared to be no specific benefit of pulmonary rehabilitation for anxiety. The study by Dekhuijzen and colleagues[114] found no changes in hostility, self-esteem, or feelings of social inadequacy. The only reported significant change in psychosocial outcome

Table 8.	**Effects of Pulmonary Rehabilitation on Psychosocial/Behavioral Factors: Randomized Controlled Studies***		
Source/Country	**Patients**	**Intervention/Follow-up**	**Outcome**
Gayle et al[113] (1988) United States	Sample size: 15 (9 intervention, 6 control) Gender: 60% male Age: range, 46-71 yr FEV_1: NA	Intervention: 28-wk outpatient exercise program supervised 3 times per week for 50 min per session; stretching, light resistance walking, and relaxation exercises; control group did not exercise for first 14 wk, then crossed over to exercise program. Follow-up: 28 wk	State Trait Anxiety Inventory showed reduced anxiety in both groups irrespective of exercise intervention; Zung Self-Rating Depression Scale did not change significantly in either group
Dekhuijzen et al[114] (1990) The Netherlands	Sample size: 40 (20 inspiratory muscle training with pulmonary rehabilitation, 20 pulmonary rehabilitation alone); 20 nonrandomized control group with home inspiratory muscle training Gender: 75% male Age: mean, 59 yr FEV_1: mean, 1.48 L (49% pred)	Intervention: 10-wk outpatient pulmonary rehabilitation program 5 d/wk including exercise, physiotherapy, and education; daily inspiratory muscle training at target flow with added resistance twice daily for 15 min Follow-up: 10 wk	Significant reductions in depression and anxiety components of Hopkins Symptom Checklist (SCL-90) in both groups receiving exercise, but no change in inspiratory muscle training control group; no significant changes in hostility, social inadequacy, or self-esteem components of the Dutch Personality Inventory in any group
Ries et al[33] (1995) United States	Sample size: 119 (57 rehabilitation intervention, 62 education control) Gender: 73% male Age: mean, 63 yr FEV_1: mean, 1.23 L	Intervention: 8-wk outpatient comprehensive rehabilitation program (12 4-h sessions with treadmill/walking exercise, education, and psychosocial support) + monthly visits for 1 yr vs education control program (four 2-h sessions) Follow-up: 6 yr	Significant improvement in rehabilitation group in self-efficacy for walking up to 18 mo; no change in education control subjects; no change in QWB or CES-D depression scale for either group

*CES-D = Center for Epidemiological Studies-Depression Scale.

measures from pulmonary rehabilitation in these randomized studies was an increased self-efficacy for walking.[33] Other researchers have confirmed the apparently robust finding of increased self-efficacy associated with exercise training.[116]

Interestingly, the results of observational studies differ substantially from those of the randomized studies. Two of the observational studies found re-

ductions in depression and anxiety,[82,98] although only one of those studies used validated outcome measures.[98] The other two studies found reductions in affective distress, as measured by the Multiple Affect Adjective Checklist[115] and a visual analog scale (VAS),[97] but no change on a standardized measure of depression (Beck Depression Inventory).[97] Positive indicators of well-being (ie, patients reporting

Table 9. Effects of Pulmonary Rehabilitation on Psychosocial/Behavioral Factors: Observational Studies*

Source/Country	Patients	Intervention/Follow-up	Outcome
Fishman and Petty[115] (1971) United States	Sample size: 30 Gender: 100% male Age: NA FEV$_1$: mean, 0.97 L	Intervention: 1-yr program of outpatient and home care, providing individualized education and medical management	Significant decrease in affective distress in MAACL; no change in MMPI
Agle et al[62] (1973) United States	Sample size: 21 Gender: 100% male Age: mean, 51 yr FEV$_1$: NA	Intervention: 4-wk inpatient pulmonary rehabilitation program with exercise, group therapy, vocational and social counseling; monthly outpatient group counseling for 1 yr Follow-up: 1 yr	Serial psychiatric interveiws: most patients with depression and anxiety at baseline improved
Emery et al[96] (1991) United States	Sample size: 64 Gender: 55% male Age: mean, 67 yr (range, 53-82 yr) FEV$_1$: mean, 1.01 L	Intervention: 1-mo outpatient pulmonary rehabilitation program, 5 d/wk, 4 h per session including exercise (walking, cycle ergometry, strength training, pool), education, stress management Follow-up, 1 mo	Significant reductions in SCL-90 measures of depression, anxiety, and psychiatric symptoms; significant improvement in all six dimensions of PGWB—depression, anxiety, well-being, self-control, health, vitality, and total score; improved psychomotor speed and mental flexibility on cognitive testing; no change in memory or concentration
Ojanen et al[97] (1993) Finland	Sample size: 40 Gender: 95% male Age: mean, 63 yr (range, 52-107 yr) FEV$_1$ mean, 0.97 L	Intervention: 3-wk inpatient pulmonary rehabilitation program including education, breathing retraining, bronchial hygiene, and exercise 2 times per day, 6 d/wk (treadmill walking for up to 15 min per session) Follow-up: 6 mo	No change in Beck Depression Inventory at 6-mo follow-up; significant improvement in VAS ratings of mood and well-being after rehabilitation program; at 6 mo, improved well-being but not mood; no significant change in self-related coping skills for daily activities

*MAACL = Multiple Affect Adjective Checklist; MMPI = Minnesota Multiphasic Personality Inventory; PGWB = Psychological General Well-Being Index; SCL-9O = Hopkins Symptom Checklist.

affirmative feelings, not simply the absence of distress) were found to increase in two of the studies,[97,98] and one of the studies also found enhanced functioning on tests of cognitive functioning.[98] Review of the studies listed in Tables 8 and 9 indicates that psychological distress was generally greater in the studies in which significant decreases were observed. Thus, pulmonary rehabilitation may reduce psychological distress among subjects who enter with higher levels of distress, but this assertion has not been empirically confirmed in a randomized study.

Conclusions

Findings to date suggest that depression and anxiety may be concomitants of COPD, but that they are not pervasive. Other psychosocial concerns, such as low self-esteem, poor social relations, and marital conflict may be sequelae of psychological distress or may be more directly associated with the disease process. However, to our knowledge, no studies have evaluated the complex interaction of psychological distress with related behavioral difficulties among patients with COPD in the context of pulmonary rehabilitation. The randomized controlled intervention studies suggest that exercise rehabilitation is associated with increased self-efficacy for walking, but not with reduced psychological distress. The only studies suggestive of decreases in affective distress (ie, depression, anxiety) are observational studies without control groups. Hence, the evidence for psychosocial benefits of pulmonary rehabilitation is weak, although it is possible that benefits are most apparent among patients who exhibit significant distress at the outset of the program. This latter observation is consistent with the perception, which is widely held by both patients and staff associated with pulmonary rehabilitation programs, that patients with COPD reap psychological/psychosocial/behavioral benefits from their participation. To support or refute this belief, there is a need for further well-controlled studies, utilizing validated measures of psychological and behavioral functioning, in addition to subjective reports from participants, staff, and family members to clarify the nature of the changes taking place, and the extent to which psychosocial changes can be expected among patients with COPD in pulmonary rehabilitation.

DYSPNEA

Introduction

Preventing or reducing the intensity and distress of dyspnea improves the QOL of patients with pulmonary disease and is an important goal of pulmonary rehabilitation.[30,31,117] The effect of pulmonary rehabilitation on the symptom of dyspnea has only recently been measured with instruments that have been shown to be valid and reliable measures of the perception of dyspnea.[30-34,37,117] Investigators have reported the effect of pulmonary rehabilitation on the symptom response to laboratory exercise or the concomitant changes in dyspnea with ADLs.[33,34,37,118] More comprehensive multidimensional measures also have been used to assess the impact of dyspnea on overall functioning or QOL.[31,117]

Recommendation

Pulmonary rehabilitation improves the symptom of dyspnea in patients with COPD.

Strength of Evidence = A

Scientific Evidence. In all the published randomized clinical trials, comprehensive pulmonary rehabilitation programs resulted in improvement in dyspnea during laboratory exercise and with ADLs.[30-33,37,117] This conclusion is supported by a recent report of a metaanalysis including 14 clinical trials in which respiratory rehabilitation improved dyspnea and improved control over COPD.[118] There also is evidence that this reduction in the symptom of dyspnea is maintained if there is reinforcement of education and a maintenance exercise program.[33] This decrease in dyspnea after exercise training may occur because of improved exercise performance (ie, more efficient movement or physical conditioning), less ventilation, or a process of desensitization defined as less perceived dyspnea for the same ventilation.[50,119] In addition, changes in mediating cognitive, emotional, sensory, and behavioral factors, such as self-efficacy or anxiety with the symptom, may enhance the improvement in dyspnea with activity.[120] In the studies that have measured dyspnea, there is inconsistent use of instructions, instruments, or measurement overtime. Future longitudinal trials in pulmonary rehabilitation should use instruments to measure dyspnea that are established and shown to be valid, reliable, and responsive to change.

Nine published studies have measured dyspnea before and after a comprehensive pulmonary rehabilitation program. Five studies evaluated outpatient pulmonary rehabilitation programs,[26,31,33,37,121] two examined the effects of inpatient programs,[32,117] and two measured the effects of pulmonary rehabilitation in the home.[30,34] Six studies were randomized controlled trials,[26,31-34,117] one was a nonrandomized trial,[37] and two were observational studies.[26,121] Three studies measured dyspnea before and after pulmonary rehabilitation both during laboratory exercise and during ADLs.[31,33,37] One measured dyspnea only during laboratory exercise.[32] Seven studies measured dyspnea only during ADLs with a variety of different instruments. Only controlled clinical trials using valid and reliable instruments to measure dyspnea are included in Table 10.[30-34,37]

All studies have shown an improvement in dyspnea following pulmonary rehabilitation. The three randomized studies[31-33] and one nonrandomized study[37] using more recent, valid, and reliable measurements found significant decreases in dyspnea during laboratory exercise testing for the group that had completed comprehensive pulmonary rehabilitation compared to a control group. One of these studies was longitudinal and reported that the decrease in dyspnea during laboratory exercise extended for 24 months.[33]

All nine studies that measured dyspnea with ADLs found a decrease in dyspnea with activities. Earlier studies found changes in self-report or positive changes in dyspnea grades[26,121,122] with later studies demonstrating significant and clinically relevant decreases in dyspnea with psychometrically tested instruments described in the next section.[30,31,33,34,37,117]

Measurement of Dyspnea: In the context of pulmonary rehabilitation, dyspnea during exercise testing or with physical activity during a program is typically measured with either a VAS or Borg Scale that has been modified to measure breathlessness. Dyspnea with ADLs or at home has also been measured with several instruments described below. Earlier studies used self-reports, the Medical Research Council (MRC) Dyspnea Scale or Grade of Breathlessness Scale. More recently, investigators have used psychometrically tested instruments, including the following: the baseline

Table 10. Effect of Pulmonary Rehabilitation on Dyspnea

Source/Country	Patients	Intervention/Follow-up	Outcome
Randomized controlled trials			
Goldstein et al[31] (1994) Canada	Sample size: 89 (45 intervention, 44 control) Gender: 49% male Age: mean, 66 yr FEV_1: mean, 35% pred	Intervention: 8-wk inpatient multidisciplinary rehabilitation program (upper and lower extremity exercise, education) +16-wk supervised outpatient program vs conventional community care control Follow-up: 24 wk	Significantly greater improvement in CRQ (dyspnea, fatigue, emotion and mastery) and BDI/TDI for rehabilitation group compared to controls
Wijkstra et al[38] (1994) The Netherlands	Sample size: 43 (28 rehabilitation intervention, 15 control) Gender: 86% male Age: mean, 63 yr FEV_1: mean, 1.33 L (44% pred)	Intervention: 12-wk outpatient rehabilitation program (24 sessions with cycle, upper extremity, and inspiratory muscle exercise) with monthly nurse and physician visits vs control Follow-up: 12 wk	Significant improvement in all four components of the CRQ (dyspnea, fatigue, emotion, and mastery) for rehabilitation group only. Change was significantly greater than controls for dyspnea, emotion, and mastery components
Reardon et al[30] (1994) United States	Sample size: 20 (10 rehabilitation intervention, 10 control) Gender: 50% male Age: mean, 66 yr (range, 52-75 yr) FEV_1: mean, 0.87 L	Intervention: 6-wk outpatient comprehensive rehabilitation program (12 3-h sessions with education and lower/upper extremity plus inspiratory resistive exercise) vs control Follow-up: 6 wk	Dyspnea at maximal treadmill exercise (VAS) decreased 32% in rehabilitation group vs 10% increase in controls (p = 0.015). BDI/TDI improved significantly more in the rehabilitation group (+2.3) compared to controls (+0.2) (p = 0.006)

(continued)

Table 10. *(continued)*

Source/Country	Patients	Intervention/Follow-up	Outcome
Ries et al. al[33] (1995) United States	Sample size: 119 (57 rehabilitation intervention, 62 education control) Gender: 73% male Age: mean, 63 yr FEV_1: mean, 1.23 L	Intervention: 8-wk outpatient comprehensive rehabilitation program (12 4-h sessions with treadmill/walking exercise, education, and psychosocial support) + monthly visits for 1 yr vs education control program (four 2-h sessions) Follow-up: 6 yr	Borg scale ratings of perceived breathlessness during endurance exercise test improved significantly in rehabilitation group to 24 months vs no change in controls; SOBQ improved significantly in rehabilitation group up to 6 months vs no change in controls
Strijbos et al[34] (1996) The Netherlands	Sample size: 45 (15 outpatient rehabilitation, 15 home rehabilitation, 15 control) Gender: 84% male Age: mean, 61 yr FEV_1: mean, 1.23 (43% pred)	Intervention: 12-wk outpatient rehabilitation program (24 1-h exercise sessions + 3 nurse education and 3 physician visits) vs home rehabilitation program (24 1-h exercise sessions + 3 nurse and 3 physician visits) vs control Follow-up: 18 mo	Borg scale ratings of dyspnea during cycle ergometry exercise did not change at maximal exercise in any group; maximum exercise level increased significantly in outpatient and home rehabilitation groups; Borg scale ratings of dyspnea at similar exercise levels decreased significantly for the outpatient rehabilitation group up to 6 months and for the home rehabilitation group up to 18 months

Nonrandomized controlled trials

Source/Country	Patients	Intervention/Follow-up	Outcome
O'Donnell et al[37] (1995) United States	Sample size: 60 (30 intervention, 30 control: self-selected) Gender: 72% male Age: mean, 68 yr FEV_1: mean, 0.96 L (38% pred)	Intervention: 6-wk outpatient exercise program (18 2.5-h sessions with multimodality upper and lower extremity training with some education) vs control group that chose to defer exercise training Follow-up: 6 wk	Significant improvement in BDI/TDI (+2.8) and in OCD (26% increase) in rehabilitation group vs no change in control group; Borg scale ratings of perceived breathlessness at maximum exercise on cycle ergometer significantly improved in rehabilitation group (28%) vs no significant change in control group (8% improvement); slopes of Borg ratings in relation to $\dot{V}O_2$ and $\dot{V}E$ during exercise significantly improved (ie, decreased) in rehabilitation group vs no change in control group

dyspnea index (BDI) and Transitional Dyspnea Index (TDI); the dyspnea component of the Chronic Respiratory Disease Questionnaire (CRQ); the Oxygen Cost Diagram (OCD); the Pulmonary Functional Status and Dyspnea Questionnaire (PFSDQ); or the University of California, San Diego Shortness of Breath Questionnaire (SOBQ). Daily logs are an additional method that can be used to monitor dyspnea with prescribed walking regimens or to demonstrate changes in dyspnea with ADL.

Instruments used to measure dyspnea are described briefly below and have been reviewed by the Outcomes Committee of the AACVPR.[123]

Direct Measures of Dyspnea

1. Modified Borg Scale for Breathlessness: The Borg Scale rating of perceived exertion[124] has been modified to measure symptoms such as breathlessness.[125] A commonly used format is a 10-point scale with a nonlinear scaling scheme using descriptive terms to anchor responses.[125] This scale has strong and significant correlations with the VAS in patients with COPD (r = 0.99)[126] with $\dot{V}E$ (r = 0.98) and $\dot{V}O_2$ during exercise (r = 0.95).[127] It has demonstrated sensitivity to treatment effects.[126] Advantages of the Borg Scale are that the adjectives may help patients in selecting the sensation intensity, descriptors facilitate more absolute responses to stimuli and direct interindividual comparisons, and the scale has been used in several randomized clinical trials allowing comparison of findings across studies.

2. Visual Analog Scale: A VAS is a vertical or horizontal line with anchors to indicate extremes of sensation. The VAS is most commonly 100 cm in length, although some researchers have used other lengths for easier reading and rating by older exercising patients. Some researchers use a light display rather than a written form. Subjects are asked to indicate their dyspnea intensity during exercise by marking the line. Anchors have varied and included "no breathlessness" to "worst imaginable breathlessness" and "no difficulty breathing" to "extreme difficulty breathing." Concurrent validity has been established with the Borg Scale and the Grade of Breathlessness Scale. The VAS has been shown to be reproducible with the same level of exercise and at maximal exercise.[129] The correlation between a horizontal and vertical VAS is reported at 0.97.[130] Patients should be given specific instructions regard-

ing the sensation to be rated, such as shortness of breath, effort of breathing, etc. There is also evidence that the intensity of dyspnea and the distress evoked by dyspnea can be scaled differently by patients.[131]

Indirect Measures of Dyspnea Targeted to Activities

1. Baseline and Transitional Dyspnea Index: The BDI is completed by an interviewer and measures three components that are influenced by dyspnea: functional impairment (the degree to which ADLs are impaired); magnitude of effort (the overall effort exerted to perform activities); and the magnitude of task that provokes breathing difficulty. The focus is on the activity consequences of the individual's breathlessness. Content validity was established by correlation of scores of the BDI with the MRC (r = -0.70, p < 0.01) and the OCD (r = -0.54, p < 0.01).[132,133] Interobserver agreement (interrater reliability) between physician and pulmonary technician has been evaluated by weighted percentages and weighted kappa (K_w).[132] The results demonstrated a range across dimensions of 91 to 93 weighted percent agreement and a K_w ranging from 0.66 to 0.73 demonstrating creditable agreement of the two observers.[132] The TDI measures changes in dyspnea rated by the interviewer comparing patient report with baseline state. Validity was demonstrated by comparing the TDI and CRQ which showed comparable improvements in dyspnea after rehabilitation. Advantages include extensive testing and extensive use in research studies. A disadvantage is that the rating of dyspnea is performed by the health-care provider.

2. Chronic Respiratory Disease Questionnaire: The CRQ is a 20-item self-report questionnaire administered by an interviewer that measures four dimensions: dyspnea, fatigue, emotional function, and mastery of breathing.[134] The patient rates the level of dyspnea he/she has with five usual individual activities. Test-retest reliability was reported as r = 0.73. Advantages include extensive testing and extensive use in research studies. The instrument is sensitive to therapy and a level of change that can be used to judge a "clinically significant" change has been reported. Disadvantages are that it requires a structured 15-min interview and the dyspnea scale ratings are individualized.[135]

Other Relevant Questionnaires

1. St. George's Respiratory Questionnaire: The St. George's Respiratory Questionnaire (SGRQ) is a self-administered, disease-specific QOL questionnaire listing 53 questions measuring three areas of illness: "symptoms" "activity" and "impact" of disease on daily life. The "symptoms" category elicits information about cough, sputum, wheeze, and dyspnea; therefore, dyspnea is not measured separately. Test-retest reliability of the questionnaire in patients with COPD has been reported as r = 0.92.[136] Thresholds of significant clinical change are reported.

2. Pulmonary Functional Status and Dyspnea Questionnaire: The pulmonary functional status and dyspnea questionnaire (PFSDQ) elicits ratings of 79 activities in six categories (number of activities): self-care (15); mobility (14); eating (8); home management (22); social (10); and recreational (10). The activities are independently evaluated for performance, as well as in association with dyspnea. Internal consistency of the instrument has been reported as 0.91.[137] The level of dyspnea for many activities can be monitored over time and the instrument is sensitive to small changes in dyspnea with activities.

3. University of California, San Diego Shortness of Breath Questionnaire: The SOBQ was developed as a clinical evaluation tool to assess shortness of breath for various ADLs. Patients indicate on a six-point scale how frequently they experience shortness of breath during 21 ADLs that are associated with varying levels of exertion. The questionnaire includes three additional questions about limitations caused by shortness of breath, fear of harm from overexertion, and fear of shortness of breath. Responses are summed to produce a total score. Initial testing has been completed and reported.[138]

The PFSDQ and the SOBQ have been used to measure dyspnea; however, both need further evaluation at the present time.

Conclusions

In various studies using a variety of instruments, pulmonary rehabilitation has consistently been shown to reduce the symptom of dyspnea in patients with COPD. The importance of dyspnea as an outcome measure in studies of patients with chronic lung disease has gained greater recognition with the development of several established measurement instruments. Future studies should utilize these instruments.

QUALITY OF LIFE

Introduction

Health-related QOL, the degree to which a medical condition affects one's ability to function in daily life, has become increasingly recognized as an important outcome of medical interventions. The concept of QOL is based on the World Health Organization definition of health as a "state of complete physical, mental, and social well-being and not merely the absence of disease."[139] The implication of this definition is that health, and thus health-related QOL, encompasses multiple dimensions. More specifically, it has been suggested that there are five separate dimensions of QOL: physical health, mental health, social functioning, everyday functioning in role activities, and general perception of well-being.[140]

Recommendation

Pulmonary rehabilitation improves health-related QOL in patients with COPD.

Strength of Evidence = B

QOL Instruments: Earlier studies of pulmonary rehabilitation[36,122,141-146] lacked adequate control groups but nevertheless almost uniformly suggested that QOL was improved following rehabilitation. These investigations laid the foundation for later studies that more rigorously evaluated QOL. Prior to 1980, investigators generally employed interviews or simple questionnaires as QOL assessment tools, but these techniques are considered crude by current criteria.[147] Even some later studies have not used well-standardized QOL measurement instruments.[26,34,79,97,146,148] It is now well recognized that reliability, validity, and sensitivity of QOL tools should be substantiated prior to their application in research investigations.[149] QOL measures should be accurate and stable over time in patients who are not receiving interventions (reliability). Tools should accurately measure the domains of QOL of interest (validity). In addition, evaluative tools should be responsive to changes associated with therapeutic interventions (sensitivity). Health-related QOL measurement tools may be applicable to large populations of patients with a variety of medical conditions or only applicable to smaller numbers of patients with a specific medical problem. Measures that can be used with all populations are referred to as generic instruments and include the Sickness Impact Profile,[150] Quality of Well-Being Scale (QWB),[151,152] and Medical Outcomes Study—Short Form-36.[153] Measures that are used only for respiratory patients are referred to as disease-specific tools and include the CRQ[134] and the SGRQ.[136] The latter instruments usually incorporate questions about symptoms of importance to patients with an illness of a specific organ system (such as shortness of breath in patients with pulmonary disorders). Table 11 outlines key features of the most commonly used tools to assess QOL in patients with COPD.[134,136,150-153] As noted by a recent NIH Workshop on Pulmonary Rehabilitation Research,

Table 11. Commonly Used Tools to Assess Health-Related QOL in Patients With COPD*			
Tool	**No. of Questions**	**Time to Complete; Administration**	**Domain Assessed**
Disease-specific tools			
CRQ Guyatt et al[134] (1987)	15 Subject chooses five specific activities that produce dyspnea	15-30 min; trained interviewer	Dyspnea, fatigue (physical function), emotional function (anxiety, depression), mastery (sense of control over disease)
SGRQ Jones et al[136] (1992)	76	15-20 min; self-administered	Respiratory symptoms, activities (limitations due to breathlessness), impacts of disease (social functioning, psychological disturbances)
Generic tools			
Sickness Impact Profile Bergner et al[150] (1981)	235	20-30 min; self-administered	Social interaction, ambulation and location, sleep and rest, taking nutrition, usual daily work, household management, mobility and confinement, movement of the body, communication activity, leisure pastimes and recreation, intellectual functioning, interaction with family members, emotions, feelings and sensations, personal hygiene
QWB Kaplan and Anderson[151,152] (1988) (1990)	50	10-15 min; trained interviewer	Mobility, physical activity, social activity, symptoms; results weighted by general population preferences with scores from 1 (optimal function) to 0 (death); treatment effects may be expressed as well-years
SF-36 Health Survey Ware and Sherbourne[153] (1992)	36	5-10 min; self-administered	Physical functioning, role functioning, bodily pain, general health, vitality, social functioning, mental health

*SF-36 = Short Form-36.

further investigations are indicated to develop QOL tools that can be used to assess the short- and long-term benefits of pulmonary rehabilitation, and to explore the relationship among QOL, functional performance, and physiologic function.[14]

Scientific Evidence

The recommendation is based on scientific evidence from randomized and nonrandomized trials outlined in Table 12 that provide statistically significant results.[31-33,154] However, the results of these studies do not uniformly demonstrate improved QOL following pulmonary rehabilitation. As noted in Table 12, two of three randomized clinical trials of comprehensive rehabilitation employing standardized QOL

tools have demonstrated improvement in QOL. The available information on employment following pulmonary rehabilitation is inconclusive.

Among investigations of pulmonary rehabilitation outcomes in patients with COPD, 30 studies were identified that assessed some aspect of QOL as a result of pulmonary rehabilitation. The nine articles that used standardized QOL outcome measures were classified on the basis of the study design: (1) three studies used a randomized controlled design evaluating the effects of comprehensive rehabilitation (Table 12); (2) three randomized controlled studies employed only limited aspects of rehabilitation (Table 13);[102,108,155] and (3) three studies used a nonrandomized design (Table 14).[156-158] An additional six studies assessed employment fol-

Table 12. Effect of Pulmonary Rehabilitation on QOL—Randomized Controlled Trials

Source/Country	Patients	Intervention/Follow-up	Outcome
Goldstein et al[31] (1994) Canada	Sample size: 89 (45 intervention, 44 control) Gender: 49% male Age: mean, 66 yr FEV_1: mean, 35% pred	Intervention: 8-wk inpatient multidisciplinary rehabilitation (upper and lower extremity exercise program, education) + 16-wk supervised outpatient program vs conventional community care control Follow-up: 24 wk	Improvement in all four components of CRQ in rehabilitation group; dyspnea, emotional function, and mastery were significantly improved and fatigue tended to improve in rehabilitation patients compared to control subjects; mastery met established minimum change for clinical significance
Wijkstra et al[32,154] (1994) (1996) The Netherlands	Sample size: 43 (28 rehabilitation intervention, 15 control) Gender: 86% male Age: mean, 63 yr FEV_1: mean, 1.33 L (44% pred)	Intervention: 12-wk outpatient rehabilitation program (24 sessions with cycle, upper extremity, and inspiratory muscle exercise) with monthly nurse and physician visits vs control Follow-up: 18 mo	CRQ sum score was improved in patients receiving rehabilitation at 3, 6, 12, and 18 mo compared to control subjects; in patients receiving monthly follow-up, fatigue, emotion, and mastery were improved over baseline at all time points, and the CRQ sum score was improved over control subjects at all time points
Ries et al[33] (1995) United States	Sample size: 119 (57 rehabilitation intervention, 62 education control) Gender: 73% male Age: mean, 63 yr FEV_1: mean, 1.23 L	Intervention: 8-wk outpatient comprehensive rehabilitation program (12 4-h sessions with treadmill/walking exercise, education and psychosocial support)+monthly visits for 1 yr vs education control program (four 2-h sessions) Follow-up: 6 yr	No significant changes in QWB in either group

lowing pulmonary rehabilitation.[141,159-163] The only two investigations that assessed employment and that used control groups of patients not receiving comprehensive pulmonary rehabilitation were analyzed and included in the evidence table (Table 15).[141,160]

Two of the three randomized controlled studies of pulmonary rehabilitation demonstrated improved QOL (Table 12). Goldstein and coworkers[31] utilized a disease-specific measure of QOL (CRQ) and demonstrated significant benefits in patients receiving rehabilitation compared to patients receiving only conventional medical treatment. Statistically signifi-

cant benefits were achieved in emotional function and mastery, and there was an improvement that was not statistically significant in the fatigue scale of the CRQ. Although these investigators employed comprehensive rehabilitation, the program was initially conducted in an inpatient setting for 8 weeks and followed by an additional supervised outpatient program for 16 weeks. Studies by Wijkstra and coworkers[32,154] have demonstrated both short- and long-term improvements in QOL following pulmonary rehabilitation as measured by the CRQ. Ries and coworkers[33] used the QWB, a generic QOL measure, in a 6-year study of the effects of pulmonary

Table 13. Effect of Limited Pulmonary Rehabilitation on QOL—Randomized Controlled Trials

Source/Country	Patients	Intervention/Follow-up	Outcome
Atkins et al[108] (1984) United States	Sample size: 76 (4 behavioral intervention groups, 1 control group) Gender: 37% male Age: mean, 65 yr FEV_1: NA	Intervention: 3-mo home exercise program with 5 different treatment groups of behavioral/cognitive strategies to maintain compliance: behavior modification; cognitive modification; cognitive and behavior modification; attention control; and no-treatment control Follow-up: 18 mo	The 3 cognitive-behavioral treatment groups showed significant improvement over attention control group in QWB; all 4 treatment groups showed improvement over no-treatment control group in QWB
Simpson et al[135] (1992) Canada	Sample size: 28 (14 weightlifting exercise training, 14 control) Gender: 54% male Age: mean, 72 yr FEV_1: mean, 39% pred	Intervention: 8-wk outpatient weightlifting exercise training program; weightlifting; 10 repetitions of legs and arms 3 times a week; resistance progressively increased Follow-up: 8 wk	Significant improvement in CRQ components of dyspnea, mastery, and fatigue in trained subjects; no changes in control subjects
Sassi-Dambron et al[108] (1995) United States	Sample size: 89 (46 dyspnea management treatment, 43 health education control) Gender: 55% male Age: mean, 67 yr FEV_1: mean, 1.15 L (50% pred)	Intervention: 6-wk, 6-session outpatient dyspnea management treatment (lung disease and dyspnea education, progressive muscle relaxation, breathing retraining, pacing, self-talk, panic control) vs general health education control group who received lectures not directly related to lung disease Follow-up: 6 mo	No change in QWB at the end of treatment (6 wk) or at long-term follow-up (6 mo) in either group

Table 14. Effect of Pulmonary Rehabilitation on QOL—Nonrandomized Trials

Source/Country	Patients	Intervention/Follow-up	Outcome
Guyatt et al[156] (1987) Canada	Sample size: 31 Gender: 74% male Age: mean, 65 yr FEV$_1$: mean, 1.10 L (38% pred)	Intervention: 4- to 6-wk inpatient pulmonary rehabilitation program including education, breathing control, relaxation classes, occupational therapy, psychosocial counseling, and exercise trainings Follow-up: 28-30 wk	Significant improvement: in physical and emotional function and quality of life 2 wk after program completion; at 6 mo, 11 of 24 subjects (46%) who had initial improvement showed improved QOL
Vale et al[157] (1993) United States	Sample size: 51 pulmonary rehabilitation program graduates Gender: 37% male Age: mean, 64 yr FEV$_1$: mean, 1.08 L (38% pred)	Intervention: 6-wk outpatient pulmonary rehabilitation program including twice weekly education, breathing training, stress management, relaxation training, energy conservation, dyspnea control and exercise (upper body conditioning, lower extremity exercise and inspiratory resistive loading); retrospective follow-up of program graduates Follow-up: mean, 11 mo after rehabilitation program (range, 3 to 21 mo)	Significant improvement in CRQ sum score following rehabilitation program; CRQ sum declined at follow-up after the rehabilitation program but remained significantly better than prior to rehabilitation
Reardon et al[158] (1993) United States	Sample size: 44 Gender: 43% male Age: mean, 65 yr FEV$_1$: mean, 1.01 L	Intervention: 6-wk outpatient pulmonary rehabilitation program twice weekly including education, support, breathing training, dyspnea control, nutritional counseling, energy conservation, stress management, relaxation training; exercise included inspiratory resistive training, lower extremity exercise, and upper body strengthening Follow-up: 6 wk	Significant improvement in CRQ sum score and all component scores (dyspnea, fatigue, emotional function, and mastery) after rehabilitation

rehabilitation. In this study, patients receiving comprehensive pulmonary rehabilitation were compared to an education-only control group. No benefits were seen in QOL, but the authors speculated that the generic QOL tool used may have been insensitive to the changes observed after rehabilitation in patients with COPD. Because of improvement in exercise endurance and maximal exercise capacity, the authors postulated that a disease-specific QOL tool may have demonstrated benefits from pulmonary rehabilitation. It should also be noted that an earlier study using the same instrument demonstrated improved QOL in response to an exercise and behavioral modification program in patients with COPD.[108]

Two of the three randomized trials that employed only limited aspects of pulmonary rehabilitation have demonstrated improved QOL (Table 12). A weight-lifting exercise program without comprehensive rehabilitation improved QOL as measured by the CRQ.[155] Cognitive modification and a combination of cognitive and behavioral modification added to exercise training resulted in improved QOL measured by the QWB.[108] However, QOL measured by the QWB did not change in patients receiving dyspnea management interventions.[102]

All three nonrandomized trials of pulmonary rehabilitation used the CRQ and demonstrated improved QOL up to 11 months following rehabilitation (Table 14).[156-158]

Two earlier studies demonstrated increased employment following pulmonary rehabilitation (Table 15).[141,160] Since the information presented in the publications of these studies is limited and others have not been able to reproduce these findings, the ability of pulmonary rehabilitation to increase employment is considered to be inconclusive.

Conclusions

Comprehensive pulmonary rehabilitation programs have been demonstrated to improve QOL. Although the precise components of rehabilitation and the

Table 15. Effect of Pulmonary Rehabilitation on Employment			
Source/Country	**Patients**	**Intervention/Follow-up**	**Outcome**
Lustig et al[150] (1972) United States	Sample size: 45 (15 rehabilitation, 15 psychotherapy, 15 control) random assignment Gender: NA Age: NA FEV_1 80% pred	Intervention: 6- to 7-wk outpatient program; rehabilitation: 15-20 sessions of exercise and chest physiotherapy; psychotherapy: 15-20 sessions of psychotherapy; control: no treatment; all groups then received guidance and counseling on vocational activities Follow-up: 14 wk	Significantly more patients receiving rehabilitation were employed 6 wk after the program (11 of 15) compared with the psychotherapy (4 of 15) or no treatment group (3 of 15)
Haas and Cardon[141] (1969) United States	Sample size: 302 (252 rehabilitation, 50 control) Gender: 100% male Age: mean, 57 yr FEV_1: NA	Intervention: 4-wk inpatient or outpatient pulmonary rehabilitation program with relaxation exercises, postural drainage, IPPB, breathing training and exercise (walking, stair climbing, cycling), vocational counseling, and training; inpatients: 1 h twice daily; outpatients: 1 h daily; follow-up physical therapy weekly for 3 mo, then quarterly; control group selected from outpatient clinic had no pulmonary rehabilitation Follow-up: 5 yr	Compared to control group, the pulmonary rehabilitation group had more persons employed (19% vs 3%), greater self-care (19% vs 5%), and less nursing home placement (8% vs 17%) 5 yr later

method of application have varied in the published studies, comprehensive programs usually include education, breathing training, relaxation, dyspnea management, and progressive lower extremity aerobic exercise training. Further investigations are warranted to determine the most effective application of the components of pulmonary rehabilitation.

It appears that disease-specific QOL questionnaires such as the CRQ may be more sensitive to change following pulmonary rehabilitation than generic health status indexes such as the QWB. Nevertheless, further investigations are required to determine which QOL domains are most responsive to pulmonary rehabilitation and which program components are most responsible for improvement in QOL.

HEALTH-CARE UTILIZATION

Introduction

An important aspect in evaluating any type of therapy relates to the effects of that therapy on the utilization of health-care resources. Patients with COPD are heavy users of the health-care system. The effects of pulmonary rehabilitation on the utilization of health-care resources in reducing the number, days, and length of hospitalizations for pulmonary disease have been noted for several decades.[164] Given the current changes in today's health-care system, it will be important to collect additional data on the outpatient as well as inpatient utilization of health services for these chronic disease patients.

Recommendation

Pulmonary rehabilitation has reduced the number of hospitalizations and the number of days of hospitalization for patients with COPD.

Strength of Evidence = B

Scientific Evidence. A total of 11 studies have addressed the effect of a comprehensive pulmonary rehabilitation program on health-care utilization. Of these, two were randomized controlled trials, two were nonrandomized controlled trials, and seven were observational studies.

Randomized Controlled Trials: There has been one randomized controlled trial comparing the ef-

fect of education (group A) alone vs a comprehensive rehabilitation program (group B) on various outcomes in patients with COPD.[33] There were slight but not statistically significant differences in the duration of hospital stay between the two groups (group A: +1.3 days per patient per year compared to group B: -2.4 days per patient per year [p = 0.20]) during the year following the rehabilitation program. A second randomized trial showed a significant reduction in hospitalizations over 6 months for high-risk patients randomly assigned to pulmonary rehabilitation or a self-help group compared to a control group[165] (Table 16). [33,165]

Nonrandomized Controlled Trials: Two nonrandomized, controlled trials in which utilization of health-care resources was evaluated showed a reduction in the number of days the patients required hospitalization for pulmonary-related illness. In one study, Sneider and coworkers[166] examined follow-up data on patients randomly selected retrospectively from three groups: interview only; education only; and both exercise and education. During a 5-year follow-up period compared to 5 years before entry to the program, the first group had an increase in total number of days of hospitalization from 1,069 to 1,570; the second group had an increase from 586 to 946; and the third group had a decrease from 801 to 417. In the second study, two groups of patients were evaluated: one group of patients who had not yet begun comprehensive rehabilitation and one group in which the patients had completed a comprehensive rehabilitation program.[167] In the former group, an average of 6.77 days hospitalized was noted during the preceding 365 days, compared to 1.88 days while in the rehabilitation group (Table 17). [166,167]

Observational Studies: Most of the published studies evaluating the use of health-care resources are in this category. Each study used a patient as his/her own control subject with follow-up from 1 to 10 years following a comprehensive pulmonary rehabilitation program. Seven studies showed a decrease in the total number of hospital days required for a pulmonary-related illness,[164,168-173] while two showed a decrease in the total number of hospitalizations.[82,171] In each of these studies, the total number of hospital days during the year preceding entry into the rehabilitation program was compared to those year(s) following completion of the rehabilitation program (Table 18).[82,164,168-173]

Table 16. Effects of Pulmonary Rehabilitation on Health-Care Utilization: Randomized Controlled Trials

Source/Country	Patients	Intervention/Follow-up	Outcome
Jensen[155] (1983) United States	Sample size: 31 high-risk (10 pulmonary rehabilitation, 10 self-help support club, 11 control); 27 low-risk Gender: 53% male Age: mean, 64 yr FEV$_1$: NA	Intervention: 6-mo outpatient program; rehabilitation: biweekly education and respiratory care instruction; self-help: patient support group meetings on own Follow-up: 6 mo	Hospitalizations during 6-mo follow-up in high-risk group: 2 rehabilitation; 2 self-help; and 7 control; mean hospital days per patient: 0.5 rehabilitation, 0.8 self-help; and 5.0 control; one hospitalization in 27 low-risk patients
Ries et al[33] (1995) United States	Sample size: 119 (57 rehabilitation intervention, 62 education control) Gender: 73% male Age: mean, 63 yr FEV$_1$: mean, 1.23 L	Intervention: 8-wk outpatient comprehensive rehabilitation program (12 4-h sessions with treadmill/walking exercise, education and psychosocial support) + monthly visits for 1 yr vs education control program (four-2 sessions) Follow-up: 6 yr	Trend toward a decrease in number of hospitalization days per patient in the rehabilitation group (-2.4 days) vs those in the education-only group (1.3 days); these differences were not statistically significant

Table 17. Effects of Pulmonary Rehabilitation on Health-Care Utilization: Nonrandomized Controlled Trials

Source/Country	Patients	Intervention/Follow-up	Outcome
Sneider et al[166] (1988) United States	Sample size: 150 (50 randomly selected retrospectively from each of three groups) Gender: 57% male Age: mean, 65 yr FEV$_1$: mean, 1.19 L (49% pred)	Intervention: 3 groups of patients randomly selected from patients who had: (1) interview only; (2) education program; (3) 10-wk outpatient comprehensive pulmonary rehabilitation programs Follow-up: 5 yr	Hospital days during the 5-yr follow-up period compared to 5 yr prior to program: Group 1: 1,069 before, 1,570 after Group 2: 586 before, 946 after Group 3: 801 before, 417 after
Lewis and Bell[167] (1995) United States	Sample size: 30 (convenience sample of 13 not yet in rehabilitation program and 17 participating in rehabilitation program) Gender: 53% male Age: mean, 66 yr FEV$_1$: NA	Intervention: outpatient comprehensive program rehabilitation program Follow-up: 5 mo	In the previous 365 days, the prerehabilitation group spent on average of 6.77 days in the hospital due to program disease compared to 1.88 days in the postrehabilitation group

Table 18. Effects of Pulmonary Rehabilitation on Health-Care Utilization: Observational Studies

Source/Country	Patients	Intervention/Follow-up	Outcome
Petty et al[168] (1969) United States	Sample size: 182 Gender: 87% male Age: mean, 61 yr FEV$_1$: mean, 0.94 L	Intervention: 8-wk outpatient comprehensive pulmonary rehabilitation program Follow-up: 12 mo	Total hospital days during year following the program (542 days) was significantly less than during the year prior to program entry (868 days)
Agle et al[82] (1973) United States	Sample size: 24 Gender: NA Age: mean, 51 yr FEV$_1$: NA	Intervention 4-wk inpatient comprehensive pulmonary rehabilitation program Follow-up: 1 yr	Total number of hospitalizations was less (5) during the year after rehabilitation compared to the year prior to entry into the program (30)
Burton et al[173] (1975) United States	Sample size: 80 Gender: NA Age: NA FEV$_1$: NA	Intervention: outpatient comprehensive pulmonary rehabilitation program Follow-up: 1 yr	Reduction of 9 hospital days per patient between the year prior to and the year following entry into the program
Dunham et al[164] (1984) United States	Sample size: 80 Gender: NA Age: NA FEV$_1$: NA	Intervention: outpatient comprehensive pulmonary rehabilitation program Follow-up: 8 yr	Maintained reduction in the number of hospital days per patient per year during the 8-yr follow-up; as described in reference 174
Hudson et al[169] (1976) United States	Sample size: 44 patients alive 4 yr after pulmonary rehabilitation (14 hospitalized during year prior to program, 30 not hospitalized) Gender: NA Age: NA FEV$_1$: mean, 1.12 L	Intervention: outpatient comprehensive pulmonary rehabilitation program Follow-up: 4 yr	Significant reduction in the number of days of hospitalization in each of 4 yr following program entry, compared to the year prior to rehabilitation Prior to entry: 529 hospital days in 14 patients After program: Year 1: 145 days in 11 patients Year 2: 270 days in 13 patients Year 3: 278 days in 13 patients Year 4: 207 days in 12 patients
Sahn et al[170] (1980) United States	Sample size: 182 Gender: 87% male Age: mean, 61 yr (range, 33-81 yr) FEV$_1$: mean, 0.94 L	Intervention: outpatient comprehensive pulmonary rehabilitation program Follow-up: 10 yr	Significant reduction in pulmonary hospital days for both a group of 54 patients who survived 5 yr and 44 who survived 6 yr
Johnson et al[172] (1980) United States	Sample size: 96 Gender: NA Age: 65 yr FEV$_1$: mean, 0.87 L	Intervention: 2- to 4-wk inpatient comprehensive pulmonary rehabilitation program Follow-up: 1 yr	Hospital days in the year before compared to the year after pulmonary rehabilitation were 4,081 vs 1,313 in all 96 patients and 2,808 vs 730 in 74 surviving patients

(continued)

Source/Country	Patients	Intervention/Follow-up	Outcome
Wright et al[171] (1983) United States	Sample size: 57 Gender: NA Age: NA FEV_i: NA	Intervention: 10-wk (18 visit) outpatient comprehensive pulmonary rehabilitation program Follow-up: 1 yr	Significant reduction in the total number of hospitalizations (42 vs 5) and total number of hospital days (497 vs 34) comparing the year prior to the rehabilitation program and the year following program completion

Conclusions

There is currently little information available from randomized controlled studies that evaluate the utilization of health-care resources for patients completing a comprehensive pulmonary rehabilitation program. It has been shown, however, in several nonrandomized and observational studies that there is a trend toward a decrease in the total number of hospitalization days as well as the total number of hospitalizations required for a patient with COPD in the years following completion of a comprehensive pulmonary rehabilitation program compared to the year preceding rehabilitation. Further studies are necessary, especially with the currently changing health-care environment.

SURVIVAL

Introduction

Most studies of pulmonary rehabilitation have focused on outcomes related to morbidity, QOL, exercise capacity, and health-care utilization of patients with chronic lung disease. This section reviews those articles that have included information on the survival of individuals following pulmonary rehabilitation.

Recommendation

Pulmonary rehabilitation may improve survival in patients with COPD.

Strength of Evidence = C

Scientific Evidence. Six studies have assessed the effect of comprehensive pulmonary rehabilitation on survival in patients with COPD. One was a randomized controlled trial, one was a nonrandomized controlled trial, and four were observational studies. Survival in the six studies reviewed was also compared with survival in a historical control study that predated pulmonary rehabilitation programs.[174,175]

Randomized Controlled Trials: One randomized controlled trial compared the effect of a pulmonary rehabilitation program with a group education program in 119 patients with COPD.[33] Survival at 6 years was slightly better in the group participating in the comprehensive pulmonary rehabilitation program, ie, 67%, compared with 56% for the education-only group. The difference in survival between the two groups was not statistically significant (p = 0.32) (Table 19).[33]

Nonrandomized Controlled Trials: There was one nonrandomized controlled trial that was reviewed.[166] Sneider and colleagues[166] reported a 10-year survival of 66% in patients completing a pulmonary rehabilitation program, 60% in patients evaluated by a nurse coordinator but who did not complete the program, and 53% in a group of patients with COPD who were not referred to the pulmonary rehabilitation program but who were followed up at the same hospital (Table 20).[166]

Observational Studies: Four observational studies were found and reviewed. The study by Sahn and colleagues[170] reported survival of 41% at 5 years and 17% at 10 years. The patients in this study resided at high altitude (Denver). Survival at 2.5 years was compared with that of the only other available study of patients with COPD residing at an equivalent altitude,[176] ie, patients in the Veterans Affairs (VA) Cooperative Study who did not participate in a pulmonary rehabilitation program. Survival in the Colorado study was 67% compared with 50% survival in the VA study (p < 0.05). In another

Table 19. Effect of Pulmonary Rehabilitation on Survival-Randomized Controlled Trials

Source/Country	Patients	Intervention/Follow-up	Outcome
Ries et al[33] (1995) United States	Sample size: 119 (57 rehabilitation intervention, 62 education control) Gender: 73% male Age: mean, 63 yr FEV$_1$: mean, 1.23 L	Intervention: 8-wk outpatient comprehensive rehabilitation program (12 4-h sessions with treadmill/walking exercise, education and psychosocial support) + monthly visits for 1 yr vs education control program (four 2-h sessions) Follow-up: 6 yr	Survival: Pulmonary rehabilitation 3 yr: 86% 5 yr: 67% 6 yr: 67% Education only 3 yr: 77% 5 yr: 66% 6 yr: 56% Group differences not statistically significant

Table 20. Effect of Pulmonary Rehabilitation on Survival—Nonrandomized Controlled Trials

Source/Country	Patients	Intervention/Follow-up	Outcome
Sneider et al[165] (1988) United States	Sample size: 1,133 (212 pulmonary rehabilitation, 921 no pulmonary rehabilitation) Gender: 57% male (rehabilitation) Age: mean, 65 yr (range, 40-83 yr) FEV$_1$: mean, 1.19 L (rehabilitation)	Intervention: 10-wk outpatient comprehensive pulmonary rehabilitation program; nonrehabilitation patients seen at hospital but not enrolled in rehabilitation program Follow-up: 10 yr	Survival: Pulmonary rehabilitation 3 yr: 93% 5 yr: 86% 10 yr: 66% No pulmonary rehabilitation 5 yr: 67% 10 yr: 60%

comparison of patients participating in the University of Colorado pulmonary rehabilitation program with similar patients living in the Denver area who received their medical care primarily from private physicians within the community,[177] the patients participating in the pulmonary rehabilitation program had slightly better survival (p = 0.08).

A landmark study started by Burrows and colleagues[174,175] in 1960 at a clinic established at the University of Chicago Hospitals has been used by subsequent groups as a historical control to compare survival for patients with COPD. Burrows and colleagues enrolled 200 patients (89% male/11% female) in this study. The mean age was 59 years, and the mean FEV$_1$ was 1.04 L (33.5% of predicted). Therapy for these patients was not standardized, and

patients did not participate in a pulmonary rehabilitation program. Survival in these patients was 67% at 3 years, 52% at 5 years, 23% at 10 years, and 12% at 15 years.

In a report by Bebout and associates,[178] patients who participated in a pulmonary rehabilitation program had a 5-year survival of 86% and a 10-year survival of 64%. Patients enrolled in this study had milder obstructive airway disease than those in the other studies reporting on survival. However, patients with an FEV$_1$ above 1.24 L from this study were compared with patients with a similar level of pulmonary impairment from the Burrows et al[174,175] historical control group.

Patients participating in the study by Bebout et al had significantly better survival (p < 0.01) at up to 7 years of follow-up than patients with similar impairment in the Burrows et al historical control group.

The largest study to suggest that good comprehensive care may improve survival in patients with COPD is the NIH Intermittent Positive Pressure Breathing (IPPB) trial.[179,180] Although these patients were enrolled in a multicenter collaborative study, the type of assessment, education, and training were similar to that found in pulmonary rehabilitation programs. The age and level of pulmonary impairment in patients enrolled in this study were similar to those of subjects in the Burrows et al[174,175] historical control group. A comparison of patients from the NIH IPPB study was made with those from the Burrows et al historical control group.[180] Survival was similar in patients with the least obstruction (postbronchodilator FEV_1 above 42.5% of predicted); however, in the more obstructed patients, survival was greater in the NIH IPPB patients than in the historical control group. It is possible that survival was better in the patients enrolled in the NIH IPPB study because of the careful assessment, education, training, and intense follow-up they received as being part of this clinical trial. Patients in

the NIH IPPB study were followed up for 3 years, and survival at 3 years was 77%. Survival at 3 years in the Burrows et al historical control group was 67%.

The last observational study reviewed was that from the pulmonary rehabilitation program of Burns and colleagues.[181] Five-year survival in this study was 58% compared to 52% in the Burrows et al study; 10-year survival in the Burns et al study was 32% compared to 23% in the Burrows et al study (Table 21).[171,178-181]

Conclusions

Although many factors have been shown to relate to survival in patients with COPD, the patient's age and baseline FEV_1 are the best predictors of mortality.[180] Other factors also have to be taken into consideration when attempting to compare survival curves in patients with COPD. Patients with reactive airway disease have a better prognosis than those with typical COPD (emphysema and chronic bronchitis).[182] Patients should be matched closely for age and severity of impairment since younger individuals and those with milder impairment are

Table 21. Effects of Pulmonary Rehabilitation on Survival—Observational Studies

Source/Country	Patients	Intervention/Follow-up	Outcome
Sahn et al[170] (1980) United States	Sample size: 182 Gender: 87% male Age: mean, 61 yr (range, 33-81 yr) FEV_1: mean, 0.94 L	Intervention: outpatient comprehensive pulmonary rehabilitation program Follow-up: 10 yr	Survival: 2.5 yr: 67% 3 yr: 64% 5 yr: 41% 10 yr: 17%
Bebout et al[178] (1983) United States	Sample size: 75 Gender: 61% male Age: mean, 60 yr (range, 32-82 yr) FEV_1: mean, 1.53 L	Intervention: 2-wk inpatient pulmonary rehabilitation program Follow-up: 10 yr	Survival: 3 yr: 100% 5 yr: 86% 10 yr: 64%
IPPB Trial Group[179] (1983) Anthonisen et al[180] (1986) United States	Sample size: 985 Gender: 79% male Age: mean, 61 yr FEV_1: mean, 1.03 L (36% pred)	Intervention: outpatient intensive assessment and education initially, with monthly follow-up Follow-up: 3 yr	Survival: 3 yr: 77%
Burns et al[181] (1989) United States	Sample size: 240 Gender: 54% male Age: mean, 65 yr FEV_1: mean, 0.89 L	Intervention: 4- to 5.5-wk outpatient pulmonary rehabilitation program Follow-up: 10 yr	Survival: 3 yr: 75% 5 yr: 58% 10 yr: 32%

likely to live longer. Patients who stop smoking are likely to survive longer than those who continue to smoke.[183] Oxygen therapy improves survival in patients with COPD with significant hypoxemia.[184,185] The studies reviewed in this section suggest that the type of comprehensive care provided by pulmonary rehabilitation programs may improve survival in patients with COPD. Further studies would be of value to help clarify this issue.

FUTURE RECOMMENDATIONS FOR RESEARCH

As the field of pulmonary rehabilitation has matured over the past several decades, much has been learned about the effectiveness and benefits of such programs. The practice of rehabilitation for persons with chronic lung diseases was founded in the physiology and pathophysiology of pulmonary medicine but has grown to encompass also the behavioral and social consequences that are important in understanding the impairments, disabilities, and handicaps of individuals with chronic disease. Pulmonary rehabilitation remains an art of medical practice, but one that is increasingly built on a foundation of scientific research—research that now embraces traditional outcome measures such as mortality and physiologic indexes of lung and exercise function as well as psychosocial measures such as symptoms (eg, dyspnea), health-related QOL, and economic analyses of costs and benefits.

The scientific literature highlighted in this document summarizes much of the past work in pulmonary rehabilitation. In the future, there are many potential opportunities for research in this discipline. The following are a few of the key questions and problems that present avenues for fruitful investigation:

1. What is the role of pulmonary rehabilitation in diseases other than COPD and in the increasingly popular surgical treatments for chronic lung disease (eg, transplantation, lung volume reduction surgery)?

2. How does the practice of pulmonary rehabilitation differ for the growing number of women with chronic lung disease?

3. What are the long-term benefits of pulmonary rehabilitation? How should such programs be structured to produce the greatest benefits?

4. What are the essential components of an effective pulmonary rehabilitation program (eg, exercise, education, breathing retraining, psychosocial support)?

5. How should the individual program components be designed and how might they differ when applied to individuals with different lung diseases? For instance, what are the principles of exercise training for patients with chronic lung disease? What are the benefits of lower vs upper extremity training? What, if any, is the role of VMT? Is nutritional supplementation important?

6. What are the optimal methods for measuring outcomes in pulmonary rehabilitation? How should one measure dyspnea or health-related QOL in pulmonary patients?

7. What is the cost-effectiveness of pulmonary rehabilitation in the current and future world of medical practice and health-care reimbursement?

These are but a few of the many questions that may be posed in future investigation. As an established, effective, noninvasive, and low-cost preventive health-care strategy for patients with chronic lung disease, pulmonary rehabilitation is an ideal subject for legitimate scientific inquiry within the context of the changing health-care system.

ACKNOWLEDGMENT

The authors thank Dr. Sydney Parker, Director of the ACCP Health and Science Policy Department, for organizational assistance, and Barbi Mathesius and Beth Welch from ACCP for their administrative assistance.

REFERENCES

1. Higgins MW, Thom T. Incidence, prevalence, and mortality: intra- and intercountry differences. In: Hensley MJ, Saunders NA, eds. Clinical epide-

miology of chronic obstructive pulmonary disease. New York: Marcel Dekker, 1989;23–43.

2. Feinleib M, Rosenberg HM, Collins JG, et al. Trends in COPD morbidity and mortality in the United States. Am Rev Respir Dis 1989;140:S9–S18.

3. Verbrugge LM, Patrick DL. Seven chronic conditions: their impact on US adults' activity levels and use of medical services. Am J Public Health 1995;85:173–82.

4. National Center for Health Statistics. Current estimates from the National Health Interview Survey, 1993. Vital and Health Statistics, series 10, No. 190. USDHHS (PHS), 95-1518.

5. American Thoracic Society. Standards for the diagnosis and care of patients with chronic obstructive pulmonary disease (COPD) and asthma. Am J Rev Respir Crit Care Med 1995;152:S77–121.

6. Massachusetts Medical Society. Mortality patterns—United States, 1993. MMWR 1996; 45:161–64.

7. Siafakas NM, Vermeire P, Pride NB, et al. Optimal assessment and management of chronic obstructive pulmonary disease (COPD): the European Respiratory Society Task Force. Eur Respir J 1995;8:1398–1420.

8. Ries AL. Position paper of the American Association of Cardiovascular and Pulmonary Rehabilitation: scientific basis of pulmonary rehabilitation. J Cardiopulmonary Rehabil 1990;10:418–41.

9. American Association of Cardiovascular and Pulmonary Rehabilitation. Guidelines for pulmonary rehabilitation programs. Champaign, Ill: Human Kinetics, 1993.

10. Casaburi R, Petty TL. Principles and practice of pulmonary rehabilitation. Philadelphia: WB Saunders, 1993.

11. Hodgkin JE, Connors GL, Bell CW. Pulmonary rehabilitation: guidelines to success. 2nd ed. Philadelphia: JB Lippincott, 1993.

12. Fishman AP, ed. Pulmonary rehabilitation: lung biology in health and disease (vol 91). New York: Marcel Dekker, 1996.

13. American Thoracic Society. Pulmonary rehabilitation. Am Rev Respir Dis 1981; 124: 663–66.

14. Fishman AP. Pulmonary rehabilitation research. Am J Respir Crit Care Med 1994; 149: 825–33.

15. Agency for Health Care Policy and Research. Cardiac rehabilitation: clinical practice guideline, No. 17. US Dept of Health and Human Services, 1995.

16. Casaburi R. Exercise training in chronic obstructive lung disease. In: Casaburi R, Petty TL, eds.

Principles and practice of pulmonary rehabilitation. Philadelphia: WB Saunders, 1993; 204–24.

17. Carter R, Coast JR, Idell S. Exercise training in patients with chronic obstructive pulmonary disease. Med Sci Sports Exerc 1992;24:281–91.

18. Olopade CO, Beck KC, Viggiano RW, et al. Exercise limitation and pulmonary rehabilitation in chronic obstructive pulmonary disease. Mayo Clin Proc 1992;67:144–57.

19. Celli BR. Exercise training in pulmonary rehabilitation. Semin Respir Med 1993;14:132–38.

20. Belman MJ. Exercise in patients with chronic obstructive pulmonary disease. Thorax 1993; 48:936–46.

21. Cooper CB. Determining the role of exercise in patients with chronic pulmonary disease. Med Sci Sports Exerc 1995;27:147–57.

22. Celli BR. Pulmonary rehabilitation in patients with COPD. Am J Respir Crit Care Med 1995; 152:861–64.

23. Casaburi R. Deconditioning. In: Fishman AP, ed. Pulmonary rehabilitation: lung biology in health and disease (vol 91). New York: Marcel Dekker, 1996; 213–30.

24. Chester EH, Belman MJ, Bahler RC, et al. Multidisciplinary treatment of chronic pulmonary insufficiency: III. The effect of physical training on cardiopulmonary performance in patients with chronic obstructive pulmonary disease. Chest 1977;72:695–702.

25. McGavin CR, Gupta SP, Lloyd EL, et al. Physical rehabilitation for the chronic bronchitic: results of a controlled trial of exercises in the home. Thorax 1977;32:307–11.

26. Cockcroft AE, Saunders MJ, Berry G. Randomised controlled trial of rehabilitation in chronic respiratory disability. Thorax 1981;36:200–03.

27. Busch AJ, McClements JD. Effects of a supervised home exercise program on patients with severe chronic obstructive pulmonary disease. Phys Ther 1988;68:469–74.

28. Lake FR, Henderson K, Briffa T, et al. Upper-limb and lower-limb exercise training in patients with chronic airflow obstruction. Chest 1990;97:1077–82.

29. Weiner P, Azgad Y, Ganam R. Inspiratory muscle training combined with general exercise reconditioning in patients with COPD. Chest 1992; 102:1351–56.

30. Reardon J, Awad E, Normandin E, et al. The effect of comprehensive outpatient pulmonary rehabilitation on dyspnea. Chest 1994;105:1046–52.

31. Goldstein RS, Gort EH, Stubbing D, et al. Randomised controlled trial of respiratory rehabilitation. Lancet 1994;344:1394–97.

32. Wijkstra PJ, Van Altena R, Kraan J, et al. Quality of life in patients with chronic obstructive pulmonary disease improves after rehabilitation at home. Eur Respir J 1994;7:269–73.

33. Ries AL, Kaplan RM, Limberg TM, et al. Effects of pulmonary rehabilitation on physiologic and psychosocial outcomes in patients with chronic obstructive pulmonary disease. Ann Intern Med 1995;122:823–32.

34. Strijbos JH, Postma DS, van Altena R, et al. A comparison between an outpatient hospital-based pulmonary rehabilitation program and a home-care pulmonary rehabilitation program in patients with COPD: a follow-up of 18 months. Chest 1996;109:366–72.

35. Berry MJ, Adair NE, Sevensky KS, et al. Inspiratory muscle training and whole-body reconditioning in chronic obstructive pulmonary disease: a controlled randomized trial. Am J Respir Crit Care Med 1996;153:1812–16.

36. Sinclair DJ, Ingram CG. Controlled trial of supervised exercise training in chronic bronchitis. BMJ 1980;280:519–21.

37. O'Donnell DE, McGuire M, Samis L, et al. The impact of exercise reconditioning on breathlessness in severe chronic airflow limitation. Am J Respir Crit Care Med 1995; 152: 2005–13.

38. Pollock ML, Wilmore JH. Exercise in health and disease. 2nd ed. Philadelphia: WB Saunders, 1990.

39. Davies CTM, Knibbs AV. The training stimulus: the effects of intensity, duration, and frequency of effort on maximum aerobic power output. Int Z Angew Physiol 1971;29:299–305.

40. American College of Sports Medicine position stand. The recommended quantity and quality of exercise for developing and maintaining cardiorespiratory and muscular fitness in healthy adults. Med Sci Sports Exerc 1990;22:265–74.

41. Ries AL, Archibald CJ. Endurance exercise training at maximal targets in patients with chronic obstructive pulmonary disease. J Cardiopulmonary Rehabil 1987;7:594–601.

42. Steele B. Timed walking tests of exercise capacity in chronic cardiopulmonary illness. J Cardiopulmonary Rehabil 1996;16:25–33.

43. Vyas MN, Banister EW, Morton JW, et al. Response to exercise in patients with chronic airway obstruction: I. Effects of exercise training. Am Rev Respir Dis 1971;103:390–400.

44. Holten K. Training effect in patients with severe ventilatory failure. Scand J Respir Dis 1972;53:65–76.

45. Alison JA, Samios R, Anderson SD. Evaluation of exercise training in patients with chronic airway obstruction. Phys Ther 1981;61:1273–77.

46. Mohsenifar Z, Horak D, Brown HV, et al. Sensitive indices of improvement in a pulmonary rehabilitation program. Chest 1983;83:189–92.

47. Casaburi R, Patessio A, Ioli F, et al. Reductions in exercise lactic acidosis and ventilation as a result of exercise training in patients with obstructive lung disease. Am Rev Respir Dis 1991; 143:9–18.

48. Niederman MS, Clemente PH, Fein AM, et al. Benefits of a multidisciplinary pulmonary rehabilitation program; improvements are independent of lung function. Chest 1991;99:798–804.

49. Casaburi R. Mechanisms of the reduced ventilatory requirement as a result of exercise training. Eur Respir Rev 1995;5:42–46.

50. Maltais F, LeBlanc P, Simard C, et al. Skeletal muscle adaptation to endurance training in patients with chronic obstructive pulmonary disease. Am J Respir Crit Care Med 1996;154:442–47.

51. Belman MJ, Kendregan BA. Exercise training fails to increase skeletal muscle enzymes in patients with chronic obstructive pulmonary disease. Am Rev Respir Dis 1981;123:256–61.

52. Clark CJ. The role of physical training in asthma. In: Casaburi R, Petty TL, eds. Principles and practice of pulmonary rehabilitation. Philadelphia: WB Saunders, 1993;424–38.

53. Orenstein DM, Noyes BE. Cystic fibrosis. In: Casaburi R, Petty TL, eds. Principles and practice of pulmonary rehabilitation. Philadelphia: WB Saunders, 1993;439–58.

54. Novitch RS, Thomas HM. Rehabilitation of patients with chronic ventilatory limitation from nonobstructive lung disease. In: Casaburi R, Petty TL, eds. Principles and practice of pulmonary rehabilitation. Philadelphia: WB Saunders, 1993;416–23.

55. Novitch RS, Thomas HM III. Pulmonary rehabilitation in chronic pulmonary interstitial disease. In: Fishman AP, ed. Pulmonary rehabilitation: lung biology in health and disease (vol 91). New York: Marcel Dekker, 1996;683–700.

56. Bach JR. Pulmonary rehabilitation in musculoskeletal disorders. In: Fishman AP, ed. Pulmonary rehabilitation: lung biology in health disease (vol 91). New York: Marcel Dekker, 1996;701–24.

57. Haas F, Salazar-Schicchi J, Axen K. Desensitization to dyspnea in chronic obstructive pulmonary disease. In: Casaburi R, Petty TL, eds. Principles and practice of pulmonary rehabilitation. Philadelphia: WB Saunders, 1993;241–51.

58. Casaburi R. Physiologic responses to training. Clin Chest Med 1994;15:215–27.

59. Criner GJ, Celli BR. Effect of unsupported arm exercise on ventilatory muscle recruitment in patients with severe chronic airflow obstruction. Am Rev Respir Dis 1988;138:856–61.

60. Martinez FJ, Couser JI, Celli BR. Factors influencing ventilatory muscle recruitment in patients with chronic airflow obstruction. Am Rev Respir Dis 1990;142:276–82.

61. Banzett RB, Topulos GP, Leith DE, et al. Bracing arms increases the capacity for hyperpnea. Am Rev Respir Dis 1988;138:106–09.

62. Keens GT, Krastins IRB, Wannamaker EM, et al. Ventilatory muscle endurance training in normal subjects and patients with cystic fibrosis. Am Rev Respir Dis 1977;116:853–60.

63. O'Hara WJ, Lasachuk KE, Matheson PC, et al. Weight training and backpacking in COPD. Respir Care 1984;29:1202–10.

64. Ries AL, Ellis B, Hawkins RW. Upper extremity exercise training in chronic obstructive pulmonary disease. Chest 1988;93:688–92.

65. Martinez FJ, Vogel PD, Dupont DN, et al. Supported arm exercise vs unsupported arm exercise in the rehabilitation of patients with severe chronic airflow obstruction. Chest 1993;103:1397–1402.

66. Estenne M, Knoop C, Vanvaerenbergh J, et al. The effect of pectoralis muscle training in tetraplegic subjects. Am Rev Respir Dis 1989;139:1218–22.

67. Couser JI, Martinez FJ, Celli BR. Pulmonary rehabilitation that includes arm exercise reduces metabolic and ventilatory requirements for simple arm elevation. Chest 1993;103:37–41.

68. Killian KJ, Jones NL. Respiratory muscles and dyspnea. Clin Chest Med 1988;9:237–48.

69. Mahler DA, Wells CK. Evaluation of clinical methods for rating dyspnea. Chest 1988;93:580–86.

70. Smith K, Cook D, Guyatt GH, et al. Respiratory muscle training in chronic airflow limitation: a meta-analysis. Am Rev Respir Dis 1992;145:533–39.

71. American Association of Cardiovascular and Pulmonary Rehabilitation Outcomes Committee (Pashkow P, Chair). Outcome measurement in cardiac and pulmonary rehabilitation. J Cardiopulmonary Rehabil 1995;15:394–405.

72. Pardy RL, Rivington RN, Despas PJ, et al. Inspiratory muscle training compared with physiotherapy in patients with chronic airflow limitation. Am Rev Respir Dis 1981;123:421–25.

73. Larson JL, Kim MJ, Sharp JT, et al. Inspiratory muscle training with a pressure threshold breathing device in patients with chronic obstructive pulmonary disease. Am Rev Respir Dis 1988;138:689–96.

74. Harver A, Mahler DA, Daubenspeck JA. Targeted inspiratory muscle training improves respiratory muscle function and reduces dyspnea in patients with chronic obstructive pulmonary disease. Ann Intern Med 1989;111:117–24.

75. Guyatt G, Keller J, Singer J, et al. Controlled trial of respiratory muscle training in chronic airflow limitation. Thorax 1992;47:598–602.

76. Lisboa C, Muñoz V, Beroiza T, et al. Inspiratory muscle training in chronic airflow limitation: comparison of two different training loads with a threshold device. Eur Respir J 1994;7:1266–74.

77. Preusser BA, Winningham ML, Clanton TL. High-vs low-intensity inspiratory muscle interval training in patients with COPD. Chest 1994;106:110–17.

78. Goldstein R, De Rosie J, Long S, et al. Applicability of a threshold loading device for inspiratory muscle testing and training in patients with COPD. Chest 1989;96:564–71.

79. Dekhuijzen PN, Folgering HTM, van Herwaarden CLA. Target-flow inspiratory muscle training during pulmonary rehabilitation in patients with COPD. Chest 1991;99:128–33.

80. Wanke T, Formanek D, Lahrmann H, et al. Effects of combined inspiratory muscle and cycle ergometer training on exercise performance in patients with COPD. Eur Respir J 1994;7:2205–11.

81. Belman MJ, Botnick WC, Nathan SD, et al. Ventilatory load characteristics during ventilatory muscle training. Am J Respir Crit Care Med 1994;149:925–29.

82. Agle DP, Baum GL, Chester EH, et al. Multidiscipline treatment of chronic pulmonary insufficiency: I. Psychologic aspects of rehabilitation. Psychosom Med 1973;35:41–49.

83. Borak J, Sliwinski P, Piasecki Z, et al. Psychological status of COPD patients on long term oxygen therapy. Eur Respir J 1991;4:59–62.

84. Light RW, Merrill EJ, Despars JA, et al. Prevalence of depression and anxiety in patients with COPD. Chest 1985;87:35–38.

85. Morgan AD, Peck DF, Buchanan DR, et al. Effect of attitudes and beliefs on exercise tolerance in chronic bronchitis. Br Med J 1983;286:171–73.

86. Porzelius J, Vest M, Nochomovitz M. Respiratory function, cognitions, and panic in chronic obstructive pulmonary patients. Behav Res Ther 1992;30:75–77.

87. Nicholas PK, Leuner JD. Relationship between body image and chronic obstructive pulmonary disease. Appl Nurs Res 1992;5:83–88.

88. Keele-Card G, Foxall MJ, Barron CR. Loneliness, depression, and social support of patients with COPD and their spouses. Public Health Nurs 1993;10:245–51.

89. Kersten L. Changes in self-concept during pulmonary rehabilitation, part 1. Heart Lung 1990; 19:456–62.

90. Beck JG, Scott SK, Teague RB, et al. Correlates of daily impairment in COPD. Rehab Psychol 1988;33:77–84.

91. Graydon JE, Ross E. Influence of symptoms, lung function, mood, and social support on level of functioning of patients with COPD. Res Nurs Health 1995;18:525–33.

92. Weaver TE, Narsavage GL. Physiological and psychological variables related to functional status in chronic obstructive pulmonary disease. Nurs Res 1992;41:286–91.

93. Kaplan RM, Ries AL, Prewitt LM, et al. Self-efficacy expectations predict survival for patients with chronic obstructive pulmonary disease. Health Psychol 1994;13:366–68.

94. Incalzi RA, Gemma A, Marra C, et al. Chronic obstructive pulmonary disease: an original model of cognitive decline. Am Rev Respir Dis 1993; 148:418–24.

95. Grant I, Heaton RK, McSweeny AJ, et al. Neuropsychologic findings in hypoxemic chronic obstructive pulmonary disease. Arch Intern Med 1982;142:1470–76.

96. Fix AJ, Golden CJ, Daughton D, et al. Neuropsychological deficits among patients with chronic obstructive pulmonary disease. Int J Neurosci 1982;16:99–105.

97. Ojanen M, Lahdensuo A, Laitinen J, et al. Psychosocial changes in patients participating in a chronic obstructive pulmonary disease rehabilitation program. Respiration 1993;60:96–102.

98. Emery CF, Leatherman NE, Burker EJ, et al. Psychological outcomes of a pulmonary rehabilitation program. Chest 1991;100:613–17.

99. Tandon MK. Adjunct treatment with yoga in chronic severe airways obstruction. Thorax 1978;33:514–17.

100. Renfroe KL. Effect of progressive relaxation on dyspnea and state anxiety in patients with chronic obstructive pulmonary disease. Heart Lung 1988;17:408–13.

101. Blake RL Jr, Vandiver TA, Braun S, et al. A randomized controlled evaluation of a psychosocial intervention in adults with chronic lung disease. Fam Med 1990;22:365–70.

102. Sassi-Dambron DE, Eakin EG, Ries AL, et al. Treatment of dyspnea in COPD: a controlled clinical trial of dyspnea management strategies. Chest 1995;107:724–29.

103. Janelli LM, Scherer UK, Schmieder LE. Can a pulmonary health teaching program alter patients' ability to cope with COPD? Rehab Nurs 1991;16:199–202.

104. Gift AG, Moore T, Soeken K. Relaxation to reduce dyspnea and anxiety in COPD patients. Nurs Res 1992;41:242–46.

105. Kanner RE. Early intervention in chronic obstructive pulmonary disease: a review of the Lung Health Study results. Med Clin North Am 1996;80:523–47.

106. Pederson LL, Wanklin JM, Lefcoe NM. The effects of counseling on smoking cessation among patients hospitalized with chronic obstructive pulmonary disease: a randomized clinical trial. Int J Addict 1991;26:107–19.

107. Turner SA, Daniels JL, Hollandsworth JG. The effects of a multicomponent smoking cessation program with chronic obstructive pulmonary disease outpatients. Addict Behav 1985;10:87–90.

108. Atkins CJ, Kaplan RM, Timms RM, et al. Behavioral exercise programs in the management of chronic obstructive pulmonary disease. J Consult Clin Psychol 1984;52:591–603.

109. Hopp JW, Lee JW, Hills R. Development and validation of a pulmonary rehabilitation knowledge test. J Cardiopulmonary Rehabil 1989;9:273–78.

110. Rosser R, Denford J, Heslop A, et al. Breathlessness in and psychiatric morbidity in chronic bronchitis and emphysema: a study of psychotherapeutic management. Psychol Med 1983;13:93–110.

111. Frith P, Walker P, Rowland S, et al. Using an education program for improving quality of life in patients with chronic obstructive pulmonary disease [abstract]. Chest 1993;103:180S.

112. Scherer YK, Janelli LM, Schmieder LE. Chronic obstructive pulmonary disease: does participating in a help yourself to better breathing program make a difference? J Cardiopulmonary Rehabil 1989;9:492–96.

113. Gayle RC, Spitler DL, Karper WB, et al. Psychological changes in exercising COPD patients. Int J Rehab Res 1988;11:335–42.

114. Dekhuijzen PN, Beek MM, Folgering HT, et al. Psychological changes during pulmonary rehabilitation and target-flow inspiratory muscle training in COPD patients with a ventilatory limitation during exercise. Int J Rehab Res 1990;13:109–17.

115. Fishman DB, Petty TL. Physical, symptomatic and psychological improvement in patients receiving comprehensive care for chronic airway obstruction. J Chronic Dis 1971;24:775–85.

116. Gormley JM, Carrieri-Kohlman V, Douglas MK, et al. Treadmill self-efficacy and walking performance in patients with COPD. J Cardiopulmonary Rehabil 1993;13:424–31.

117. Strijbos JH, Sluiter HJ, Postma DS, et al. Objective and subjective performance indicators in COPD. Eur Respir J 1989;2:666–69.

118. Lacasse Y, Wong E, Guyatt GH, et al. Meta-analysis of respiratory rehabilitation in chronic obstructive pulmonary disease. Lancet 1996;348:1115–19.

119. Belman MJ. Exercise in chronic obstructive pulmonary disease. Clin Chest Med 1986;7:585–97.

120. Carrieri-Kohlman V, Douglas MK, Gormley JM, et al. Desensitization and guided mastery: treatment approaches for the management of dyspnea. Heart Lung 1993;22:226–34.

121. Mall RW, Madeiros M. Objective evaluation of results of a pulmonary rehabilitation program in a community hospital. Chest 1988;94:1156–60.

122. Moser KM, Bokinsky GE, Savage RT, et al. Results of a comprehensive rehabilitation program: physiologic and functional effects on patients with chronic obstructive pulmonary disease. Arch Intern Med 1980;140:1596–1601.

123. AACVPR Outcomes Committee. Outcome measurement in cardiac and pulmonary rehabilitation. J Cardiopulmonary Rehabil 1995;15:394–405.

124. Borg GA. Psychophysical bases of perceived exertion. Med Sci Sports Exerc 1982;14:377–81.

125. Burdon JGW, Juniper EF, Killian KJ, et al. The perception of breathlessness in asthma. Am Rev Respir Dis 1982;126:825–28.

126. Lush MT, Janson-Bjerklie S, Carrieri VK, et al. Dyspnea in the ventilator-assisted patient. Heart Lung 1988;17:528–35.

127. Adams L, Chronos N, Lane R, et al. The measurement of breathlessness induced in normal patients: validity of two scaling techniques. Clin Sci 1985;69:7–16.

128. Mahler DA, Farynlarz K, Lentine T, et al. Measurement of breathlessness during exercise in asthmatics: predictor variables, reliability and responsiveness. Am Rev Respir Dis 1991;144:39–44.

129. Mador MJ, Kufel TJ. Reproducibility of visual analog scale measurement of dyspnea in patients with chronic obstructive pulmonary disease. Am Rev Respir Dis 1992;146:82–87.

130. Gift AG. Validation of a vertical visual analogue scale as a measure of clinical dyspnea. Rehab Nurs 1989;14:323–25.

131. Carrieri-Kohlman V, Gormley JM, Douglas M, et al. Patients with chronic obstructive pulmonary disease can differentiate between dyspnea and the anxiety and distress associated with it. West J Nurs Res 1996;18:626–42.

132. Mahler DA, Weinberg DM, Wells CK, et al. The measurement of dyspnea: contents, interobserver agreement, and physiologic correlates of two new clinical indexes. Chest 1984;85:751–58

133. Stoller JK, Ferranti R, Feinstein AR. Further specification and evaluation of a new clinical index for dyspnea. Am Rev Respir Dis 1986;134:1129–34.

134. Guyatt GH, Berman LB, Townsend M, et al. A measure of quality of life for clinical trials in chronic lung disease. Thorax 1987;42:773–78.

135. Wijkstra PJ, TenVergert EM, Van Altena R, et al. Reliability and validity of the chronic respiratory questionnaire (CRQ). Thorax 1994;49:465–67.

136. Jones PW, Quirk FH, Baveystock CM, et al. A self-complete measure of health status for chronic airflow limitation: the St. George's respiratory questionnaire. Am Rev Respir Dis 1992; 145:1321–27.

137. Lareau S, Kohlman-Carrieri V, Janson-Bjerklie S, et al. Development and testing of the pulmonary functional status and dyspnea questionnaire (PFSDQ). Heart Lung 1994;23:242–50.

138. Eakin EG, Sassi-Dambron DE, Ries AL, et al. Reliability and validity of dyspnea measures in patients with obstructive lung disease. Int J Behav Med 1995;2:118–34.

139. World Health Organization: constitution of the World Health Organization: basic documents. Geneva: World Health Organization, 1948.

140. Ware E Jr. Standards for validating health measures: definition and content. J Chronic Dis 1987; 40:473–80.

141. Haas A, Cardon H. Rehabilitation in chronic obstructive pulmonary disease: a 5-year study of 252 patients. Med Clin North Am 1969;53:593–606.

142. Bass H, Whitcomb JF, Forman R. Exercise training: therapy for patients with chronic obstructive pulmonary disease. Chest 1970;57:116–21.

143. Nicholas JJ, Gilbert R, Gabe R, et al. Evaluation of an exercise therapy program for patients with chronic obstructive pulmonary disease. Am Rev Respir Dis 1970;102:1–9.

144. Mertens DJ, Shephard RJ, Kavanagh T. Long-term exercise therapy for chronic obstructive lung disease. Respiration 1978;35:96–107.

145. White B, Andrews JL Jr, Mogan JJ, et al. Pulmonary rehabilitation in an ambulatory group practice setting. Med Clin North Am 1979;63:379–90.

146. Booker HA. Exercise training and breathing control in patients with chronic airflow limitation. Physiotherapy (London) 1984;70:258–60.

147. McSweeny AJ. Quality of life in relation to COPD. In: McSweeny AJ, Grant I, eds. Chronic obstructive pulmonary disease: a behavioral perspective: lung biology in health and disease (vol 36). New York: Marcel Dekker, 1988;59–85.

148. Cox NJM, Hendricks JC, Binkhorst RA, et al. A pulmonary rehabilitation program for patients with asthma and mild chronic obstructive pulmonary diseases (COPD). Lung 1993;171:235–44.

149. Make BJ, Glenn K. Outcomes of pulmonary rehabilitation. In: Bach JR, ed. Pulmonary rehabilitation: the obstructive and paralytic conditions. Philadelphia: Hanley & Belfus, 1996;173–91.

150. Bergner M, Bobbitt RA, Carter WB, et al. The sickness impact profile: development and final revision of a health status measure. Med Care 1981;19:787–805.

151. Kaplan RM, Anderson JP. A general health model policy: update and applications. Health Serv Res 1988;23:203–35.

152. Kaplan RM, Anderson JP. A general health policy model: an integrated approach. In: Spiker B, ed. Quality of life assessments in clinical trials. New York: Raven Press, 1990;131–49.

153. Ware JE Jr, Sherbourne CD. The MOS 36-item short form health survey (SF-36): I. Conceptual framework and item selection. Med Care 1992;30:473–83.

154. Wijkstra PJ. Pulmonary rehabilitation at home [editorial]. Thorax 1996;51:117–18.

155. Simpson K, Killian K, McCartney N, et al. Randomised controlled trial of weightlifting exercise in patients with chronic airflow limitation. Thorax 1992;47:70–75.

156. Guyatt GH, Berman LB, Townsend M. Long-term outcome after respiratory rehabilitation. Can Med Assoc J 1987;137:1089–95.

157. Vale F, Reardon JZ, ZuWallack RL. The long-term benefits of outpatient pulmonary rehabilitation on exercise endurance and quality of life. Chest 1993;103:42–45.

158. Reardon J, Patel K, ZuWallack RL. Improvement in quality of life is unrelated to improvement in exercise endurance after outpatient pulmonary rehabilitation. J Cardiopulm Rehabil 1993;13:51–54.

159. Petty TL, MacIlroy ER, Swigert MA, et al. Chronic airway obstruction, respiratory insufficiency, and gainful employment. Arch Environ Health 1970;21:71–78.

160. Lustig FM, Haas A, Castillo R. Clinical and rehabilitation regime in patients with chronic obstructive pulmonary diseases. Arch Phys Med Rehabil 1972;53:315–22.

161. Kass I, Dyksterhuis JE, Rubin H, et al. Correlation of psychophysiologic variables with vocational rehabilitation outcome in patients with chronic obstructive pulmonary disease. Chest 1975;67:433–40.

162. Fix AJ, Daughton D, Kass I, et al. Personality traits affecting vocational rehabilitation success in patients with chronic obstructive pulmonary disease. Psychol Rep 1978;43:939–44.

163. Holle RHO, Williams DV, Vandree JC, et al. Increased muscle efficiency and sustained benefits in an outpatient community hospital-based pulmonary rehabilitation program. Chest 1988;94:1161–68.

164. Dunham JL, Hodgkin JE, Nicol J, et al. Cost effectiveness of pulmonary rehabilitation programs. In: Hodgkin JE, Zorn EG, Connors GL, eds. Pulmonary rehabilitation: guidelines to success. Boston: Butterworth, 1984;389–402.

165. Jensen PS. Risk, protective factors, and supportive interventions in chronic airway obstruction. Arch Gen Psychiatry 1983;40:1203–07.

166. Sneider R, O'Malley JA, Kahn M. Trends in pulmonary rehabilitation at Eisenhower Medical Center: an 11-years' experience (1976–1987). J Cardiopulmonary Rehabil 1988;8:453–61.

167. Lewis D, Bell SK. Pulmonary rehabilitation, psychosocial adjustment, and use of healthcare services. Rehabil Nurs 1995;20:102–07.

168. Petty TL, Nett LM, Finigan MM, et al. A comprehensive care program for chronic airway obstruction: methods and preliminary evaluation of symptomatic and functional improvement. Ann Intern Med 1969;70:1109–20.

169. Hudson LD, Tyler ML, Petty TL. Hospitalization needs during an outpatient rehabilitation program for severe chronic airway obstruction. Chest 1976;70:606–10.

170. Sahn SA, Nett LM, Petty TL. Ten-year follow-up of a comprehensive rehabilitation program for severe COPD. Chest 1980;77(suppl):311–14.

171. Wright RW, Larsen DF, Monie RG, et al. Benefits of a community-hospital pulmonary rehabilitation program. Respir Care 1983;28:1474–79.

172. Johnson NR, Tanzi F, Balchum OJ, et al. Inpatient comprehensive pulmonary rehabilitation in severe COLD: Barlow Hospital Study. Respir Ther 1980;May/June:15–19.

173. Burton GG, Gee GN, Hodgkin JE, et al. Respiratory care warrants studies for cost-effectiveness. Hospitals 1975;49:61–71.

174. Burrows B, Earle RH. Course and prognosis of chronic obstructive lung disease. N Engl J Med 1969;280:397–404.

175. Traver GA, Cline MG, Burrows B. Predictors of mortality in chronic obstructive pulmonary disease: a 15-year follow-up study. Am Rev Respir Dis 1979;119:895–902.

176. Renzetti AD Jr, McClement JH, Litt BD. The Veterans Administration cooperative study of pulmonary function: III. Mortality in relation to respiratory function in chronic obstructive pulmonary disease. Am J Med 1966;41:115–29.

177. Petty TL. Pulmonary rehabilitation. Am Rev Respir Dis 1980;122(suppl):159–61.

178. Bebout DE, Hodgkin JE, Zorn EG, et al. Clinical and physiological outcomes of a university-hospital pulmonary rehabilitation program. Respir Care 1983;28:1468–73.

179. Intermittent Positive Pressure Breathing Trial Group. Intermittent positive pressure breathing therapy of chronic obstructive pulmonary disease. Ann Intern Med 1983;99:612–20.

180. Anthonisen NR, Wright EC, Hodgkin JE, et al. Prognosis in chronic obstructive pulmonary disease. Am Rev Respir Dis 1986;133:14–20.

181. Burns MR, Sherman B, Madison R, et al. Pulmonary rehabilitation outcome. RT: J Respir Care Practitioners 1989;2:25–30.

182. Burrows B, Bloom JW, Traver GA, et al. The course and prognosis of different forms of chronic airways obstruction in a sample from the general population. N Engl J Med 1987; 317: 1309–14.

183. Postma DS, Sluiter HJ. Prognosis of chronic obstructive pulmonary disease: the Dutch experience. Am Rev Respir Dis 1989;140(suppl):S100–05.

184. Nocturnal Oxygen Therapy Trial Group. Continuous or nocturnal oxygen therapy in hypoxemic chronic obstructive lung disease: a clinical trial. Ann Intern Med 1980;93:391–98.

185. Medical Research Council Working Party. Long-term domiciliary oxygen therapy in chronic hypoxic cor pulmonale complicating chronic bronchitis and emphysema. Lancet 1981; 1:681–86.

Training Resources

A special "thank you" to the volunteers of pulmonary rehabilitation at Mt. Diablo Medical Center, for compiling and editing the Appendix, especially Beverly Striplin, PR volunteer coordinator. "Thank you" also to the following students who assisted with this project: Jeri Bruno, Toni Hiscox, and Sara Mackle.

The appendix is current as of October 1997. For additional resources, contact your local or national home medical equipment supplier, pharmaceutical company, or the American Lung Association.

A.V. Equipment

Key:

AARC: American Association for Respiratory Care
ALA: American Lung Association
BO: Booklet
E-M: E-mail address
HTTP: Website address
S/T: Slides and tape
Tape: Cassette tape
VHS: Videotape

NAME	TYPE	COMPANY	ADDRESS/PHONE
Arm-Chair Conditioning for Better Breathing	Tape	ALA	(800) LUNG-USA*
Arterial Blood Gas Studies & PFT	VHS	Krames Communication	1100 Grundy Ln. San Bruno, CA 94066-3030 (800) 333-3032 FAX (650) 244-4512 HTTP://www.krames.com
The Asthma Handbook	S/T & BO	ALA, NY	(800) LUNG-USA or (212) 315-8700
Be in Control of Your Lungs (Patient Discharge Teaching)	Tape/BO	Gretchen Peske, Pul. Rehab. Ed.	Pulmonary Therapy Group RD #7, Box 148 Greensburg, PA 15601 (412) 837-8899 FAX (412) 837-8997
Better Breathers Panic Control Workbook 2nd Edition	Tape/BO	California College for Health Sciences, Allied Health Publishers (AHP)	222 W. 24th St. National City, CA 91950 (800) 221-7374 FAX (619) 477-5202 E-M: ahp@cchs.edu

*Dialing (800) LUNG-USA will connect you with your local American Lung Association office. If there is no office in your region you will hear a message stating that the number has been disconnected. In such a case, you should call ALA's National Office in New York at (212) 315-8700 for information.

NAME	TYPE	COMPANY	ADDRESS/PHONE
Better Breathing Today	Tape/BO	Health Communication Services, Inc.	249 S. Hwy 101, Ste. 434 Solano Beach, CA 92075 (619) 755-2459 FAX (619) 477-5202 E-M: ahp@cchs.edu
Beyond Stress Series: *Breathing Away Stress* *Relaxing Muscle Tension* *The Relaxation Response* *Focusing the Mind* *Maximizing Performance* *The Session*	VHS	TVO Video	1140 Kildaire Farm Rd. Cary, NC 27511 (800) 331-9566 FAX (919) 380-0961 E-M: ussales@tvo.org
Breath of Life: Pulmonary *Rehabilitation*	VHS	UCSD Medical Center, Pulmonary Rehab. Program	200 W. Arbor Dr. San Diego, CA 92103-8377 (619) 294-6066 FAX (619) 296-9542
Breathe Correctly, Getting *a Second Wind*	Tape	PN Medical, Inc.	214 N. Goldenrod Rd. Ste. #6 Orlando, FL 32807 (407) 898-1775 FAX (407) 894-7100
Chairobics—Home Pulmonary *Rehab*	VHS	Chairobics—Home Pulmonary Rehab	2611 W. Fanbrook Tucson, AZ 85741 (800) 521-7303
Choices—The Key Is You	VHS	Dorothy DeBolt	1931 Hidden Springs Dr. El Cajon, CA 92019 (619) 444-7757 FAX (619) 401-4061
Clearing Your Airways	Tape	Training Edge, Inc.	201 E. Dundee Rd. Palatine, IL 60067 (800) 292-4375 FAX (800) 776-0072 E-M: tei@interaccess.com
Clearing Your Airways	VHS	Encyclopaedia Britannica	310 S. Michigan Ave. Chicago, IL 60604 (312) 347-7000 FAX (312) 347-7966 E-M: info@ebec.com
COPD	VHS	Milner-Fenwick, Inc.	2125 Greenspring Dr. Timonium, MD 21093 (800) 432-8433 FAX (410) 252-6316 HTTP://www.milner-fenwick.com

NAME	TYPE	COMPANY	ADDRESS/PHONE
COPD Specialty Exercise Tape	Tape	Sit and Be Fit, Inc.	P. O. Box 8033 Spokane, WA 99203-0033 (509) 448-9438 FAX (509) 448-5078
Daydreams	Tape	Whole Person Assoc., Inc.	210 W. Michigan Duluth, MN 55802-1908 (800) 247-6789 FAX (218) 727-0505 E-M: books@wholeperson.com
Death in the West	VHS	Pyramid Film & Video	P. O. Box 1048 Santa Monica, CA 90406-1048 (800) 421-2304 FAX (310) 453-9083
Fat Stuff	VHS	Coronet MTI Film & Video	Columbus Customer Service Ctr. P. O. Box 2649 Columbus, OH 43216 (800) 321-3106 FAX (614) 771-7360
Feminine Mistake: The Next Generation	VHS	Pyramid Film & Video	P. O. Box 1048 Santa Monica, CA 90406-1048 (800) 421-2304 FAX (310) 453-9083
From Stress to Strength: How to Lighten Your Load and Save Your Life	VHS	Institute of Stress Management, Inc.	P. O. Box 279 Wilson, WY 83014-0279 (307) 733-0037 FAX (307) 734-1557
Help Yourself to Better Breathing	VHS	ALA	(800) LUNG-USA
How to Beat Cigarettes	VHS	Milner-Fenwick, Inc.	2125 Greenspring Dr. Timonium, MD 21093 (800) 432-8433 FAX (410) 252-6316 HTTP://www.milner-fenwick.com
How You Can Help Patients Stop Smoking: Opportunities for Respiratory Care Practitioners	VHS/BO	AARC	11030 Ables Ln. Dallas, TX 75229-4593 (972) 243-2272 FAX (972) 484-2720 HTTP://www.aarc.org
I Am Joe's Heart: New Version *I Am Joe's Lung: New Version*	VHS VHS	Pyramid Film & Video	P. O. Box 1048 Santa Monica, CA 90406-1048 (800) 421-2304 FAX (310) 453-9083

NAME	TYPE	COMPANY	ADDRESS/PHONE
Is It Worth Dying For (Stress)	Tape/BO	Institute of Stress Management, Inc.	P. O. Box 279 Wilson, WY 83014-0279 (307) 733-0037 FAX (307) 734-1557
Learning to Breathe Better	VHS	Encyclopaedia Britannica	310 S. Michigan Ave. Chicago, IL 60604 (312) 347-7000 FAX (312) 347-7966 E-M: info@ebec.com
Living With Asthma	VHS	Milner-Fenwick, Inc.	2125 Greenspring Dr. Timonium, MD 21093 (800) 432-8433 FAX (410) 252-6316 HTTP://www.milner-fenwick.com
Living With a Breathing Problem	VHS	Encyclopaedia Britannica	310 S. Michigan Ave. Chicago, IL 60604 (312) 347-7000 FAX (312) 347-7966 E-M: info@ebec.com
Living With Emphysema Five-part series: *1. Development and Detection* *2. Diagnosis* *3. Treatment* *4. Rehabilitation* *5. Family Support*	VHS	Aims Media Film	9710 DeSoto Ave. Chatsworth, CA 91311 (800) 367-2467 x443 FAX (818) 341-6700
Living With Stress	VHS	Milner-Fenwick, Inc.	2125 Greenspring Dr. Timonium, MD 21093 (800) 432-8433 FAX (410) 252-6316 HTTP://www.milner-fenwick.com
Making a Difference, *Opportunities for Smoking* *Cessation Counseling*	VHS	National Heart, Lung, and Blood Institution, Smoking Education Program	P. O. Box 30105 Bethesda, MD 30824-0105 (301) 251-1222
Nicotine Intervention Kit	VHS	AARC	11030 Ables Ln. Dallas, TX 75229-4593 (972) 243-2272 FAX (972) 484-2720 HTTP://www.aarc.org
Nutrition for Better Health	VHS	Milner-Fenwick, Inc.	2125 Greenspring Dr. Timonium, MD 21093 (800) 432-8433 FAX (410) 252-6316 HTTP://www.milner-fenwick.com

NAME	TYPE	COMPANY	ADDRESS/PHONE
Nutrition: Eat and Be Healthy *Overweight: Who's in Control*	VHS VHS	Milner-Fenwick, Inc.	2125 Greenspring Dr. Timonium, MD 21093 (800) 432-8433 FAX (410) 252-6316 HTTP://www.milner-fenwick.com
PEP Series: *How the Lungs Work* *What Is COPD?* *Chronic Bronchitis* *What Is Emphysema?* *Understanding Asthma* *Drug Therapy of COPD* *Inhalation Therapy* *Oxygen Therapy* *Breathing Exercises* *General Health Measures*	VHS & S/T	ALA, Florida	Gulfcoast Lung Division 15438 N. Florida Ave. Ste. 102 Tampa, FL 33613-1221 (904) 743-2933
Pulmonary Rehabilitation	VHS	AARC	11030 Ables Ln. Dallas, TX 75229 (972) 243-2272 FAX (972) 484-2720 HTTP://www.aarc.org
Pulmonary Rehabilitation: *A Success Story*	Tape	Pulmonary Education Research Foundation PERF - Mary Burns	P. O. Box 1133 Lomita, CA 90717-5133 (310) 539-8390
Pulmonary Self-Care Four-part series: *Living With a Breathing Problem* *Learning to Breathe Better* *Clearing Your Airways* *Building Your Strength and* *Endurance*	VHS	Training Edge, Inc.	201 E. Dundee Rd. Palatine, IL 60067 (800) 292-4375 FAX (847) 776-7031 E-M: tei@interaccess.com
Relaxation/Panic Control	Tape	PN Medical, Inc.	214 N. Goldenrod Rd. Ste. #6 Orlando, FL 32807 (407) 898-1775 FAX (407) 894-7100
Relaxation Techniques *for Better Breathing*	Tape	California College for Health Sciences	222 W. 24th St. National City, CA 91950 (800) 221-7374 x315 FAX (619) 477-5202 E-M: ahp@cchs.edu
Scenes: Coping With COPD	VHS	Vermont Lung Assoc.	30 Farrel St. S. Burlington, VT 05403 (802) 863-6817

NAME	TYPE	COMPANY	ADDRESS/PHONE
Secondhand Smoke	VHS	Pyramid Film & Video	P. O. Box 1048 Santa Monica, CA 90406-1048 (800) 421-2304 FAX (310) 453-9083

Self-Help: Your Strategy for Living With COPD
  1. COPD: What Is It?
  2. Learning Helpful Ways to Breathe
  3. Clearing Your Lungs to Help You Breathe Easier, Parts 1 & 2
	VHS/BO	Bull Publishing Co.	P. O. Box 208
			Palo Alto, CA 94302
			(800) 676-2855
			FAX (650) 327-3300

Smoking: Everything You and Your Family Need to Know	VHS	Ambrose Video Publishing	28 W. 44th St., Ste. 2100 New York, NY 10036 (800) 526-4663 FAX (212) 768-9282

St. John's Hospital Series
  Breathing Easier
  Chronic Lung Disease
  Living With It: Asthma
	VHS	St. John's Hospital	c/o Care Video Productions
			1650 Crossings Pkwy, Ste. F
			Westlake, OH 44145
			(216) 835-5872

Stressbreak *Relaxation* *Relaxation—Changing Behavior* *Healing Journey* *Rainbow Butterfly* (Formerly *Stress Management Series*)	VHS VHS VHS Tape	Source Cassett Learning Systems	(800) 52TAPES
Take a Deep Breath With Terry Bradshaw	VHS	Shumpert Medical Center, Pulmonary Rehabilitation	1 St. Mary Pl. Shreveport, LA 71101 (318) 681-6645 FAX (318) 681-6854
A Touch in the Night: Maintaining Intimacy for the Short of Breath	Tape	California College for the Health Sciences	222 W. 24th St. National City, CA 91950 (800) 221-7374 FAX (619) 477-5202 E-M: ahp@cchs.edu
Traveling With Lung Disease (by Dr. Joel Seidman)	VHS	Medical Center of Central Massachusetts Memorial, Pulmonary Rehabilitation	119 Belmont St. Worchester, MA 01605 (508) 793-6637

Booklets

Key:

AACVPR: American Association of Cardiovascular and Pulmonary Rehabilitation
AARC: American Association of Respiratory Care
ALA: American Lung Association
BO: Booklet
E-M: E-mail address
HTTP: Website address

NAME	TYPE	COMPANY	ADDRESS/PHONE
Airways	BO	Herc Publishing	Box 30090 Lincoln, NE 68503 (800) 676-0321
Around the Clock With COPD	BO	ALA, NY	1740 Broadway New York, NY 10019 (800) LUNG-USA (212) 315-8700
Being Close	BO	National Jewish Ctr.	1400 Jackson St. Denver, CO 80206 (800) 222-LUNG
Better Breathers Club Travel Guide	BO	ALA, San Diego	(619) 297-3901

Bronchoscopy
   Pre- and Post-Op Instructions
   Brushing, Biopsy, Extraction
     of Foreign Objects
	BO	Krames Communications	Order Department
			1100 Grundy Ln.
			San Bruno, CA 94066-9821
			(800) 333-3032
			FAX (650) 244-4512

The Choice Is Yours
   Patient Education on Artificial
   Life Support
	BO	Calif. Thoracic Society	202 Fashion Ln., Ste. 219
			Tustin, CA 92780
			(714) 730-1944
			FAX (714) 730-4057
			E-M: ctslung@aol.com

COPD
   Effects of COPD
   Breathing techniques
   Exercise and nutrition
   Treatments and medications
   Oxygen therapy
   Smoking cessation
	BO	Krames Communications	Order Department
			1100 Grundy Ln.
			San Bruno, CA 94066-9821
			(800) 333-3032
			FAX (650) 244-4512

COPD and You *A Patient Education Manual*	BO	California College for Health Sciences, Allied Health Publishers (AHP)	222 W. 24th St. National City, CA 91950 (800) 221-7374 FAX (619) 477-5202 E-M: ahp@cchs.edu
COPD Resource Guide	BO	ALA	(800) LUNG-USA

NAME	TYPE	COMPANY	ADDRESS/PHONE
Educational Resource Guide	BO	AACVPR	7611 Elmwood Ave., #201 Middleton, WI 53562-3128 (608) 831-6989 FAX (608) 831-5122 E-M: aacvpr@tmahq.com HTTP://www.aarc.org
Essentials of Pulmonary *Rehabilitation* 3-part series	BO	Pulmonary Education Research Foundation PERF - Mary Burns	P. O. Box 1133 Lomita, CA 90717-5133 (510) 539-8390
Guide for the Traveler With COPD	BO	ALA	(800) LUNG-USA
How to Use Your Metered *Dose Inhaler*	BO	ALA	(800) LUNG-USA
Lung Surgery *Lung Anatomy* *Evaluation: Imaging, Biopsy,* *Function tests* *Cancer Staging and Treatment Options* *Thoracoscopy* *Thoracotomy*	BO	Krames Communications	Order Department 1100 Grundy Ln. San Bruno, CA 94066-9821 (800) 333-3032 FAX (650) 244-4512
Self-Help: Your Strategy *for Living With COPD*	BO	Bull Publishing Co.	P. O. Box 208 Palo Alto, CA 94302 (650) 322-2855 FAX (650) 327-3300
To Air Is Human	BO	Pritchett & Hull Associates, Inc.	3440 Oakcliff Rd., NE Ste. 110 Atlanta, GA 30340 (800) 241-4925
Traveling With Oxygen	BO	AARC	11030 Ables Ln. Dallas TX 75229 (972) 243-2272 FAX (972) 484-2720 HTTP://www.aarc.org

Books/Newsletters

Key:

   AACVPR: American Association of Cardiovascular and Pulmonary Rehabilitation
   AARC: American Association for Respiratory Care
   E-M: E-mail address
   HTTP: Website address
   Nsltr: Newsletter

NAME	TYPE	COMPANY	ADDRESS/PHONE
Alpha1 News	Nsltr	Alpha 1 National Association	4220 Old Shakopee Rd., Ste. 101 Minneapolis, MN 55437-2974 (800) 521-3025 FAX (612) 885-0133 E-M: brandley@winternet.com HTTP://www.alpha1.org
Enjoying Life With Emphysema	Book	Lea & Febiger	351 West Camden Baltimore, MD 21201 (800) 638-0672
Enjoying Life With Emphysema	Book	Thomas Petty, M.D.	Williams & Wilkins Attn: Editorial Department 428 E. Preston St. Baltimore, MD 21202
FAN Newsletter	Nsltr	The Food Allergy Network	10400 Eaton Place, Ste. 107 Fairfax, VA 22030-2208 (703) 691-3179 FAX (703) 691-2713
Guide to Occupational Respiratory Disease in California	Book	CMA Publications	P. O. Box 7690 San Francisco, CA 94120-7690 (415) 882-5175 FAX (415) 882-5195
Guidelines for Pulmonary Rehabilitation Programs, AACVPR	Book	Human Kinetics	P. O. Box 5076 Champaign, IL 61825-5076 (800) 747-4457
Living Well With Emphysema and Bronchitis	Book	Doubleday & Co.	1540 N. Broadway New York, NY 10036 (800) 223-6834
The MA Report	Nsltr	Allergy & Asthma Network/Mothers of Asthmatics, Inc.	3554 Chain Bridge Rd., Ste. 200 Fairfax, VA. 22030 (800) 878-4403 or (703) 385-4403
Mainstay	Nsltr	Well Spouse Foundation	610 Lexington Ave., #814 New York, NY 10022 (212) 644-1241 FAX (212) 644-1338
Principles/Practices: Pulmonary Rehabilitation	Book	W.B. Saunders Co.	The Curtis Center, Ste. 300 Independence Square West Philadelphia, PA 19106-3399 (215) 238-7800 FAX (215) 238-8772

NAME	TYPE	COMPANY	ADDRESS/PHONE
Pulmonary Nursing Care	Book	C.V. Mosby	11830 Westline Industrial Dr. St. Louis, MO 63146 (314) 872-8370
The Pulmonary Paper	Nsltr	The Pulmonary Paper	P. O. Box 877 Ormond Beach, FL 32175 (800) 950-3698
Pulmonary Rehabilitation, Guidelines to Success	Book	J.B. Lippincott Co./Raven Press	227 E. Washington Square Philadelphia, PA 19106 (215) 238-4200
Shortness of Breath "A Guide to Better Living and Breathing" (3rd Edition)	Book	C.V. Mosby	11830 Westline Industrial Dr. St. Louis, MO 63146 (314) 872-8370
Take Care	Nsltr	National Family Caregivers Association	9621 E. Bexhill Dr. Kensington, MD 20895 (800) 896-3650 or (301) 942-6463

Agencies/Organizations

Key:
   E-M: E-mail address
   HTTP: Website address

NAME	DESCRIPTION	ADDRESS/PHONE
Alpha 1 National Association	Alpha 1 antitrypsin deficiency	4220 Old Shakopee Rd., Ste. 101 Minneapolis, MN 55437-2974 (800) 521-3025 FAX (612) 885-0133 E-M: brandley@winternet.com HTTP://www.alpha1.org
American Association of Retired Persons (AARP)	Member special benefits and services, i.e., prescriptions, insurance, volunteer opportunities and information on day-to-day living	601 E. St. NW Washington, DC 20049 (800) 424-2277
American Disability Association	Provides a quality information network for people of diverse disabilities, their care providers, and support professionals, promoting worldwide disability culture and providing forums for creating and refining social policy enhancing the quality of life for all people with disabilities. (Listed on the webnet.)	2201 6th Ave. S. Birmingham, AL 35233 (205) 323-0088 FAX (205) 251-7417 HTTP://www.adanet.org

NAME	DESCRIPTION	ADDRESS/PHONE
American Lung Association (ALA)	Educational materials—audio, booklets, etc.	1740 Broadway New York, NY 10019-4374 (800) LUNG-USA or (212) 315-8700
Asbestos Victims of America	A.V.A.	P. O. Box 66594 Scotts Valley, CA 95067 (408) 438-5864
Asthma and Allergy Foundation of America	Research, patient advocacy, getting news out to public. Has videos, programs to medical profession as well as patients.	1125 15th St. NW, Ste. 502 Washington, DC 20005 (202) 466-7643
Eldercare Locator (Aging)	In conjunction with the U.S. Administration on Aging, provides referrals to local community agencies for home care, respite services, adult day-care, senior centers, legal assistance, transportation, etc.	(800) 677-1116
MedicAlert	MedicAlert provides bracelet or necklace engraved with your medical condition, personal ID number, and MedicAlert's hotline number.	(800) 344-3226
Medicare Hotline	Hotline	(800) 638-6833
National Allergy and Asthma Network	Support and practical advice for parents	3554 Chain Bridge Rd., Ste. 200 Fairfax, VA 22030-2709 (703) 385-4403
National Assoc. of Meal Programs	Professionals and volunteers who provide congregate and home-delivered meals to elderly.	204 E. Street NE Washington, DC 20002
National Council on Aging	Directory of Adult Day Care in America	409 3rd St. SW, #200 Washington, DC 20024 (800) 424-9046 or (202) 479-1200
National Family Caregivers Association	"Take Care" quarterly newsletter, cards to caregivers three times a year. Matches them up with similar caregivers.	9621 E. Bexhill Dr. Kensington, MD 20895 (800) 896-3650 or (301) 942-6463
National Heart, Lung and Blood Institute (NHLB)	Section of National Institutes of Health, government's principal agency for research on diseases of the heart, lung, blood. A list of information is available upon request for high blood pressure, heart disease, cholesterol, smoking, lung diseases, and blood diseases, etc.	Information Center P. O. Box 30105 Bethesda, MD 20824-0105 (301) 251-1222 FAX (301) 251-1223

NAME	DESCRIPTION	ADDRESS/PHONE
National Institute on Aging Information Center	Clearing house. Call for free publications on health and aging	P. O. Box 8057 Gaithersburg, MD 20898-8057 (800) 222-2225
National Jewish Center for Immunology and Respiratory Medicine	Research and education in chronic respiratory diseases	1400 Jackson St. Denver, CO 80206 (800) 222-LUNG
National Jewish Lung Line Information Service	Updated recorded information on lung disease	(800) 222-LUNG
National Lung Association	This voluntary organization funds research and conducts educational programs on lung diseases. Has local chapters in all major cities and offers smoking cessation programs as well as educational programs about lung diseases, including influenza, pneumonia, emphysema, chronic bronchitis, and lung cancer. The association offers a variety of excellent free publications—a list is available upon request.	1740 Broadway New York, NY 10019 (212) 315-8700
Social Security Administration	Hotline	(800) 772-1213 (800) 325-0778 (TTD)
The Well Spouse Foundation	Newsletters, conferences	610 Lexington Ave. #814 New York, NY 10022 (212) 644-1241 FAX (212) 644-1338

Catalogs

Key:
    ALA: American Lung Association
    BO: Booklet
    E-M: E-mail address
    HTTP: Website address
    VHS: Videotape

NAME	DESCRIPTION	ADDRESS/PHONE
ALA	COPD, Resource Guide	(800) LUNG-USA
Bull Publishing Co.	Audio and booklet material	P. O. Box 208 Palo Alto, CA 94302 (800) 676-2855 FAX (650) 327-3300
Healthcare Advances Div. of Nimco, Inc.	Occupational Training, Nursing, Patient Education	P. O. Box 9 102 Hwy, 81 North Calhoun, KY 42327-0009 (800) 962-6662 FAX (502) 273-5844 E-M: support@nimcoinc.com HTTP://www.nimcoinc.com

NAME	DESCRIPTION	ADDRESS/PHONE
Health Edco, Div. of WRS Group, Inc.	Lifestyle education: alcohol, tobacco, drugs, nutrition, breast health	P. O. Box 21207 Waco, TX 76702-1207 (800) 299-3366, x295 FAX (888) 977-7653 E-M: sales@wrsgroup.com HTTP://www.wrsgroup.com
Herc Publishing	Patient Education Catalog	P. O. Box 30090 Lincoln, NE 68503 (800) 676-0321
Journeyworks Publishing	Health promotion and health education publishing	P. O. Box 8466 Santa Cruz, CA 95061-8466 (800) 775-1998 FAX (408) 423-8102
Krames Communications	Designed for the practice of medicine and patient education	1100 Grundy Ln. San Bruno, CA 94066-3030 (800) 333-3032 FAX (650) 244-4512 HTTP://www.krames.com
Milner & Fenwick, Inc.	Patient Education VHS & BO	2125 Greenspring Dr. Timonium, MD 21093 (800) 432-8433 FAX (410) 252-6316 HTTP://www.milner-fenwick.com
Positive Promotions	Health, wellness, safety, promotions	40-01 168th St. Flushing, NY 11358 (800) 635-2666 FAX (800) 635-2329
Pritchett & Hull Assoc., Inc.	Health education materials	3440 Oakcliff Rd. NE, Ste. 110 Atlanta, GA 30340-3079 (800) 241-4925 FAX (800) 752-0510
Tobacco Education Clearinghouse of California	Tobacco Education Materials	P. O. Box 1830 Santa Cruz, CA 95061-1830 (408) 438-4822 FAX (408) 438-3618
Whole Person Associates	Creative tools for change—books, audio, video, and more	210 West Michigan Duluth MN 55802-1908 (800) 247-6789 FAX (218) 727-0505 E-M: books@wholeperson.com HTTP://www.wholeperson.com

AACVPR Outcome Tools Resource Guide

Compiled by the American Association of Cardiovascular and Pulmonary Rehabilitation Outcomes Committee

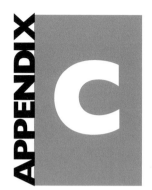

TABLE OF CONTENTS

INTRODUCTION

Within this booklet, the American Association of Cardiovascular and Pulmonary Rehabilitation (AACVPR) Outcomes Committee has compiled a synopsis of the tools currently available for measuring outcomes in cardiac and pulmonary rehabilitation (updated 12/97). After reviewing many areas of outcome, the Committee suggests selecting and measuring change in each of three general areas: Health, which includes morbidity, mortality, and quality of life; Clinical, which includes physical, psychological, and social functions; and Behavioral, which includes those behaviors patients attempt to change in order to reduce risk.

The tools have been divided into three sections. The Health section contains the quality of life tools. Functional activity and exercise-related measures, psychological measures, and psychosocial measures are found in the Clinical section. The third section contains Behavioral tools. While most of the tools listed are related to dietary change, measurement of adherence to any behavioral change that reduces risk for the patient is acceptable. We recommend that each rehabilitation program measure at least one quality of life measure, one functional activity or exercise-related measure, and one behavioral measure.

As you begin measuring outcomes, please follow the administration, scoring, and interpretation instructions carefully for each tool to ensure that the results of the measurement are valid.

While we have attempted to include all standardized, validated, and reliable tools, we know there will be some that we have missed. Further, you may have additional information about a tool which we were unable to obtain. There are several tools included with incomplete information listed. If you have additional information, please complete the template provided at the end of the Resource Guide and mail the information to the National Office. The template may also be used for additional tools with which you may be familiar. Please consider mailing a copy of this information to the AACVPR National Office for the next edition of this Guide.

The value of evaluating the outcomes of patients and programs is well established. We wish you success as you proceed in the measurement process to improve your patient and program outcomes.

—The AACVPR Outcomes Committee

HEALTH-RELATED TOOLS

GENERAL QUALITY OF LIFE TOOLS

Dartmouth Primary Care Cooperative (COOP) Information

Tool measures	Functional status: Physical, emotional, and social role function, pain, overall health, health change, quality of life, and social support
Author(s)	Dartmouth COOP Project
Reference	Wasson J, Keller A, Rubenstein L, et al: Benefits and obstacles of health status assessment in ambulatory settings: The clinician's point of view. *Med Care* 1992; 30(5)ms42-49.
Does this test measure change?	Yes
Cost to use this instrument	$15.00 administration fee for comprehensive packet with camera-ready charts.
Test method	Charts completed by interviewer or self-administered
Language of the test	English and other languages are available
Grade level for which the test is written	Simple; pictures make it useful for those with limited vocabulary
Number of items	Nine charts
Estimated time for patient	5-7 minutes
Number of patients who can take the test simultaneously	One
Level of staff needed to administer	Technician
Number of staff needed to administer test	One
Estimated time for staff to administer	5-7 minutes
Level of staff needed to score	Self-scoring
Estimated time for staff to score	None
Level of staff needed to interpret	None
Estimated time for staff to interpret	None
Equipment needed	Pencil and paper
Time and cost for equipment use per test	N/A
Applicable patient populations	Adult and geriatric populations. New charts are available for adolescent populations.
Comments	Reliable and valid but may lack sensitivity of longer instruments. Dr. Wasson has also developed Dartmouth COOP Clinical Improvement Systems with software and computer which is more comprehensive.
Source	Debbie Johnson or John Wasson, M.D., Dartmouth COOP Project, Dartmouth Medical School, Hanover, NH 03755; Phone: 603-650-1220 or 800-369-6669

DUKE Health Profiles

Tool measures	Five health measures (physical, mental, social, general, and perceived), a self-esteem measure, and four measures of dysfunction (anxiety, depression, pain, and disability)
Author(s)	George Parkerson, Jr., M.D., M.P.H.
Reference	Parkerson GR Jr, Broadhead WE, Tse-C-KJ: The Duke Health Profile, a 17-item measure of health and dysfunction. *Med Care* 1990;28:1056-1072.
Does this test measure change?	Yes
Cost to use this instrument	None for noncommercial use
Test method	Self-administered
Language of the test	English and nine translations
Grade level for which the test is written	Simple for even less educated adults (interviewer administered for those with less than a ninth grade education)
Number of items	63
Estimated time for patient	2-4 minutes
Number of patients who can take the test simultaneously	Unlimited
Level of staff needed to administer	Secretary or aide
Number of staff needed to administer test	One
Estimated time for staff to administer	Only distribution time
Level of staff needed to score	Trained to score manually or by computer
Estimated time for staff to score	Minutes
Level of staff needed to interpret	Trained
Estimated time for staff to interpret	Minutes
Equipment needed	Calculator or computer
Time and cost for equipment use per test	Minutes
Applicable patient populations	Adults with acute or chronic illness or well adults
Comments	
Source	George Parkerson, M.D., Dept. of Community and Family Medicine, Box 3886, Duke University Medical Center, Durham, NC 27710; Phone: 919-684-3620 ext. 452

Illness Effects Questionnaire

Tool measures	Biological, psychological, and social aspects of disease from patient's perspective
Author(s)	Glen Greenberg, Ph.D.; Rolf Peterson, Ph.D.; Robert Heilbronner, Ph.D.
Reference	Copyrighted in 1989

Does this test measure change?	It is a "state" measure.
Cost to use this instrument	None
Test method	Paper and pencil; self-administered
Language of the test	English
Grade level for which the test is written	Eighth grade and above
Number of items	20
Estimated time for patient	20 minutes
Number of patients who can take the test simultaneously	No limit
Level of staff needed to administer	N/A
Number of staff needed to administer test	None
Estimated time for staff to administer	5-10 minutes to give patients directions and follow-up for missing data
Level of staff needed to score	N/A
Estimated time for staff to score	N/A
Level of staff needed to interpret	N/A
Estimated time for staff to interpret	15 minutes
Equipment needed	None
Time and cost for equipment use per test	N/A
Applicable patient populations	Physical medicine, chronic pain, dialysis, cancer, and cardiac patients.
Comments	
Source	Glen D. Greenberg, M.D., Children's Rehabilitation Hospital, Thomas Jefferson University Hospital, Ford Road and Fairmount Park, Philadelphia, PA 19131; Phone: 215-879-9041

Medical Outcomes Study Short Form (MOS SF-36)

Tool measures	Health and functional status in eight areas under three categories: 1) functional status (physical functioning, social functioning, and role limitations attributed to physical and emotional problems), 2) well-being (mental health, energy/fatigue, pain), and 3) general health perception
Author(s)	J.E. Ware and C.D. Sherbourne
Reference	Stewart AL, Hays RD, Ware JE: The MOS Short Form General Health Survey: Reliability and validity in a patient population. *Med Care* 1988;724-735.
Does this test measure change?	Yes
Cost to use this instrument	$145.00
Test method	Self-administered
Language of the test	English and Spanish

Grade level for which the test is written	
Number of items	36 (covers eight health concepts from MOS surveys)
Estimated time for patient	10-15 minutes
Number of patients who can take the test simultaneously	Unlimited
Level of staff needed to administer	None
Number of staff needed to administer test	None
Estimated time for staff to administer	None
Level of staff needed to score	Different recoding for Pain and Health Perception Scales; training in data entry or scanning for computer scoring needed
Estimated time for staff to score	Minutes
Level of staff needed to interpret	
Estimated time for staff to interpret	2 minutes
Equipment needed	Computer for scoring
Time and cost for equipment use per test	Royalty-free upon completion of user agreement
Applicable patient populations	U.S. adults with mild to severe chronic medical and psychiatric problems
Comments	The Rand 36 Item Health Survey: Contains the same 36 items as SF-36; Scoring has been recoded so high score indicates a better state of health. Pain & Health Perception scored differently from SF-36; Survey costs nothing, but there is a $3 shipping/handling charge; The RAND Corporation, 1700 Main Street, P. O. Box 2138, Santa Monica, CA 90407-2138; Phone: 310-451-7002; FAX: 310-451-6915.
	HSQ (Health Status Questionnaire): Contains the same 36 items plus 3 to screen for depression; Scoring has been recoded so high score indicates a better state of health. Pain & Health Perception scored differently from SF-36. Questionnaire costs $22; The Health Outcomes Institute, 2001 Killebrew Dr., Ste. 122, Bloomington, MN 55425; Phone: 612-858-9188; FAX: 612-858-9189.
Source	Medical Outcomes Trust, 20 Park Plaza, Ste. 1014, Boston, MA 02116; Phone: 617-426-4046; Fax: 617-426-4131

Multidimensional Health Locus of Control Inventory (MHLOC)

Tool measures	Perceived control over health and health care
Author(s)	Wallston, Wallston, and DeVellis
Reference	Health Education Monograph (1978)
Does this test measure change?	Yes
Cost to use this instrument	Photocopying costs
Test method	Paper and pencil

Language of the test	English
Grade level for which the test is written	Eighth grade
Number of items	18
Estimated time for patient	10 minutes
Number of patients who can take the test simultaneously	Unlimited
Level of staff needed to administer	Technician
Number of staff needed to administer test	One
Estimated time for staff to administer	
Level of staff needed to score	Technician
Estimated time for staff to score	
Level of staff needed to interpret	Technician
Estimated time for staff to interpret	
Equipment needed	Test form
Time and cost for equipment use per test	Minimal
Applicable patient populations	Used extensively in research studies including studies of cardiac and pulmonary patients. Clinical utility is not clear.
Comments	
Source	Health Education Monographs

Nottingham Health Profile (NHP)

Tool measures	Quality of life including energy, pain, emotional reaction, physical mobility, sleep, social isolation, and activities of daily living.
Author(s)	Sonja Hunt and Carlos Martini
Reference	Hunt SM, McEwen J, McKenna SP: A quantitative approach to perceived health. *J Epid Com Health* 1980;34:281-295.
Does this test measure change?	Yes
Cost to use this instrument	No cost
Test method	Pencil and paper; interview or self-administered
Language of the test	English (has been translated to other languages)
Grade level for which the test is written	N/A
Number of items	45
Estimated time for patient	10 minutes
Number of patients who can take the test simultaneously	Unlimited
Level of staff needed to administer	No special training required. Permission to administer test from authors only.

Number of staff needed to administer test	Patient-administered
Estimated time for staff to administer	N/A
Level of staff needed to score	Basic data entry skills
Estimated time for staff to score	10 minutes manually or 2 minutes by computer
Level of staff needed to interpret	Basic patient counseling skills are required.
Estimated time for staff to interpret	5 minutes to explain test results
Equipment needed	None
Time and cost for equipment use per test	N/A
Applicable patient populations	Multiple patient populations, including cardiac patients
Comments	Easy to use and extensively tested. It addresses Score/Scale 1-100 (1 = no impact; 100 = major impact). 1977, revised 1981.
Source	Marilyn Berhner, Ph.D., Professor, Health Policy and Management, School of Hygiene and Public Health, The Johns Hopkins University, 624 North Broadway, Baltimore, MD 21205

Quality of Life Systemic Inventory (QLSI)

Tool measures	The gap between the patient's actual condition and his/her goal for 30 life domains, taking into account the priority of each life domain and the actual dynamic process of evolution within each one (this represents the QOL score)
Author(s)	Gilles Dupuis, Ph.D.
Reference	Dupuis G, Perrault J, Lambany MC, Kennedy E, David P: A new tool to assess quality of life: The Quality of Life System Inventory. *Quality of Life and Cardiovascular Care* 1989; Spring:36-45.
Does this test measure change?	Yes and allows comparison with normal subjects
Cost to use this instrument	$100 for two 1-hour sessions of training (interview, scoring, and interpreting), $3.00 or $5.00 per copy for automated scoring, depending on the level of scoring asked, or $250 to buy scoring material and diskette
Test method	Interview
Language of the test	English and French
Grade level for which the test is written	
Number of items	30
Estimated time for patient	45-60 minutes
Number of patients who can take the test simultaneously	Individual or small group of 5-10
Level of staff needed to administer	Undergraduate (psychology, nursing, social worker) with experience in interviewing or patient contact
Number of staff needed to administer test	One

Estimated time for staff to administer	45-60 minutes
Level of staff needed to score	Undergraduate (psychology, nursing, social worker)
Estimated time for staff to score	15 minutes to score and 5 minutes of data entry
Level of staff needed to interpret	Undergraduate (psychology, nursing, social worker)
Estimated time for staff to interpret	Scores are immediately interpretable in terms of changes or comparison to normal subjects.
Equipment needed	Macintosh and Excel software. IBM will soon be available.
Time and cost for equipment use per test	N/A
Applicable patient populations	Any population, including normal subjects
Comments	
Source	Gilles Dupuis, Ph.D., Montreal Heart Institute, 5000 Belanger East, Montreal, Quebec Canada H1T 1C8; Phone: 514-376-3330, ext. 3441

Quality of Well-Being Scale (QWB)

Tool measures	Mobility, physical activity, social activity, self-care, and symptoms
Author(s)	Robert M. Kaplan
Reference	Kaplan RM, Atkins CJ, Timms RM: Validity of a quality of well-being scale as an outcome measure in chronic obstructive pulmonary disease. *Journal of Chronic Disease* 1984;37(2):85-95.
Does this test measure change?	Yes
Cost to use this instrument	$69.00 includes instrument, taped interview, interview instructions, coding and scoring interview
Test method	Structured interview
Language of the test	English, French, Spanish, Navajo, and Indonesian
Grade level for which the test is written	Ninth grade
Number of items	18-62
Estimated time for patient	10-15 minutes
Number of patients who can take the test simultaneously	One
Level of staff needed to administer	Research associate or someone trained by formal training session
Number of staff needed to administer test	One
Estimated time for staff to administer	10-15 minutes
Level of staff needed to score	
Estimated time for staff to score	15-20 minutes by hand (computerized version available)
Level of staff needed to interpret	Trained
Estimated time for staff to interpret	

Equipment needed

Time and cost for equipment use per test   See above

Applicable patient populations   Adults with disease or injury

Comments

Source   Holly Teetzel, Hope Outcomes Assessment Project; Phone: 619-543-5496

Sickness Impact Profile (SIP)

Tool measures   Perceived health status in physical, psychological, and five independent factors

Author(s)   B.S. Gibson, M. Bergner, R.A. Bobbitt, and W.B. Carter

Reference   Gibson BS, Gibson JS: The Sickness Impact Profile—Development of an outcome. *Annals of Internal Medicine* 1975;65(12):1304-1310.

Does this test measure change?   Yes

Cost to use this instrument $100 administration and training manual on diskette

Test method   Interview or self-administered

Language of the test   English and Spanish

Grade level for which the test is written

Number of items   136 (12 categories, 2 dimensions [physical and psychosocial])

Estimated time for patient   30 minutes

Number of patients who can take the test simultaneously   Unlimited if self-administered

Level of staff needed to administer   Trained staff to explain

Number of staff needed to administer test   If self-administered, none. If interviewed, one staff member to each patient.

Estimated time for staff to administer   If interview, 30 minutes

Level of staff needed to score   Trained staff

Estimated time for staff to score   5-10 minutes

Level of staff needed to interpret   Psychologist

Estimated time for staff to interpret

Equipment needed   Calculator

Time and cost for equipment use per test   Photocopying costs

Applicable patient populations   Relevant to all types and severities of illnesses

Comments   1976, revised 1981

Source   Julia Bouie, School of Hygiene and Public Health, Room 607, The Johns Hopkins University, 624 North Broadway, Baltimore, MD 21205; Phone: 410-955-5660; Fax: 410-955-0470

Symptom Questionnaire

Tool measures	Depression, anxiety, somatic symptoms, and anger-hostility
Author(s)	Robert Kellner, M.D., Ph.D.
Reference	
Date	1987
Does this test measure change?	No, it measures the present condition of the above four variables. If repeated postrehab, change can be assessed.
Cost to use this instrument	$10.00-$25.00
Test method	Yes/No questions and answers
Language of the test	English (has been translated to other languages)
Grade level for which the test is written	Unknown
Number of items	92
Estimated time for patient	2-5 minutes
Number of patients who can take the test simultaneously	Unlimited
Level of staff needed to administer	No special training required
Number of staff needed to administer test	One
Estimated time for staff to administer	5-10 minutes
Level of staff needed to score	Office staff
Estimated time for staff to score	2 minutes
Level of staff needed to interpret	Office staff
Estimated time for staff to interpret	2 minutes
Equipment needed	Stenciled score sheet
Time and cost for equipment use per test	Minimal
Applicable patient populations	Psychiatric patient populations
Comments	Limited use in patients with pulmonary disease and has not been used in cardiac patients. One advantage to the test is that it is quick and easy to score.
Source	University of New Mexico, Health Sciences Center; Phone: 505-272-1724

Psychosocial Adjustment to Illness Scale

Tool measures	Coping with illness; handicap
Author(s)	G.R. Morrow, R. Chiarello, and L. Derogatis
Reference	*Psychological Medicine,* 1978; 8:605-610.
Does this test measure change?	Yes

Cost to use this instrument	Initial fee for questionnaire approximately $35
Test method	Self-report questionnaire
Language of the test	English
Grade level for which the test is written	Sixth grade
Number of items	45
Estimated time for patient	15 minutes
Number of patients who can take the test simultaneously	Unlimited
Level of staff needed to administer	Technician
Number of staff needed to administer test	One
Estimated time for staff to administer	None
Level of staff needed to score	Technician
Estimated time for staff to score	5 minutes
Level of staff needed to interpret	Health care worker
Estimated time for staff to interpret	5 minutes
Equipment needed	Pencil
Time and cost for equipment use per test	None
Applicable patient populations	Chronic illness (e.g., COPD)
Comments	Has been used to assess COPD patients and to monitor outcome following rehabilitation
Source	Clinical Psychometric Research, Inc., P.O. Box 619, Riderwood, MD 21139

CARDIAC-SPECIFIC QUALITY OF LIFE TOOLS

Outcomes Institute Angina TyPE Specification

Tool measures	Outcomes of patients with possible or proven coronary artery disease. It also can be used to evaluate important changes.
Author(s)	David B. Pryor, M.D.
Reference	
Date	1993
Does this test measure change?	Yes
Cost to use this instrument	$8.00 administrative fee
Test method	Self-administered
Language of the test	English
Grade level for which the test is written	

Number of items	9.1 = 14 (all patients at entry); 9.8 = 12 (all patients at follow-up); 9.2 - 9.6 (short questionnaires completed by physician based on patient's course of care)
Estimated time for patient	Few minutes
Number of patients who can take the test simultaneously	Unlimited
Level of staff needed to administer	Clinical
Number of staff needed to administer test	One
Estimated time for staff to administer	Few minutes
Level of staff needed to score	Office staff
Estimated time for staff to score	Few minutes
Level of staff needed to interpret	
Estimated time for staff to interpret	
Equipment needed	
Time and cost for equipment use per test	Photocopying costs and equipment
Applicable patient populations	Patients with angina chest pain
Comments	This tool is to be used in conjunction with the SF-36.
Source	Health Outcomes Institute, 2001 Killebrew Drive, Suite 122, Bloomington, MN 55425; Phone: 612-858-9188; Fax: 612-858-9189

Minnesota Living With Heart Failure Questionnaire (LHFQ)

Tool measures	Quality of life, including physical, socioeconomic, and psychological impairments in patients with congestive heart failure
Author(s)	T.S. Rector, S.H. Kubo, J.N. Cohn
Reference	Rector, TS, Kubo SH, Cohn JN: Patients' self-assessment of their congestive heart failure. *Heart Failure* 1987;Oct/Nov:198-209.
Does this test measure change?	Yes
Cost to use this instrument	Free of charge
Test method	Self-administered test
Language of the test	English
Grade level for which the test is written	Approximately sixth grade level
Number of items	21
Estimated time for patient	10-15 minutes
Number of patients who can take the test simultaneously	Unlimited
Level of staff needed to administer	Office staff; instructions are provided and are minimal.
Number of staff needed to administer test	One

Estimated time for staff to administer	15 minutes
Level of staff needed to score	Office staff
Estimated time for staff to score	3-5 minutes
Level of staff needed to interpret	Office staff
Estimated time for staff to interpret	3-5 minutes
Equipment needed	None
Time and cost for equipment use per test	None
Applicable patient populations	Congestive heart failure patients
Comments	
Source	Thomas Rector, Ph.D., Dept. of Medicine, Cardiovascular Division, University of Minnesota, Box 508 UMHC, 420 Delaware Street, SE, Minneapolis, MN 55455

Quality of Life After Myocardial Infarction

Tool measures	Health-related quality of life
Author(s)	Neil Oldridge, Ph.D.
Reference	Oldridge N, Guyatt G, Jones NL, et al: Effects on quality of life with comprehensive rehabilitation after acute myocardial infarction. *Am J Cardiol* 1991;67:1084-1089.
Does this test measure change?	Yes
Cost to use this instrument	Free of charge
Test method	Self-administered or interviewed questionnaire
Language of the test	English
Grade level for which the test is written	
Number of items	26
Estimated time for patient	10 minutes
Number of patients who can take the test simultaneously	Unlimited
Level of staff needed to administer	N/A
Number of staff needed to administer test	N/A
Estimated time for staff to administer	N/A
Level of staff needed to score	Office staff
Estimated time for staff to score	N/A
Level of staff needed to interpret	N/A
Estimated time for staff to interpret	N/A
Equipment needed	Paper questionnaire

Time and cost for equipment use per test	None
Applicable patient populations	MI patient populations
Comments	None
Source	For information, contact Diane at 414-229-6568.

Ferrans and Powers Quality of Life Index (QLI)—Cardiac Version

Tool measures	Measures four dimensions of quality of life: health and functioning, socioeconomic, psychological/spiritual, and family
Author(s)	Carol Ferrans and Marjorie Powers
Reference	Ferrans CE, Powers MJ: Psychometric assessment of the quality of life index. *Research in Nursing and Health* 1992;15:29-38.
Does this test measure change?	Yes
Cost to use this instrument	Nominal administrative fee then cost of copying for test-taking
Test method	Self-administered questionnaire
Language of the test	English, Spanish, Mandarin Chinese, and other translations
Grade level for which the test is written	Fourth grade
Number of items	72
Estimated time for patient	10 minutes
Number of patients who can take the test simultaneously	Unlimited
Level of staff needed to administer	Office staff
Number of staff needed to administer test	None
Estimated time for staff to administer	None if self-administered, 10-20 minutes if interviewed
Level of staff needed to score	Statistician
Estimated time for staff to score	Coding takes approximately 15 minutes with computer, 30 minutes manually.
Level of staff needed to interpret	Masters level
Estimated time for staff to interpret	Varies
Equipment needed	Calculator or computer
Time and cost for equipment use per test	Time and expense of copying tool
Applicable patient populations	Cardiac patients. A version has also been developed for respiratory patients.
Comments	First part measures satisfaction with 39 aspects of life and the second part measures importance of those aspects to the patients.
Source	Carol Estwing Ferrans, Ph.D., R.N., FAAN, Dept. of Medical-Surgical Nursing, College of Nursing (M/C 802), University of Illinois at Chicago, 845 South Damen Avenue, Chicago, IL 60612-7350; Phone: 312-996-7900; Fax: 312-996-4979

PULMONARY-SPECIFIC QUALITY OF LIFE TOOLS

Chronic Respiratory Disease Questionnaire (CRQ)

Tool measures	Dyspnea, fatigue, emotional function, mastery of disease
Author(s)	G. H. Guyatt, L. B. Berman, M. Townsend, et al.
Reference	Guyatt GH, Berman LB, Townsend M, et al: A measure of quality of life for clinical trials in chronic lung disease. *Thorax* 1987;42:773-778.
Does this test measure change?	Yes
Cost to use this instrument	$50
Test method	Interview
Language of the test	English
Grade level for which the test is written	
Number of items	123
Estimated time for patient	15-30 minutes
Number of patients who can take the test simultaneously	One
Level of staff needed to administer	Respiratory nurse/RCP
Number of staff needed to administer test	One per patient
Estimated time for staff to administer	Up to 30 minutes
Level of staff needed to score	Respiratory nurse/RCP
Estimated time for staff to score	30 minutes
Level of staff needed to interpret	Respiratory nurse/RCP
Estimated time for staff to interpret	Included in score time
Equipment needed	Pencil and paper
Time and cost for equipment use per test	Minimal
Applicable patient populations	Chronic obstructive pulmonary disease
Comments	Measures items of change associated with dyspnea and life functions. Limitation is time as this is not a self-administered test. This is a hallmark of pulmonary disease questionnaires.
Source	Dr. Gordon Guyatt, Dept. of Clinical Epidemiology, McMaster University Medical Center, 1200 Main Street, Hamilton, Ontario, Canada L8N 3Z5; Phone: 905-525-9140, ext. 22900

The Living With Asthma Questionnaire

Tool measures	Quality of life in patients with asthma
Author(s)	Michael Hyland, Ph. D.
Reference	Hyland, ME: The living with asthma questionnaire: *Respiratory Medicine* 1991;85(suppl B):13-16.

Does this test measure change?	Yes
Cost to use this instrument	
Test method	Self-administered, paper and pencil or interviewer assisted
Language of the test	English
Grade level for which the test is written	Unknown
Number of items	68
Estimated time for patient	20 minutes
Number of patients who can take the test simultaneously	Unlimited if self-administered
Level of staff needed to administer	
Number of staff needed to administer test	At least one
Estimated time for staff to administer	20 minutes
Level of staff needed to score	Physician, nurse, professional
Estimated time for staff to score	A few minutes
Level of staff needed to interpret	Physician, nurse, professional
Estimated time for staff to interpret	Minutes
Equipment needed	
Time and cost for equipment use per test	
Applicable patient populations	Asthmatics
Comments	Designed to be a screening device to assist in individual patient management and as an outcome evaluation for use in clinical trials (e.g., steroid use). Use as a pulmonary rehabilitation program outcome measurement instrument is questionable.
Source	M. E. Hyland, Ph.D., Professor of Psychology, Dept. of Psychology, University of Plymouth, Plymouth, Deron PL4 8AA United Kingdom; Phone: 44-1752-233238; Fax: 44-1752-233176

Pulmonary Functional Status and Dyspnea Questionnaire (PFSDQ)

Tool measures	Dyspnea and functional status in patients with respiratory disease
Author(s)	Suzanne C. Lareau, R.N., M.S.
Reference	Lareau S, Carrieri-Kohlman V, Janson-Bjerklie S, Roos P: Development and testing of the Pulmonary Functional Status and Dyspnea Questionnaire (PFSDQ). *Heart and Lung* 1994;23(3):242-250.
Does this test measure change?	Yes
Cost to use this instrument	
Test method	Self-administered questionnaire
Language of the test	English

Grade level for which the test is written	Unknown
Number of items	82 dyspnea questions and 76 activity questions
Estimated time for patient	15 minutes
Number of patients who can take the test simultaneously	Unlimited
Level of staff needed to administer	Office staff
Number of staff needed to administer test	One
Estimated time for staff to administer	Minimal
Level of staff needed to score	Minimal math skills
Estimated time for staff to score	10 minutes
Level of staff needed to interpret	
Estimated time for staff to interpret	Few minutes
Equipment needed	
Time and cost for equipment use per test	
Applicable patient populations	Those with moderate to severe chronic obstructive pulmonary disease
Comments	Strong emphasis on ADLs plus a comprehensive dyspnea measure. This tool has promise.
Source	Suzanne Lareau, R.N., M.S. (111-P), Jerry L. Pettis VA Hospital, 11201 Benton Street, Loma Linda, CA 93457; Phone: 909-422-3098, ext. 2656; Fax: 909-777-3214

Pulmonary Functional Status Scale (PFSS)

Tool measures	Activities of daily living in respiratory patients including self care, transportation, household tasks, grocery shopping, meal prep, daily activities, relationships, dyspnea anxiety, depression
Author(s)	Terri Weaver, Ph.D., R.N., C.S.
Reference	Weaver TE, Narsavage GL: Physiological and psychological variables related to functional status in chronic obstructive pulmonary disease. *Nursing Res* 1992;41:286-291.
Does this test measure change?	Pre- and post-ADLs can be measured
Cost to use this instrument	None
Test method	Questionnaire can be completed at home by patient
Language of the test	English
Grade level for which the test is written	Seventh grade (Flesch-Kincaid Grade Level)
Number of items	82 dyspnea questions and 79 activity questions
Estimated time for patient	15-30 minutes

Number of patients who can take the test simultaneously	One
Level of staff needed to administer	Office staff
Number of staff needed to administer test	N/A
Estimated time for staff to administer	N/A
Level of staff needed to score	
Estimated time for staff to score	20 minutes manually, less with a computer
Level of staff needed to interpret	Minimal arithmetic required to obtain scores
Estimated time for staff to interpret	
Equipment needed	Questionnaire
Time and cost for equipment use per test	N/A
Applicable patient populations	Chronic obstructive pulmonary disease
Comments	Not widely tested, but it has face validity and concurrent validity with Sickness Impact Profile (r = 0.54). Test-retest reliability was r = 0.67.
Source	Suzanne Lareau, R.N., M.S. (111-P), Jerry L. Pettis VA Hospital, 11201 Benton Street, Loma Linda, CA 93457; Phone: 909-422-3098, ext. 2656; Fax: 909-777-3214

The Saint George's Respiratory Questionnaire (SGRQ)

Tool measures	Symptoms, activity, impact
Reference	Jones PW, Quirk FH, Baveystock CM, Littlejohn P: A self-complete measure of health status for chronic airflow limitation. ARRD 1992;145:1321-1327.
Does this test measure change?	Yes
Cost to use this instrument	N/A
Test method	Paper and pencil, self-administered questionnaire
Language of the test	English, Finnish, Dutch, Italian, French, Spanish, Portuguese, German, Swedish, Norwegian, Danish, and Japanese
Grade level for which the test is written	Unknown
Number of items	50 (76 responses)
Estimated time for patient	10-15 minutes
Number of patients who can take the test simultaneously	Unlimited
Level of staff needed to administer	Basic training level required
Number of staff needed to administer test	One
Estimated time for staff to administer	Self-administered (supervised)

Level of staff needed to score	Computer program
Estimated time for staff to score	5 minutes
Level of staff needed to interpret	Experienced
Estimated time for staff to interpret	
Equipment needed	Pencil
Time and cost for equipment use per test	Minimal
Applicable patient populations	Asthmatics and patients with chronic obstructive pulmonary disease
Comments	Suitable for a wide range of treatments
Source	Dr. Paul Jones, St. George Hospital Medical School, Dept. of Physiological Medicine, Granmor Terrace, London SW17, United Kingdom; Phone: 44-1817-255371

CLINICAL TOOLS

PHYSICAL-FUNCTIONAL ACTIVITY AND EXERCISE-RELATED MEASURES

Baseline Dyspnea Index and Transitional Dyspnea Index (BDI/TDI)

Tool measures	Baseline and transitional dyspnea
Author(s)	Donald Mahler, D.H. Weinberg, C.K. Wells, A.R. Feinstein
Reference	Mahler DA, Weinberg DH, Wells CK, Feinstein AR: The measurement of dyspnea: Contents, interobserver agreement and physiologic correlates of two new clinical indexes. *Chest* 1984;85:751-758.
Does this test measure change?	Specifically designed to measure changes in functional impairment, magnitude of task needed to evoke dyspnea, and magnitude of effort needed to evoke dyspnea.
Cost to use this instrument	Personnel time only
Test method	Interview
Language of the test	English
Grade level for which the test is written	
Number of items	47 (3 categories with 5 possible choices in each)
Estimated time for patient	5-10 minutes
Number of patients who can take the test simultaneously	One per interviewer
Level of staff needed to administer	Physician, nurse, or respiratory therapist with advanced knowledge of chronic dyspnea
Number of staff needed to administer test	One
Estimated time for staff to administer	5-10 minutes

Level of staff needed to score	Physician, nurse, or respiratory therapist with advanced knowledge of chronic dyspnea
Estimated time for staff to score	Done simultaneously during interview
Level of staff needed to interpret	Physician, nurse, or respiratory therapist with advanced knowledge of chronic dyspnea
Estimated time for staff to interpret	Done simultaneously during interview
Equipment needed	Paper and pencil
Time and cost for equipment use per test	Personnel time
Applicable patient populations	Applicable to patients with chronic dyspnea and respiratory disease
Comments	At first intimidating to do, but this can soon easily become incorporated into the interview and follow-up process.
Source	Pulmonary and Critical Care Medicine School, Dartmouth Hitchcock Medical Center, 1 Medical Center Drive, Lebanon, NH 03756-0001; Phone 603-650-5533; Fax: 603-650-4437

Borg Scale

Tool measures	Severity of dyspnea on a 1-1 0 category scale (with ratio properties)
Author(s)	Gunnar Borg
Reference	Borg, G: Perceived exertion as an indicator of somatic stress. *Scandinavian Journal of Rehabilitation Medicine* 1970;2:92-98.
Does this test measure change?	Yes (perceived exertion)
Cost to use this instrument	Personnel time only
Test method	Patient is asked to rate his/her perception of exertion. The non-linear spacing of verbal descriptions of severity anchored to specific numbers provides that this scale has ratio properties of sensation intensities.
Language of the test	English
Grade level for which the test is written	
Number of items	
Estimated time for patient	Seconds
Number of patients who can take the test simultaneously	Up to 10
Level of staff needed to administer	Staff with specific instructions on how to use test
Number of staff needed to administer test	One
Estimated time for staff to administer	Seconds
Level of staff needed to score	Staff with specific instructions on how to use test
Estimated time for staff to score	Done simultaneously during interview
Level of staff needed to interpret	Physician, nurse, or respiratory therapist with advanced knowledge of chronic dyspnea

Estimated time for staff to interpret	Done simultaneously during questioning
Equipment needed	Copy of Borg Scale readily visible during exercise
Time and cost for equipment use per test	None additional to exercise equipment
Applicable patient populations	Applicable to cardiac and pulmonary patients
Comments	May be used during multistage testing or any rehabilitation activity to rate perceived exertion
Source	See reference.

Duke Activity Status Index (DASI)

Tool measures	Functional Status
Author(s)	M. Hlatky, R. Boineau, M. Higgenbotham
Reference	Hlatky M, Boineau R, Higgenbotham M, et al: A brief self-administered questionnaire to determine functional capacity (the Duke Activity Status Index). *Am J Cardiol* 1989;64:651-654.
Does this test measure change?	Yes (perceived exertion)
Cost to use this instrument	
Test method	Self-administered
Language of the test	English
Grade level for which the test is written	Eighth grade
Number of items	12
Estimated time for patient	Less than 5 minutes
Number of patients who can take the test simultaneously	Unlimited
Level of staff needed to administer	Anyone
Number of staff needed to administer test	One
Estimated time for staff to administer	Minutes
Level of staff needed to score	Anyone
Estimated time for staff to score	Less than one minute
Level of staff needed to interpret	Medical
Estimated time for staff to interpret	Less than one minute
Equipment needed	
Time and cost for equipment use per test	
Applicable patient populations	Applicable to cardiac and pulmonary patients
Comments	

Source   Mark Hlatky, M.D., Stanford University School of Medicine, Health
                                        Services Research, HRP Redwood Building, Room 150, Stanford, CA
                                        94305-5092; Phone: 415-723-6426

Functional Status Questionnaire

Tool measures   Physical, psychological, social, and role function in ambulatory patients

Author(s)   A.M. Jette, A.R. Davies, P.D. Cleary

Reference   Jette AM, Davies AR, Cleary PD, et al: The Functional Status Question-
                                        naire: Reliability and validity when used in primary care. *Journal of Gen-
                                        eral Internal Medicine* 1986;1:143-149.

Does this test measure change?   Yes

Cost to use this instrument

Test method   Self-administered

Language of the test   English

**Grade level for which the test
is written**

Number of items   34

Estimated time for patient   15 minutes

**Number of patients who can take   Unlimited
the test simultaneously**

Level of staff needed to administer Clerical

**Number of staff needed to   One
administer test**

**Estimated time for staff to   Minutes
administer**

Level of staff needed to score   Trained in data entry

Estimated time for staff to score   Minutes

Level of staff needed to interpret Trained

**Estimated time for staff to   Computer scored in minutes. Computer generated report summary
interpret**   gives patients "status" in each scale.

Equipment needed   Computer and software

**Time and cost for equipment
use per test**

Applicable patient populations   Adults (oriented to time and place)

Comments   Six scores of functional status to screen for disability and monitor clini-
                                        cal change in function

Source   Alan Jette, Ph.D., Massachusetts General Hospital, Institute of Health
                                        Professions, Boston, MA 02114

Graded Exercise Test (GXT)

Tool measures   Using treadmill or cycle ergometer, this tool measures workload, oxygen
                                        consumption (direct or indirect), heart rate, arrhythmias, and blood pres-
                                        sure responses with exertion.

Author(s)

Reference   *Guidelines for Graded Exercise Testing and Exercise Prescription.* American College of Sports Medicine. Baltimore, MD: Williams & Wilkins; 1991.

Does this test measure change?   Yes, if done pre- and post-rehabilitation

Cost to use this instrument   Moderately expensive

Test method   Single user test

Language of the test

Grade level for which the test is written

Number of items

Estimated time for patient   1 hour

Number of patients who can take the test simultaneously   One

Level of staff needed to administer   Exercise physiologist, nurse, therapist, and/or physician

Number of staff needed to administer test   One or two

Estimated time for staff to administer   1 hour

Level of staff needed to score   Exercise physiologist, nurse, therapist, and/or physician

Estimated time for staff to score   30 minutes

Level of staff needed to interpret   Physician

Estimated time for staff to interpret   30 minutes

Equipment needed   Treadmill, monitor, gas analyzer (optional, but recommended), oximeter

Time and cost for equipment use per test   Moderately expensive

Applicable patient populations   Applicable to cardiac and pulmonary patients

Comments   Useful as a pre-rehabilitation test to pick up ischemia, abnormal blood pressure response, arrhythmias, and for prescribing exercise

Source   See reference; Phone: 800-358-3583

Human Activity Profile (HAP)

Tool measures   Activity level based on estimated METs

Author(s)   A. James Fix and David M. Daughton

Reference   Psychological Assessment Resources (PAR), Inc.

Does this test measure change?   Yes

Cost to use this instrument $42.90 for 50 test booklets

Test method   Self-report

Language of the test   English

Grade level for which the test is written   Fourth grade

Number of items	94
Estimated time for patient	30 minutes
Number of patients who can take the test simultaneously	Unlimited
Level of staff needed to administer	Good communicator to explain the procedure
Number of staff needed to administer test	One
Estimated time for staff to administer	30 minutes
Level of staff needed to score	High school
Estimated time for staff to score	10 minutes
Level of staff needed to interpret	College degree
Estimated time for staff to interpret	10 minutes
Equipment needed	Pencil, table, chair
Time and cost for equipment use per test	
Applicable patient populations	Applicable to cardiac and pulmonary rehabilitation patients, ages 20-79
Comments	Contains other scales and subscales, dyspnea, activity subscales (self-care, personal/household work, entertainment/social, independent exercise), and muscle group subscales (hand use, leg effort, back effort, wheelchair activities)
Source	Psychological Assessment Resources, Inc., 10500 University Center Drive, Suite 270, Tampa, FL 33612; Phone: 800-331-8378

NYHA Functional Classification

Tool measures	Grades limitations of ability to perform physical activity
Author(s)	R. Harvey, E. Doyle, K. Ellis
Reference	Harvey R, Doyle E, Ellis K, et al: Major changes made by the Criteria Committee of the New York Heart Association. *Circulation* 1974;49:390.
Does this test measure change?	Yes
Cost to use this instrument	Free of charge
Test method	Physician-given
Language of the test	N/A
Grade level for which the test is written	N/A
Number of items	4
Estimated time for patient	Minutes
Number of patients who can take the test simultaneously	One
Level of staff needed to administer	Physician

Number of staff needed to administer test	One
Estimated time for staff to administer	Minutes
Level of staff needed to score	Scored simultaneously with administration
Estimated time for staff to score	Minutes
Level of staff needed to interpret	Basic
Estimated time for staff to interpret	Minutes
Equipment needed	None
Time and cost for equipment use per test	None
Applicable patient populations	Applicable to cardiac patients
Comments	Contains other scales and subscales, dyspnea, activity subscales (self-care, personal/household work, entertainment/social, independent exercise), and muscle group subscales (hand use, leg effort, back effort, wheelchair activities)
Source	See reference.

Six or Twelve Minute Walk

Tool measures	Exercise endurance (area of function)
Author(s)	C.R. McGavin, S.P. Gupta, G.J.R. McHardy
Reference	McGavin CR, Gupta SP, McHardy GJR: Twelve minute walking test for assessing disability in chronic bronchitis. *British Medical Journal* 1976;1:822-823.
Does this test measure change?	Yes, usually performed before and after exercise intervention
Cost to use this instrument	Free of charge
Test method	Observed distance covered in 6 or 12 minute period with number and duration of rest periods. Noted VIS, oximetry, and Borg RPE measured during and after walk.
Language of the test	
Grade level for which the test is written	
Number of items	
Estimated time for patient	30 minutes
Number of patients who can take the test simultaneously	Unlimited
Level of staff needed to administer	BLS certification needed
Number of staff needed to administer test	One
Estimated time for staff to administer	30 minutes
Level of staff needed to score	No special education

Estimated time for staff to score	5 minutes
Level of staff needed to interpret	
Estimated time for staff to interpret	
Equipment needed	Flat, indoor walking area; chairs; sphygmomanometer; stethoscope; clock; oximeter; counting device
Time and cost for equipment use per test	
Applicable patient populations	Patients with respiratory impairment, some cardiac patients
Comments	Reliable, valid test. Easily performed with minimal staff and equipment resources. Performed before and immediately after rehabilitation at 1, 3, 6, and 12 month intervals to determine sustained effects. Patients using oxygen do the walk with staff person carrying the cylinder.
Source	See reference.

Specific Activity Scale

Tool measures	Functional class
Author(s)	L. Goldman, B. Hashimoto, E.F. Cook, et al.
Reference	Goldman L, Hashimoto B, Cook EF, et al: Comparative reproducibility and validity of systems for assessing cardiovascular functional class: Advantages of a new Specific Activity Scale. *Circulation* 1981;64:1227-1234.
Does this test measure change?	Yes
Cost to use this instrument	Free of charge
Test method	Self-administered
Language of the test	English
Grade level for which the test is written	
Number of items	21
Estimated time for patient	3-5 minutes
Number of patients who can take the test simultaneously	Unlimited
Level of staff needed to administer	Clinician to explain
Number of staff needed to administer test	1
Estimated time for staff to administer	3-5 minutes if patient needs assistance
Level of staff needed to score	Office staff
Estimated time for staff to score	Less than one minute
Level of staff needed to interpret	Office staff
Estimated time for staff to interpret	Less than one minute
Equipment needed	Forms

Time and cost for equipment use per test

Applicable patient populations   Adult population

Comments   Reliable and easily reproduced scale based on number of metabolic equivalents of the activities the patient can perform

Source   See reference.

Visual Analog Scale (VAS)

Tool measures	Severity of dyspnea with a 100 mm vertical line during exercise
Author(s)	A.G. Gift
Reference	Gift AG: Validation of a vertical visual analog scale as a measure of clinical dyspnea. *Rehab Nurse* 1989;14:323-325.
Does this test measure change?	Yes, quantifies the severity of dyspnea before, during, and after exercise
Cost to use this instrument	Free of charge
Test method	Patient asked to rate severity of dyspnea on a 100 mm vertical straight line with two anchor points, one at each extreme
Language of the test	N/A
Grade level for which the test is written	N/A
Number of items	N/A
Estimated time for patient	Seconds
Number of patients who can take the test simultaneously	Up to 10
Level of staff needed to administer	Respiratory therapist, physical therapist, or nurse familiar with VAS
Number of staff needed to administer test	One
Estimated time for staff to administer	Seconds
Level of staff needed to score	Respiratory therapist, physical therapist, or nurse familiar with VAS
Estimated time for staff to score	Seconds
Level of staff needed to interpret	Respiratory therapist, physical therapist, or nurse familiar with VAS
Estimated time for staff to interpret	Seconds
Equipment needed	Copy of scale and ruler in mm measure
Time and cost for equipment use per test	Staff time only
Applicable patient populations	Cardiac and pulmonary patients
Comments	Simple, brief and minimal expense. Study concludes that maximal VAS ratings are reproducible while submax VAS ratings and relationship between VAS ratings and physiologic variables vary quite a bit.
Source	Audrey Gift, University of Pennsylvania; Phone: 215-898-6395

PSYCHOLOGICAL TOOLS

Beck Depression Inventory (BDI)

Tool measures	Depressive symptomatology
Author(s)	Aaron Beck
Reference	Beck A: *The Beck Depression Inventory.* ed. Philadelphia, PA: Center for Cognitive Therapy; 1978.
Does this test measure change?	Yes
Cost to use this instrument	$45.00 for 25 tests.
Test method	Paper and pencil
Language of the test	English
Grade level for which the test is written	Eighth grade
Number of items	21
Estimated time for patient	5-10 minutes
Number of patients who can take the test simultaneously	Unlimited
Level of staff needed to administer	Technician
Number of staff needed to administer test	One
Estimated time for staff to administer	10 minutes
Level of staff needed to score	Technician
Estimated time for staff to score	5 minutes
Level of staff needed to interpret	Clinical psychologist
Estimated time for staff to interpret	N/A
Equipment needed	Test
Time and cost for equipment use per test	
Applicable patient populations	12-86 years
Comments	Useful for assessing depressive symptoms in any patients participating in cardiopulmonary rehabilitation. Particularly useful because it is quite brief and has been utilized in a number of clinical and research settings. Revised 1996.
Source	The Psychological Corporation, Order Service Center, P.O. Box 839954, San Antonio, TX 78283-3954; Phone: 800-228-0752

Cardiac Depression Scale (CDS)

Tool measures	Depression
Author(s)	David Hare, M.D.

Reference	Hare D, Davis C: Validation of a new depression scale for cardiac patients in quality of life assessment. *Australia New Zealand Journal of Medicine* 1993;23:630.
Does this test measure change?	Theoretically it should, but not enough data to be sure
Cost to use this instrument	
Test method	Self-administered questionnaire
Language of the test	English
Grade level for which the test is written	Eighth grade
Number of items	26
Estimated time for patient	10 minutes
Number of patients who can take the test simultaneously	Unlimited
Level of staff needed to administer	Technician
Number of staff needed to administer test	One
Estimated time for staff to administer	10 minutes
Level of staff needed to score	Technician
Estimated time for staff to score	15 minutes
Level of staff needed to interpret	
Estimated time for staff to interpret	15 minutes
Equipment needed	Test forms
Time and cost for equipment use per test	
Applicable patient populations	Cardiac patients
Comments	This is a new measure with limited data on reliability and validity. Although the scale is designed for cardiac patients, the items are not specific to cardiac disease and the scale could be used with other populations. However, it should be viewed as an experimental instrument until further data are available.
Source	David Hare, M.D., Cardiology Dept. at Austin Hospital, Heidelberg, Victoria 3084 Australia

Center for Epidemiological Studies—Depression Mode Scale (CES-D)

Tool measures	Depression symptomatology
Author(s)	L. Radloff
Reference	Radloff L: The CES-D scale: A self-report depression scale for research in the general population. *Applied Psychological Measurement* 1977;1:385-401.
Does this test measure change?	Yes
Cost to use this instrument	Free of charge

Test method	Paper and pencil
Language of the test	English
Grade level for which the test is written	Eighth grade
Number of items	20
Estimated time for patient	10 minutes
Number of patients who can take the test simultaneously	Unlimited
Level of staff needed to administer	Technician
Number of staff needed to administer test	One
Estimated time for staff to administer	10 minutes
Level of staff needed to score	Technician
Estimated time for staff to score	5 minutes
Level of staff needed to interpret	Technician
Estimated time for staff to interpret	
Equipment needed	Photocopied test
Time and cost for equipment use per test	None
Applicable patient populations	Applicable to any patient participating in cardiopulmonary rehabilitation. This test is especially good for older adult patients because items weigh less heavily on somatic symptoms of depression.
Comments	Quite brief and has been utilized in a number of clinical and research settings.
Source	Helen Lejner, Program Assistant, Epidemiology and Psychopathology Branch, Division of Clinical Research, National Institute for Mental Health, 5600 Fishers Lane, Room 10C-09, Rockville, MD 20857; Phone: 301-443-3774

Cook Medley Hostility Scale

Tool measures	Hostility
Author(s)	W.W. Cook and D.M. Medley
Reference	Cook WW, Medley DM: Proposed hostility and pharisaic-virtue scales for the MMPI. *J Appl Psych* 1954; 38:414-418.
Does this test measure change?	
Cost to use this instrument	
Test method	
Language of the test	
Grade level for which the test is written	

Number of items

Estimated time for patient

Number of patients who can take the test simultaneously

Level of staff needed to administer

Number of staff needed to administer test

Estimated time for staff to administer

Level of staff needed to score

Estimated time for staff to score

Level of staff needed to interpret

Estimated time for staff to interpret

Equipment needed

Time and cost for equipment use per test

Applicable patient populations

Comments

Source   See reference.

COPD Self-Efficacy Scale

Tool measures	Confidence level
Author(s)	Joan Wigel, Thomas Creer, Harry Kotses
Reference	Wigel J, Creer T, Kotses H: The COPD Self-Efficacy Scale. *Chest* 1991;99:1193-1196.
Does this test measure change?	Yes
Cost to use this instrument	None
Test method	Paper and pencil
Language of the test	English
Grade level for which the test is written	Estimated at sixth to eighth grade
Number of items	34
Estimated time for patient	5-10 minutes
Number of patients who can take the test simultaneously	Unlimited
Level of staff needed to administer	Professional
Number of staff needed to administer test	One
Estimated time for staff to administer	5-10 minutes

Level of staff needed to score	Secretarial/Clerical
Estimated time for staff to score	3-5 minutes
Level of staff needed to interpret	Professional
Estimated time for staff to interpret	25 minutes
Equipment needed	Paper and pencil
Time and cost for equipment use per test	None
Applicable patient populations	COPD patients
Comments	Seems limiting as it only measures a person's confidence level prior to patient trying physical activities. Assumes that the COPD patient does not participate in activities due to a limited amount of confidence in successfully completing the activity. This is only a measure of self-efficacy.
Source	Dr. Joan Wigel, Dept. of Psychology, Ohio University, Athens, OH 45701; Phone: 614-593-1023.

COPE Inventory

Tool measures	Different ways in which people respond to stress
Author(s)	D.S. Carver, M.P. Scheier, S.K. Weintraub
Reference	Carver DS, Scheier MP, Weintraub SK: Assessing coping strategies: A theoretically based approach. *Journal of Personality and Social Psychology* 1989;56:267-283.
Does this test measure change?	Possibly
Cost to use this instrument	Test must be purchased from author
Test method	Paper and pencil
Language of the test	English
Grade level for which the test is written	Eighth grade
Number of items	60
Estimated time for patient	20 minutes
Number of patients who can take the test simultaneously	Unlimited
Level of staff needed to administer	Technician
Number of staff needed to administer test	One
Estimated time for staff to administer	
Level of staff needed to score	Technician
Estimated time for staff to score	
Level of staff needed to interpret	Professional
Estimated time for staff to interpret	

Equipment needed	Purchase forms and scoring materials from author
Time and cost for equipment use per test	
Applicable patient populations	Those who participate in cardiopulmonary rehabilitation
Comments	Helps to assess patients' style of coping with stress, including physical illness.
Source	See reference.

Face Scale

Tool measures	Mood
Author(s)	C. Lorish and R. Maisiak
Reference	Lorish C, Maisiak R: The Face Scale: A brief, nonverbal method for assessing patient mood. *Arthritis and Rheumatism* 1986;29(7):906-910.
Does this test measure change?	Yes
Cost to use this instrument	
Test method	Interview
Language of the test	Nonverbal
Grade level for which the test is written	N/A
Number of items	20 drawings
Estimated time for patient	Less than 2 minutes
Number of patients who can take the test simultaneously	One
Level of staff needed to administer	Trained
Number of staff needed to administer test	One-on-one
Estimated time for staff to administer	Less than 2 minutes
Level of staff needed to score	
Estimated time for staff to score	
Level of staff needed to interpret	Psychologist
Estimated time for staff to interpret	
Equipment needed	
Time and cost for equipment use per test	
Applicable patient populations	Originally used with arthritic patients but applicable across all patient populations.
Comments	None
Source	Christopher Lorish, Ph.D., Office of Educational Development, Volker Hall, L21O-C, Birmingham, AL 35294; Phone: 205-934-4011 (main number), 205-934-5909 (Dr. Lorish)

Jenkins Activity Survey (JAS)

Tool measures	Four common components of Type A behavior
Author(s)	C. Jenkins, R. Rosenman, M. Friedman
Reference	Jenkins C, Rosenman R, Friedman M: Development of an objective psychological test for the determination of the coronary prone behavior pattern in employed men. *J Chronic Dis* 1976;20:371-379 or Rosenman R, Brand R, Jenkins C, et al: Coronary heart disease in the Western Collaborative Group Study: Final follow-up experience of 8 1/2 years. *JAMA* 1975; 233:872-877.
Does this test measure change?	Yes
Cost to use this instrument	Test must be purchased
Test method	Paper and pencil
Language of the test	English
Grade level for which the test is written	Eighth grade
Number of items	20
Estimated time for patient	20 minutes
Number of patients who can take the test simultaneously	Unlimited
Level of staff needed to administer	Technician
Number of staff needed to administer test	One
Estimated time for staff to administer	20 minutes
Level of staff needed to score	Technician
Estimated time for staff to score	15 minutes
Level of staff needed to interpret	Professional
Estimated time for staff to interpret	15 minutes
Equipment needed	Forms and scoring materials must be purchased
Time and cost for equipment use per test	$26 manual only, $27.25 preview package (manual, questionnaire, and one question service sheet)
Applicable patient populations	Patients participating in cardiopulmonary rehabilitation. Most widely used measure of Type A behavior pattern in clinical and research settings.
Comments	None
Source	Psychological Corporation, Order Service, P.O. Box 839954, San Antonio, TX 78283-3954; Phone: 800-228-0752

Minnesota Multiphasic Personality Inventory (MMPI)-2

Tool measures	Personality functioning, including depression, anxiety, psychosis, and personality disorders
Author(s)	W. Dahlstrom, G. Walsh, L. Dahlstrom

Reference	Dahlstrom W, Walsh G, Dahlstrom L: *An MMPI Handbook. Clinical interpretation* (rev ed.) Minneapolis, MN: University of Minnesota; 1975 or Greene RL: *The MMPI, an interpretive manual.* New York: Grune & Stratton, 1980.
Does this test measure change?	No
Cost to use this instrument	Test forms and scoring materials need to be purchased
Test method	Paper and pencil
Language of the test	English
Grade level for which the test is written	Eighth grade
Number of items	366
Estimated time for patient	3 hours
Number of patients who can take the test simultaneously	Unlimited
Level of staff needed to administer	Technician
Number of staff needed to administer test	One
Estimated time for staff to administer	3 hours
Level of staff needed to score	Technician
Estimated time for staff to score	
Level of staff needed to interpret	Psychologist
Estimated time for staff to interpret	
Equipment needed	Forms and scoring materials
Time and cost for equipment use per test	
Applicable patient populations	Useful for assessing personality functioning in any patients participating in cardiopulmonary rehabilitation. Particularly useful because it has been used in numerous research studies. Well validated, especially in revised form.
Comments	None
Source	See reference.

Profile of Mood States (POMS)

Tool measures	Various mood states (e.g., tension, anger, depression, confusion)
Author(s)	D. McNair, M. Lorr, L. Droppleman
Reference	McNair D, Lorr M, Droppleman L (eds): *Profile of Mood States.* San Diego, CA: Educational and Industrial Testing Service; 1971.
Does this test measure change?	Yes
Cost to use this instrument	
Test method	Paper and pencil

Language of the test	English
Grade level for which the test is written	Eighth grade
Number of items	65
Estimated time for patient	3-5 minutes
Number of patients who can take the test simultaneously	Unlimited
Level of staff needed to administer	Technician
Number of staff needed to administer test	One
Estimated time for staff to administer	3-5 minutes
Level of staff needed to score	Technician
Estimated time for staff to score	1 minute per sheet; can be sent to testing service for scoring.
Level of staff needed to interpret	Psychologist
Estimated time for staff to interpret	15 minutes
Equipment needed	Photocopied test forms
Time and cost for equipment use per test	
Applicable patient populations	Useful for assessing mood in any patient participating in cardiopulmonary rehabilitation
Comments	
Source	Educational and Industrial Testing Service, P.O. Box 7234, San Diego, CA 92107; Phone: 619-222-1666

Psychological General Well-Being Index (PGWB)

Tool measures	Both negative (e.g., depression, anxiety) and positive (e.g., vitality, health) mood states
Author(s)	H. Dupuy
Reference	National conference on evaluation in alcohol, drug abuse, and mental health programs, 1974.
Does this test measure change?	Yes
Cost to use this instrument	Cost of photocopying
Test method	Paper and pencil
Language of the test	English
Grade level for which the test is written	Eighth grade
Number of items	22
Estimated time for patient	15 minutes
Number of patients who can take the test simultaneously	Unlimited

Level of staff needed to administer	Technician
Number of staff needed to administer test	One
Estimated time for staff to administer	15 minutes
Level of staff needed to score	Technician
Estimated time for staff to score	10 minutes
Level of staff needed to interpret	Professional
Estimated time for staff to interpret	
Equipment needed	Photocopied test forms
Time and cost for equipment use per test	None
Applicable patient populations	Any patient participating in cardiopulmonary rehabilitation
Comments	Has been used in past studies of exercise and psychological functioning
Source	Wenger N, Mattson M, Furbewrg C (eds): Assessment of quality of life in clinical trials of cardiovascular therapies. *LeJacq*, 1984; 170-173.

Sixteen Personality Factor Questionnaire (16PF)

Tool measures	Sixteen different personality factors including emotional stability, self-sufficiency, tension, rigidity
Author(s)	Raymond Cattell, Karen Cattell, and Heather Cattell
Reference	
Does this test measure change?	Possibly
Cost to use this instrument	$107.50 includes administration manual, 10 reusable booklets, 25 answer sheets, individual record forms, and scoring template.
Test method	Paper and pencil
Language of the test	English
Grade level for which the test is written	Eighth grade
Number of items	185
Estimated time for patient	35-50 minutes
Number of patients who can take the test simultaneously	Unlimited
Level of staff needed to administer	Technician
Number of staff needed to administer test	One
Estimated time for staff to administer	60 minutes
Level of staff needed to score	Technician
Estimated time for staff to score	15 minutes
Level of staff needed to interpret	Professional

Estimated time for staff to interpret

Equipment needed	Scoring materials and forms
Time and cost for equipment use per test	
Applicable patient populations	Any patient participating in cardiopulmonary rehabilitation
Comments	Has been used in past studies of exercise and psychological functioning.
Source	Joyce Brown, Director of Sales, Institute for Personality and Ability Testing, P. O. Box 1188, Champaign, IL 61824-1188; Phone: 800-225-4728

State Trait Anger Expression Inventory

Tool measures	State and trait anger
Author(s)	Charles D. Spielberger, Ph.D.
Reference	
Does this test measure change?	State anger
Cost to use this instrument	$74 for manual and 50 booklets
Test method	Self-administered
Language of the test	English (other languages are available)
Grade level for which the test is written	Fifth grade
Number of items	44
Estimated time for patient	15 minutes
Number of patients who can take the test simultaneously	Unlimited
Level of staff needed to administer	Trained
Number of staff needed to administer test	One
Estimated time for staff to administer	15 minutes
Level of staff needed to score	Anyone can be trained
Estimated time for staff to score	5 minutes
Level of staff needed to interpret	Psychologist or someone with experience with tests and measures
Estimated time for staff to interpret	10-15 minutes
Equipment needed	
Time and cost for equipment use per test	
Applicable patient populations	All populations
Comments	No software, but has mail-in service; offers scannable answer sheet
Source	Psychological Assessment Resources, Inc., P.O. Box 998, Odessa, FL 33556-9901; Phone: 800-331-TEST

State Trait Anxiety Scale

Tool measures	State anxiety and trait anxiety
Author(s)	C. Spielberger, R. Gonsuch, R. Luschene
Reference	Spielberger C, Gonsuch R, Luschene R (eds): *Manual for the State-Trait Anxiety Inventory.* Palo Alto, CA: Consulting Psychologists Press; 1970.
Does this test measure change?	Yes, in anxiety
Cost to use this instrument	$25 for sampler set; $90 for complete set (200 cases and permission package)
Test method	Self-administered
Language of the test	English with some translations available
Grade level for which the test is written	High school and above
Number of items	40
Estimated time for patient	15 minutes
Number of patients who can take the test simultaneously	Unlimited
Level of staff needed to administer	Untrained
Number of staff needed to administer test	One
Estimated time for staff to administer	Depends on reading level of participant
Level of staff needed to score	Anyone with training
Estimated time for staff to score	5 minutes
Level of staff needed to interpret	Not difficult; may use a psychologist if preferred
Estimated time for staff to interpret	5 minutes
Equipment needed	None
Time and cost for equipment use per test	None
Applicable patient populations	Unspecified
Comments	
Source	Mind Garden, P. O. Box 60669; Palo Alto, CA 94306; Phone: 415-424-8493.

Symptom Checklist-90-Revised (SCL-90-R)

Tool measures	Subjective indicators of psychological well-being, including depression, anxiety, hostility, somatization
Author(s)	R. Derogatis, R. Brand, C. Jenkins
Reference	Derogatis R, Brand R, Jenkins C, et al: *Administration, Scoring and Procedures Manual II.* Towson, MD: Clinical Psychometric Research; 1983.
Does this test measure change?	Yes

Cost to use this instrument	$49
Test method	Paper and pencil
Language of the test	English
Grade level for which the test is written	Eighth grade
Number of items	90
Estimated time for patient	20 minutes
Number of patients who can take the test simultaneously	Unlimited
Level of staff needed to administer	Technician
Number of staff needed to administer test	One
Estimated time for staff to administer	20 minutes
Level of staff needed to score	Technical
Estimated time for staff to score	10 minutes
Level of staff needed to interpret	Psychologist
Estimated time for staff to interpret	
Equipment needed	Purchase of forms and computerized scoring procedure from author
Time and cost for equipment use per test	
Applicable patient populations	Any patient participating in cardiopulmonary rehabilitation
Comments	Quite brief and has been utilized in a number of clinical and research settings
Source	NCS Assessments, 5605 Green Circle Drive, Minnetonka, MN 55343; Phone: 800-627-7271

Ways of Coping Questionnaire

Tool measures	Thoughts and actions people use to handle stressful situations
Author(s)	Folkman and Lazarus
Reference	*Journal of Personality and Social Psychology* 1985;48:150-170
Does this test measure change?	Possibly
Cost to use this instrument	$25 for 25 tests; $25 for samplers; $90 for permission, manual, and scoring test
Test method	Paper and pencil
Language of the test	English
Grade level for which the test is written	Eighth grade
Number of items	
Estimated time for patient	10 minutes
Number of patients who can take	Unlimited

the test simultaneously

Level of staff needed to administer	Technician
Number of staff needed to administer test	One
Estimated time for staff to administer	10 minutes
Level of staff needed to score	Technical
Estimated time for staff to score	10 minutes
Level of staff needed to interpret	Professional
Estimated time for staff to interpret	
Equipment needed	Scoring materials and forms
Time and cost for equipment use per test	
Applicable patient populations	Cardiopulmonary, but also available for other diagnoses
Comments	Helps to assess patients' style of coping with stress. Widely used and validated.
Source	Mind Garden, P. O. Box 60669, Palo Alto, CA 94306; Phone: 415-424-8493

PSYCHOSOCIAL TOOLS

Locke-Wallace Marital Adjustment Test (LWMAT)

Tool measures	Marital adjustment
Author(s)	H J. Locke and K.M. Wallace
Reference	Locke HJ, Wallace KM: Short marital adjustment and prediction tests: Their reliability and validity. *Marriage and Family Living* 1959;21:251-255.
Does this test measure change?	Yes
Cost to use this instrument	
Test method	Self-administered
Language of the test	English
Grade level for which the test is written	
Number of items	
Estimated time for patient	
Number of patients who can take the test simultaneously	
Level of staff needed to administer	
Number of staff needed to administer test	

Estimated time for staff to administer	
Level of staff needed to score	
Estimated time for staff to score	
Level of staff needed to interpret	
Estimated time for staff to interpret	
Equipment needed	
Time and cost for equipment use per test	
Applicable patient populations	
Comments	
Source	See reference.

MOS Social Support Survey

Tool measures	Four dimensions of social support: emotional/informational, tangible, affectionate, and positive social interaction
Author(s)	C. Sherbourne and A. Stewart
Reference	Sherbourne C, Stewart A: The MOS Social Support Survey. *Soc Sci Med* 1991;32(6):705-714.
Does this test measure change?	Yes
Cost to use this instrument	$8.00 per questionnaire; $80.00 for all 17 measures (condition specific); $15.00 for generic health status questionnaire.
Test method	Self-administered
Language of the test	English
Grade level for which the test is written	Ninth grade
Number of items	19
Estimated time for patient	Minutes
Number of patients who can take the test simultaneously	Unlimited
Level of staff needed to administer	Trained per instructions
Number of staff needed to administer test	One
Estimated time for staff to administer	2 minutes
Level of staff needed to score	
Estimated time for staff to score	
Level of staff needed to interpret	
Estimated time for staff to interpret	
Equipment needed	

Time and cost for equipment use per test

Applicable patient populations   Patients with chronic conditions

Comments

Source   MOS Social Support Survey, Health Outcomes Institute, 2001 Killebrew Drive, Suite 122, Bloomington, MN 55425; Phone: 612-858-9188; Fax: 612-858-9189

Social Provisions Scale

Tool measures   Support from family, friends, and coworkers related to attachment, social integration, guidance, reassurance of worth, and opportunity for nurturing

Author(s)   Russell and Cutrona

Reference   *Advances in Personal Relationships,* Greenwich, CT: JAI Press Vol. 1 p. 37-67.

Does this test measure change?

Cost to use this instrument

Test method

Language of the test

Grade level for which the test is written

Number of items

Estimated time for patient

Number of patients who can take the test simultaneously

Level of staff needed to administer

Number of staff needed to administer test

Estimated time for staff to administer

Level of staff needed to score

Estimated time for staff to score

Level of staff needed to interpret

Estimated time for staff to interpret

Equipment needed

Time and cost for equipment use per test

Applicable patient populations

Comments

Source   See reference.

BEHAVIORAL TOOLS

DIET-RELATED TOOLS

Block Food Questionnaire

Tool measures	Calories, fat, fiber, protein, carbohydrate, saturated fat, linoleic and oleic acids, and 10 vitamins and minerals
Author(s)	Gladys Block
Reference	Block G: Block Food Questionnaire. *Am J Epid* 1986;124.
Does this test measure change?	Yes
Cost to use this instrument	Unknown
Test method	Interviewer-administered dietary frequency report (semi-quantitative)
Language of the test	English
Grade level for which the test is written	
Number of items	128 items or 13 items on short Fat Screener
Estimated time for patient	30-45 minutes or less with short version
Number of patients who can take the test simultaneously	One
Level of staff needed to administer	Registered dietitian
Number of staff needed to administer test	One registered dietitian
Estimated time for staff to administer	45 minutes
Level of staff needed to score	May be sent away for scoring or software may be purchased
Estimated time for staff to score	See above.
Level of staff needed to interpret	Registered dietitian
Estimated time for staff to interpret	
Equipment needed	Computer
Time and cost for equipment use per test	N/A
Applicable patient populations	Applicable to adult populations (including Asian and Hispanic populations)
Comments	Currently the Block Questionnaires seem quite popular because of the ease of use relative to the quantity of information gained.
Source	School of Public Health, University of California at Berkeley, Berkeley, CA 94710; Administration phone: 510-642-4578

Diet Habit Survey

Tool measures	Cholesterol-saturated fat intake, complex carbohydrates, and salt

Author(s)	Sonja L. Connor, Joyce R. Gustafson, et al.
Reference	Connor SL, Gustafson JR, et al: Diet Habit Survey. *J Am Diet Assoc* 1992;92.
Does this test measure change?	Yes
Cost to use this instrument	$6.00 for master copy or $30.00 for a computer disk.
Test method (2 versions)	Paper and pencil questionnaire; semi-quantitative food frequency. DHS #1 Dietician-scored—38 questions; DHS #2 Self-scored.
Language of the test	English
Grade level for which the test is written	Eighth grade
Number of items	32
Estimated time for patient	30 minutes according to literature, however, may take much less time
Number of patients who can take the test simultaneously	Unlimited
Level of staff needed to administer	N/A
Number of staff needed to administer test	N/A
Estimated time for staff to administer	N/A
Level of staff needed to score	Can be self-scored or dietitian scored. Nursing staff may also score.
Estimated time for staff to score	5 minutes
Level of staff needed to interpret	Trained dietitian or health educator (nurse could also interpret with registered dietitian consultation)
Estimated time for staff to interpret	15-30 minutes for interpretation with patient
Equipment needed	None
Time and cost for equipment use per test	N/A
Applicable patient populations	Validation obtained on white middle-class men and women.
Comments	Validated for cholesterol-saturated fat measurement—NOT for complex carbohydrates or salt
Source	Heart Studies Publications, Oregon Health Sciences University - L465, 3181 SW Sam Jackson Park Road, Portland, OR 97201-3079; Phone: 503-494-8311; Fax: 503-494-5615

Harvard-Willett Food Frequency Questionnaire

Tool measures	Calories, fat, protein, carbohydrate, saturated fat, linoleic and oleic acids, cholesterol, vitamins, and minerals
Author(s)	W.C. Willett
Reference	Willett WC, et al: Harvard-Willett Food Frequency Questionnaire. *J Am Diet Assoc* 1987;87.
Does this test measure change?	Yes, if used repeatedly over time

Cost to use this instrument	Unknown
Test method	Self-administered, paper and pencil
Language of the test	English
Grade level for which the test is written	Unknown
Number of items	116
Estimated time for patient	45-60 minutes
Number of patients who can take the test simultaneously	Unlimited
Level of staff needed to administer	Minimal
Number of staff needed to administer test	Self-administered
Estimated time for staff to administer	N/A
Level of staff needed to score	Must be sent to Harvard for computer scoring
Estimated time for staff to score	See above.
Level of staff needed to interpret	Dietitian
Estimated time for staff to interpret	See above
Equipment needed	N/A
Time and cost for equipment use per test	N/A
Applicable patient populations	Applicable to adult populations
Comments	None
Source	Laura Sampson, Channing Laboratory, Harvard Medical School, Boston, MA 02115; Phone: 508-777-0744

Quick Check (Quantitative Food Frequency Questionnaire)

Tool measures	Fat, saturated fat, and cholesterol
Author(s)	David Blankenhorn, M.D.
Reference	Blankenhorn D: Quick Check (Quantitative Food Frequency Questionnaire). *Amer Diet Assoc* 1987;87.
Does this test measure change?	Not designed to measure change, but it could be used repeatedly over time and results compared.
Cost to use this instrument	$135.00 for 100 tests
Test method	Paper and pencil
Language of the test	English
Grade level for which the test is written	Sixth grade
Number of items	74
Estimated time for patient	15 minutes

Number of patients who can take the test simultaneously	Unlimited
Level of staff needed to administer	N/A
Number of staff needed to administer test	N/A
Estimated time for staff to administer	N/A
Level of staff needed to score	Scanned by computer or data-entry level staff
Estimated time for staff to score	Unknown, but probably only minutes
Level of staff needed to interpret	Registered dietitian or specially trained health educator or nurse
Estimated time for staff to interpret	
Equipment needed	IBM Compatible
Time and cost for equipment use per test	N/A
Applicable patient populations	Applicable to English-speaking adult populations
Comments	
Source	Nutrition Scientific, 1510 Oxley Street, Suite F, South Pasadena, CA 91030; Phone: 818-441-0021

HEALTH EDUCATION TOOLS

Health Knowledge Test

Tool measures	What pulmonary rehabilitation participants have learned
Author(s)	Joyce W. Hopp, Ph.D., M.P.H.; Jerry W. Lee, Ph.D.; Renee Hills, R.N., M.S.
Reference	Hopp JW, Lee JW, Hills R: Development and validation of a pulmonary rehabilitation test. *Journal of Cardiopulmonary Rehabilitation* 1989;7:273-278.
Does this test measure change?	Yes, change in knowledge obtained from a pulmonary rehabilitation program
Cost to use this instrument	$3.50 for manual and test; may make copies after purchase
Test method	Paper and pencil
Language of the test	English
Grade level for which the test is written	Adult
Number of items	40
Estimated time for patient	30 minutes
Number of patients who can take the test simultaneously	One
Level of staff needed to administer	Clerical staff and up. Because it's a "take home test" anyone can give it to the patient to take home.

Number of staff needed to administer test	One
Estimated time for staff to administer	Minutes
Level of staff needed to score	Medical or health professional
Estimated time for staff to score	5 minutes
Level of staff needed to interpret	Medical or health professional
Estimated time for staff to interpret	15 minutes
Equipment needed	Pencil
Time and cost for equipment use per test	
Applicable patient populations	Applicable to adults in pulmonary rehabilitation programs
Comments	
Source	Joyce W. Hopp, Ph.D., M.P.H., School of Allied Health Professions, Loma Linda University, Loma Linda, CA 92350; Phone: 909-824-4932

TEMPLATE

If you are sending this to the AACVPR National Office for inclusion in a future edition of this Guide, please type or print the information below. Include your name, address, and phone number so, if necessary, you can be contacted by the Outcomes Committee. Thank you.

Name of Tool:

Tool measures

Author(s)

Reference

Does this test measure change?

Cost to use this instrument

Test method

Language of the test

Grade level for which the test is written

Number of items

Estimated time for patient

Number of patients who can take the test simultaneously

Level of staff needed to administer

Number of staff needed to administer test

Estimated time for staff to administer

Level of staff needed to score

Estimated time for staff to score

Level of staff needed to interpret

Estimated time for staff to interpret

Equipment needed

Time and cost for equipment use per test

Applicable patient populations

Comments

Source

ACKNOWLEDGMENTS

This booklet represents ongoing work of the American Association of Cardiovascular and Pulmonary Rehabilitation Outcomes Committee over the past two years under the leadership of Peg Pashkow, Committee Chair, and current chair, Cynthia L. MacDonald, R.N., C., M.S.N. Former Committee members who have contributed to this effort include David Frid, M.D.; Gretchen Peske, R.N., M.S.N.; Jane Reardon, R.N., C.; Judith Schiffert, Ed.D.; Phil Ades, M.S.N.; Charles Emery, Ph.D.; Nancy Houston Miller, R.N., B.S.N.; Richard ZuWallack, M.D.; and Douglas Southard, Ph.D., M.P.H. Current members of the outcomes committee involved in the 1997 update include Cindie Rice, R.N., C., M.S.N.; Barbara Unger, R.N.; Betty Oprian, R.N.; Deb Sanders, R.N.; and Robin Spangler, R.N. Thanks to all contributors and the AACVPR members who have assisted in recommending and evaluating these tools.

Special thanks to Lisa Nelson at the AACVPR National Office for her assistance in producing this booklet.

Clinical Competency Guidelines for Pulmonary Rehabilitation Professionals

American Association of Cardiovascular and Pulmonary Rehabilitation Position Statement

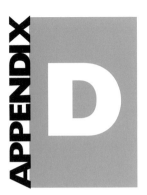

APPENDIX D

Pulmonary Clinical Competencies
Working Group:
  Douglas R. Southard, PhD, MPH, Chair*
  Lawrence P. Cahalin, MA, PT[†]
  Brian W. Carlin, MD[‡]
  Mollyn Cales, RN[§]
  Valerie K. McLeod, RRT[||]
  Kathleen Morris, RN, MS, RRT[¶]
  Edgar A. Normandin, PhD, PT[#]
  Jane Reardon, RN**
  Andrew L. Ries, MD, MPH[††]
  Alexandra J. Sciaky, PT, CCS[‡‡]

From the *Virginia Polytechnic Institute and State University, Blacksburg, Virginia; [†]Massachusetts General Hospital, Boston, Massachusetts; [‡]Allegheny General Hospital, Pittsburgh, Pennsylvania; [§]Southern West Virginia Clinic, Beckley, West Virginia; [||]McLaren Regional Medical Center, Flint, Michigan; [¶]St. Helena Hospital, Deer Park, California; [#]St. Francis Hospital and Medical Center, Hartford, Connecticut; **Hartford Hospital, Hartford, Connecticut; [††]University of California, San Diego Medical Center, San Diego, California; and [‡‡]University of Michigan Medical Center, Ann Arbor, Michigan.

Address for correspondence: Douglas R. Southard, PhD, MPH, Virginia Tech, 103 War Memorial Hall, Blacksburg, VA 24061-0351.

Reprinted, by permission, from D.R. Southard, et al, 1995, "Clinical competency guidelines for pulmonary rehabilitation professionals: American Association of Cardiovascular and Pulmonary Rehabilitation position statement," *J Cardiopulm Rehabil* 15: 173-178.

DEFINITION AND PURPOSE

This document presents an outline of the clinical competencies recommended for those providing comprehensive services in pulmonary rehabilitation. It is assumed that individuals wishing to provide such services should possess a common core of professional and clinical competencies regardless of their academic discipline. Services characteristic of a comprehensive pulmonary rehabilitation program include a multidisciplinary assessment leading to the development of an integrated treatment plan, including patient education, exercise training, psychosocial support, and follow-up. Practitioners may also serve as case managers to provide coordination of services. Individuals who commonly provide such comprehensive services include respiratory care practitioners, nurses, physical therapists, occupational therapists, exercise physiologists, and others.

In addition to the general guidelines outlined in this paper, pulmonary rehabilitation professionals should be aware of state limitations of practice acts and techniques of legal risk management as they apply to assessment, intervention, and follow-up. They should also demonstrate understanding of infection control procedures, including implications of Occupational Safety and Health Administration (OSHA) bloodborne pathogen standards and the application of universal precautions to clinical procedures.

Because of the growing recognition of the benefits of pulmonary rehabilitation for patients with chronic obstructive pulmonary disease, the application of rehabilitation principles to patients with other lung diseases are increasingly being developed and refined. These include but are not limited to individuals with asthma, cystic fibrosis, lung transplantation, interstitial/restrictive lung diseases, and ventilator dependency. This document does not specifically address these other patient populations, but does recognize the potential value of rehabilitation for all patients with chronic lung diseases and the need for further research and development.

By itself, this document conveys no approval, endorsements, or certification of either pulmonary rehabilitation professionals or their programs. Rather, it identifies and promotes common practice expectations. In doing so, the document may also serve as a self-evaluation tool for practitioners to identify continuing education needs.

During the course of its development, this manuscript underwent reviews by the American Association of Cardiovascular and Pulmonary Rehabilitation (AACVPR) Board of Directors and the Publications Committee. The document is organized into three major clinical process categories (Assessment, Intervention, and Outcome Evaluation/Follow-up) and six content categories.

Competency Guidelines

I. Assessment

 A. Pathophysiology and Co-morbidity

  1. Demonstrates a thorough knowledge of pulmonary and cardiovascular anatomy, physiology, and pathophysiology including common pulmonary and cardiovascular conditions limiting or otherwise influencing physical activity, symptom management, respiratory and chest physical therapy, dietary modification, smoking cessation, and stress management.

  2. Demonstrates an understanding of pulmonary and cardiovascular diagnostic techniques, medical and pharmacologic management, and the normal/abnormal pulmonary and cardiovascular responses to exercise.

  3. Recognizes co-morbid conditions including metabolic (e.g., diabetes, obesity), musculoskeletal (e.g., hip or knee dysfunction, osteoporosis, arthritis) and other conditions (e.g., gastroesophageal reflux with chronic aspiration, hiatal hernia, sinusitis/rhinitis, alcoholism, sleep disturbances, etc.) that may influence the prescription of physical activity, dietary intake, ventilatory muscle training, breathing retraining, smoking cessation, or stress management.

  4. Recognizes the effects of environmental factors, medication usage, and supplemental oxygen usage on the pathophysiology, treatment, and natural history of the disease process.

  5. Demonstrates a level of understanding of general anatomy, physiology, and pathophysiology equivalent to a semester length course each in anatomy/physiology and pathophysiology.

  6. Recognizes the appropriate time frame for physiologic changes to occur as well as how physiologic responses to one rehabilitation modality (i.e., breathing retraining) may influence the individual's response to other interventions (i.e., stair climbing, etc.).

 B. Professional Communication

  1. Obtains records regarding medical/health history to include diagnoses and therapeutic course.

  2. Informs patients of their rights and responsibilities within the parameters of professional ethics and legal authority, including a legally valid informed consent process, preservation of confidentiality, appropriately limiting access to patient information, and informing patients of their rights to participate (to the extent provided in state laws) in decisions regarding acceptance or refusal of medical treatment.

  3. Consults with referring physician and other health care team members to determine the need for additional assessments.

  4. Prepares a summary of patient evaluation using multidisciplinary assessment data.

  5. Develops, with active patient participation, a comprehensive plan of rehabilitation, including the establishment of reasonable and measurable goals.

tem within the context of clinical responsibilities and medicolegal norms.

5. Develops a timely and consistent system for status reports to the primary care and/or referring physician.

6. Refers to other health care professionals as appropriate.

C. Patient Education and Training

1. Uses basic educational principles, theories of learning, and methods of counseling, as well as knowledge of specific behavioral modification techniques used for breathing retraining, smoking cessation, and dietary modification.

2. Monitors clinical symptoms and laboratory data during the course of treatment that may indicate important changes relating to disease progression or lifestyle management. This would include an understanding of realistic expectations for improvement as well as circumstances during treatment that should prompt referral of the patient for consultation by specialized health professionals. Clinical domains to be monitored include: heart rate, respiratory rate, oxygen saturation, medication usage, weight loss/gain, presence of reflux, breath sounds (i.e., for secretions, etc.), dyspnea/exertion level, blood pressure, smoking status, diabetic control, and electrocardiography as indicated.

3. Develops an integrated education/training program, using a multidisciplinary approach, consisting of exercise, dyspnea management, activities of daily living training, panic control, smoking cessation, and stress management.

4. Provides patient training regarding appropriate use of medications and potential for side effects.

5. Instructs and counsels patients using a variety of methods, strategies, materials, and technologies helpful in promoting behavior change.

6. Adjusts teaching to accommodate to individual patient needs and limitations.

7. Enables patients to acquire the perspective, knowledge, and skills necessary to

independently maintain optimal health after discharge from pulmonary rehabilitation care.

8. Teaches and counsels patients regarding travel and altitude (including air travel), particularly for patients requiring supplemental oxygen therapy

9. Provides and teaches individualized respiratory care exercises to patients. These programs may include: percussion, postural drainage, vibration, controlled coughing and breathing exercises, and use of oxygen (i.e., hours of usage, liter flow at rest and with exercise).

10. Demonstrates ability to counsel regarding durable power of attorney for health care services and advanced directives.

D. Exercise

1. Develops an exercise prescription, in collaboration with the physician that will safely and effectively guide the patient toward optimal restoration and maintenance of functional capacity both on site and at home.

2. Leads, monitors, and supervises individual and group therapeutic exercise sessions appropriate to patients with varying degrees of pulmonary and cardiovascular disease.

3. Demonstrates competence to determine when ECG telemetry is indicated during exercise sessions.

4. Explains hazards of high-risk patient behaviors during exercise training (i.e., exceeding targets for dyspnea or exertional hypoxemia, exercising in excessively hot or cold weather, etc.), and how these may be reduced through patient training, supervision, and appropriate monitoring techniques.

5. Demonstrates proper techniques for performing patient's preferred avocational physical activities (i.e., golf, shopping, etc.) and for correcting faults in patient's technique.

E. Psychosocial

1. Suggests self-help techniques, materials, and resources, and/or refers the patient to

mental health professionals, support groups, community, and home care services as appropriate.

2. Provides supportive counsel to individuals experiencing mild-moderate psychological distress (i.e., depression, anxiety/panic, anger, etc.).

3. Explains and promotes appropriate relaxation skills and other stress management techniques.

4. Involves family members or significant others as appropriate in counseling to enhance social support.

5. Provides information, if needed, about techniques that can minimize disease related limitations on sexual activity.

F. Emergency Procedures

1. Maintains an emergency response capability for pulmonary rehabilitation exercise programs. This should include appropriate equipment in the exercise area along with an understanding of staff roles and the specific steps needed for various pulmonary, cardiovascular, and other emergency situations.

2. Demonstrates knowledge of medicolegal and licensing authority issues that mandate specific roles for different professionals in the making of medical decisions and in the delivery of emergency care (i.e., licensed authority to perform advanced cardiac life support [ACLS]).

3. Encourages family members to enroll in a basic cardiopulmonary resuscitation (CPR) course and identify community emergency services.

III. Outcome Evaluation and Follow-up

A. Pathophysiology and Co-morbidity

1. Evaluates whether the patient's rehabilitation program was adjusted appropriately and medical therapy provided to address any pulmonary, cardiovascular, or other medical conditions (e.g., diabetes, obesity, arthritis, etc.) that may have adversely affected the desired rehabilitation outcomes.

B. Professional Communication

1. Completes discharge summary describing client's progression in rehabilitation program in terms of: symptom changes, commitment to lifestyle changes, exercise responses, identified barriers and possible solutions to noncompliant behaviors, and achievement of personal goals (return of lost abilities such as shopping, golf, bowling, etc.) leading to an enhanced quality of life. Summary to be sent to referring physician and team members as needed.

2. Communicates to patient the degree of success in completing goals and steps that must be taken to maintain/improve gains.

3. Facilitates on-going self-care, home-care, follow-up, and support services after discharge from pulmonary rehabilitation care.

C. Patient Education and Training

1. Reassesses patient prognosis as it relates to the risk factor profile (occupational exposure, smoking, etc.).

2. Develops long-term plan to improve risk factor profile, involving both patient and family.

3. Evaluates follow-through in medication and oxygen usage and self-administration techniques.

4. Determines if client was successful in returning to desired vocation, avocational, and/or recreational activities.

5. Evaluates if interventions undertaken to accommodate the patient's verbal or written impairments, educational limitations, and visual or hearing defects have been successful.

6. Reassesses patient's self-care regimen to include activities of daily living, pulmonary hygiene skills, medication management, social/community support, and appropriate on-going medical care, and adjusts accordingly.

D. Exercise

1. Assists client to reevaluate physical activity patterns and preferences regarding specific exercise modalities (bicycle vs treadmill, etc.).

2. Reevaluates cardiopulmonary capacity for exercise, determines compliance with initial home exercise program, and updates exercise prescription and treatment regimen.

3. Reevaluates pulmonary function, cardiovascular status, body composition, strength, endurance, and flexibility in terms of ability to meet the demands of vocational, avocational, and activities of daily living (ADLs).

E. Psychosocial

1. Reassesses stress levels and modifies treatment plan accordingly.

2. Evaluates if mental health consultation and/or referrals to support groups, community, and home care services were performed based on needs determined at the initial assessment and progress through rehabilitation program.

3. Evaluates client's progress in achieving desired goals related to sexual activity.

4. Reassesses effectiveness of social support and enhances support network as needed.

F. Emergency Procedures

1. Demonstrates capability to evaluate the patient's and family's ability to monitor for signs and symptoms of respiratory infection and impending respiratory failure.

2. Modifies interventions when potential safety hazards are discovered or specific problems identified to increase margins of safety.

3. Reassesses the client's and family's knowledge of emergency procedures (i.e., CPR).

Acknowledgments

The Writing Group thanks John Hodgkin, MD, Kevin Ryan, RRT, the AACVPR Board of Directors and Publications Committee, and other rehabilitation professionals for their guidance and feedback regarding earlier drafts of this document.

Index

About the AACVPR

MISSION STATEMENT

The AACVPR is the catalyst for visibility and communication in professional education, standards, guidelines, and certification through innovative resource development. Our mission is to continually improve our products and services to meet our customers' needs, allowing us to prosper and become the preeminent association of cardiovascular and pulmonary rehabilitation professionals.

GUIDING PRINCIPLES

- Quality and integrity are never compromised;
- Customers are the focus of everything we do;
- Creating and maintaining constancy of purpose is an ongoing responsibility;
- Stewardship and creative risk taking are compatible;
- Creating and cultivating productive partnerships and alliances help position AACVPR in an ever-changing health care industry;
- Creating and maintaining a learning environment helps maintain our freshness and keeps us on the cutting edge;
- Continuous improvement is essential to our success.

PUBLICATIONS

- *Journal of Cardiopulmonary Rehabilitation* (bimonthly)
- *News and Views of AACVPR* (quarterly newsletter)
- Directory of Membership and Cardiopulmonary Rehabilitation Programs
- Position Paper: Cardiac Rehabilitation Services: A Scientific Evaluation
- Position Paper: Efficacy of Risk Factor Intervention and Psychosocial Aspects of Cardiac Rehabilitation
- Position Paper: Scientific Basis of Pulmonary Rehabilitation
- Position Paper: Core Competencies for Cardiac Rehabilitation Professionals
- Position Paper: Core Competencies for Pulmonary Rehabilitation Professionals
- Outcomes Tool Resource Guide
- Educational Resource Manual
- *Guidelines for Cardiac Rehabilitation Programs, 2nd Edition*
- *Guidelines for Pulmonary Rehabilitation Programs, 2nd Edition*
- Annual Meeting Syllabus
- Cardiac and Pulmonary Rehabilitation Weeks Media Kits
- Agency for Health Care Policy and Research *Clinical Practice Guideline for Cardiac Rehabilitation*

ANNUAL MEETING

The AACVPR has, as its primary mission, facilitation of the exchange of knowledge regarding cardiovascular and pulmonary rehabilitation among health-care professionals. To this end, the Annual National Convention is dedicated. The convention program seeks to provide the rehabilitation professional with knowledge regarding the scientific principles upon which cardiovascular and pulmonary rehabilitation is based. Furthermore, the Convention brings you the latest information regarding advances and new challenges in rehabilitation.

MEMBERSHIP BENEFITS

- Receive the *Journal of Cardiopulmonary Rehabilitation* bimonthly, keeping you updated on current research, clinical and practical information in the field of rehabilitation.
- Be part of a national network of professionals dedicated to the advancement of cardiovascular and pulmonary rehabilitation.
- Receive a quarterly newsletter about the association, affiliate societies, and practical information.
- Receive discounts to attend the AACVPR Annual Meeting.
- Be included in the national membership directory.
- Receive a complimentary copy of the AACVPR Directory of Membership and Cardiovascular and Pulmonary Rehabilitation Programs.
- For a small fee, promote your program by listing it in the AACVPR Directory of Cardiovascular and Pulmonary Rehabilitation Programs, a valuable resource for health-care professionals.
- Access to nationwide job opportunities through the Career Hotline.
- Receive up-to-date information on federal and state guidelines, reimbursement for rehabilitation services and other issues of concern to professionals in the field.
- The opportunity to publish articles in the *Journal of Cardiopulmonary Rehabilitation* and present research or educational information at the Annual Meeting.

We invite you to meet the challenge and become involved in AACVPR. Decide to join this dynamic organization today. Fill out the membership application included with this brochure and send it to AACVPR. The professional growth that you will experience by becoming a member of this Association will benefit you for years to come. We look forward to your future involvement and support.

MEMBERSHIP REQUIREMENTS

MEMBER.   Shall be any interested person of majority age who is a nurse, physician, medical scientist, allied health-care practitioner or educator, and who in his or her professional endeavors, is regularly involved in some aspect of cardiovascular and/or pulmonary rehabilitation. Members have AACVPR voting privileges.

ASSOCIATE MEMBER.   Shall be any person with an interest in cardiovascular and/or pulmonary rehabilitation, but not currently eligible for classification as a Member or Student Member. Dues are established by the Board of Directors and may be changed at its discretion. Associate Member privileges include a subscription to any AACVPR newsletter that may be published and placement on the Association mailing list.

STUDENT MEMBER.   Shall be any interested college student currently carrying the equivalent of at least one half of an academic load for one year, as defined by the university or college the person is attending, and one who is studying in a medical or allied health curriculum.

FELLOW.   Shall be qualified as a Member in good-standing for a minimum of three consecutive years; attended a minimum of two Annual Meetings; demonstrated high standards of professional development and a commitment to the goals and long-range activities of the Association; submitted evidence of outstanding performance in some aspect of cardiovascular or pulmonary rehabilitation over a period of at least five years relative to a) clinical practice, b) research and/or c) professional education in cardiovascular and pulmonary rehabilitation; received recommendations in writing by two Fellows of the Association; and received the approval of the Credentials Committee and the Board of Directors. Fellows have AACVPR voting privileges.

CODE OF ETHICAL AND PROFESSIONAL CONDUCT

A. OBJECTIVES.   This code is designed to aid the Fellows and Members of the Association, individually and collectively, to maintain a high level of ethical and professional conduct. The code may be considered a standard by which a Fellow or Member may determine the propriety of his or her conduct, relationship with colleagues, members of allied professions, the public, and all persons with whom a professional relationship has been established. These should be concordant with the principal purpose of the Association, which is the improvement of clinical practice, promotion of scientific inquiry, and advancement of education for the benefit of health-care professionals and the public in the multidisciplinary field of cardiovascular and pulmonary rehabilitation.

Fellows and Members should strive continuously to improve their knowledge and skills and to make available to their colleagues and to the public the benefits of their professional attainments.

Fellows and Members should maintain high professional and scientific standards and should not voluntarily associate professionally with those who violate this principle.

The Association should safeguard the public and itself against Fellows or Members who are deficient in ethical conduct or professional competence.

B. MAINTENANCE OF GOOD STANDING IN REGULATED PROFESSIONS.   Any Fellow or Member required by law to be licensed, certified, or otherwise regulated by any government agency or professional association in order to practice his or her profession must remain in good standing before that agency or association as a condition of continued membership in the American Association of Cardiovascular and Pulmonary Rehabilitation. Any expulsion, suspension, probation, or other sanction imposed by such government or professional body on any Fellow or Member may be grounds for disciplinary action by the Association.

C. PUBLIC DISCLOSURE OF AFFILIATION.   Any Fellow or Member may make disclosure of affiliation with the Association in an appropriate professional context, including use in curriculum vitae, in biographical descriptions, or in another professional, dignified manner. Disclosure of affiliation may not be made in connection with any commercial venture without prior written authorization of the Association. A commercial venture is defined here to mean the sale of any goods, services, or other property for a valuable consideration with the exception of books, journal articles, or other professional publications. Requests for such authorization should be made in writing to the President or the Executive Director of the Association. Fellows may list their affiliation with the Association on professional or business cards, only by the use of the initials F.A.A.C.V.P.R.: members other than Fellows may not use this affiliation on business or professional cards. Disclosure in violation of these guidelines may be grounds for disciplinary action.

The use of the name of the American Association of Cardiovascular and Pulmonary Rehabilitation as a cosponsoring or cooperating organization for professional meetings, professional education programs, and the like must follow the guidelines of the Association for these specific designations.

D. DISCIPLINE.   Any Fellow or Member of the Association may be disciplined or expelled for conduct which in the opinion of the Board of Directors, is derogatory to the dignity or inconsistent with the purposes of the Association. The expulsion of a Fellow or Member may be ordered upon the affirmative vote of two-thirds of the members of the Board of Directors present at a regular or special meeting and only after such Fellow or Member has been informed of the charges preferred and has been given an opportunity to refute such charges before the Board of Directors. Other disciplinary action such as reprimand, probation, or censure may be recommended by the Committee on Ethics and Professional Conduct and ordered following the affirmative vote of at least two-thirds of the members of the Board of Directors present at a regular or special meeting, or by mail ballot provided a quorum take action.

American Association of Cardiovascular and Pulmonary Rehabilitation (AACVPR)
Promoting Health & Preventing Disease

MEMBERSHIP APPLICATION

Name _____ Professional degree _____

(Please list no more than two)

Job title _____

Place of Employment _____

Mailing Address _____ City _____

State _____ Zip Code _____ Postal Code/Country _____

(The address above will be used for mailings and will be listed in the Membership Directory)

This address is : ❏ Home ❏ Business

Telephone Number (_____) _____ Fax Number (_____) _____

E-mail Address _____ Gender: ❏ Female ❏ Male

Birthdate: _____/_____/_____ Are you a current member of your state/regional society? ❏ Yes ❏ No

CURRENT PROGRAM INVOLVEMENT

In what area(s) do you spend the majority of your practice?
What is the emphasis of your clinical practice?

Check one:
❏ In-patient
❏ Out-patient
❏ In-patient & Out-patient

Check one:
❏ Cardiovascular
❏ Pulmonary
❏ Vascular
❏ Cardiovascular & Pulmonary

Who is your employer?
❏ Hospital
❏ Physician/Group Practice
❏ Educational Institution
❏ Other: _____

Please check here if your facility is free-standing ❏

How many new out-patients would you estimate
are seen in your program annually?
❏ Less than 100 ❏ 101-200 patients
❏ 201-300 patients ❏ Over 300 patients

How many new in-patients would you estimate are seen in your
program annually?
❏ Less than 100 ❏ 101-500 patients
❏ 501-1000 patients ❏ Over 1000 patients

Which of the following best describes the emphasis of your
work environment?
❏ 100% rehabilitation
❏ 75% rehabilitation/25% prevention
❏ 50% rehabilitation/50% prevention
❏ 25% rehabilitation/75% prevention

How many years have you been involved in rehabilitation?
❏ Less than 2 ❏ 2-4
❏ 5-7 ❏ 8+

How many health care professionals work in your program (both
full and part time)?
❏ 1-3 ❏ 4-6
❏ 7-9 ❏ 10+

Membership in the AACVPR is effective July 1
through June 30.
Members joining after March 1 will be deferred
until July 1.
Membership dues are not deductible as a charitable
contribution.
Membership dues may be deductible as an ordinary
and necessary business expense.
Consult your tax adviser for information.

Please complete both sides of this application and
send with your check or money order in U.S.
currency to:
AACVPR
7611 Elmwood Avenue, Suite 201
Middleton, WI 53562
Telephone: 608-831-6989

(continued)

MEMBERSHIP CATEGORIES *(check Member, Student Member, or Associate Member)*

❏ **MEMBER**   Membership fee: $120.00

A Member shall be any interested person of majority of age who is a nurse, exercise physiologist, educator, physician, therapist, medical scientist or allied health-care practitioner who in his or her professional endeavors is regularly involved in some aspect of cardiovascular and/or pulmonary rehabilitation.

Each of the following are professional areas represented by an AACVPR Board member. Which of these categories best represent you? Check only one.

❏ Behavioral Scientist   ❏ Cardiopulmonary Physical Therapist
❏ Cardiovascular Nurse   ❏ Cardiovascular Physician
❏ Exercise Physiologist   ❏ Exercise Rehabilitation Specialist
❏ Nutritionist/Dietitian   ❏ Pulmonary Nurse
❏ Pulmonary Physician   ❏ Respiratory Therapist
❏ Vocational Rehabilitation Counselor   ❏ Other: _____

Are you certified by a professional association?   Association Name: _____

Certification Name: _____

❏ **STUDENT MEMBER**   Membership fee: $60.00

A Student Member of AACVPR will be any interested undergraduate or graduate college student currently carrying the equivalent of at least one-half of a full-time academic load for one year, as defined by the university or college the person is attending. The area of study must be in a medical or allied health curriculum. Student Membership also applies to physicians-in-training (residents, interns). To quality as a Student Member, an individual must submit a copy of their current student identification card along with this completed application.

Educational Institution: _____

Major: _____   Year Degree Expected: _____

Advisor Signature: _____   Advisor Telephone Number: (____) _____

❏ **ASSOCIATE MEMBER**   Membership fee: $120.00

An Associate Member is any person with an interest in cardiovascular and/or pulmonary rehabilitation, but not currently eligible for classification as a Member or Student Member.

Primary Occupation: _____   Place of Employment: _____

Major Area of Interest (see descriptions under "Member") _____

GENERAL INFORMATION

Where did you hear about AACVPR?

❏ From an AACVPR Member   ❏ Have Been a Member Previously: What year(s):_____
❏ *Journal of Cardiopulmonary Rehabilitation*   ❏ Professional Colleague
❏ Received Information in the Mail   ❏ State/Regional Society
❏ University/School   ❏ Work
❏ Other: _____

If you received this application from an AACVPR member, please provide the member's name under "other."

MEMBERSHIP AGREEMENT

I certify that the above information is correct and I agree to abide by the Code of Ethics and Professional Conduct of the American Association of Cardiovascular and Pulmonary Rehabilitation as outlined on this application.

_____   _____
Signature   Date